Bandolier's Little Book of
# Making Sense of
# the Medical Evidence

# Bandolier's Little Book of
# Making Sense of the Medical Evidence

**Andrew Moore**
and
**Henry McQuay**

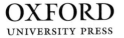

OXFORD
UNIVERSITY PRESS

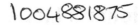

# Preface

This book is the second in a series of books that have in common the theme of evidence-based medicine (EBM). The first was *Bandolier's Little Book of Pain*, published by OUP in 2003, and the success of that book has encouraged us in the writing of this one. *Bandolier's Little Book of Pain* used the tools of EBM to look at acute and chronic pain. This book looks in a more general way at the gathering of evidence, its assessment, and the presentation of the results.

The authors of this book, Andrew Moore (RAM) and Henry McQuay (HJM), have been working together in Oxford for over 25 years on pain and anaesthesia, on investigating interesting issues around evidence, and as co-editors of *Bandolier*, a print and internet journal of evidence-based health-care information. It is the experience of sifting through clinical trials and systematic reviews to produce the monthly *Bandolier* that is distilled for this book.

This book is for any health-care professional who wants to use the best evidence available for the good of their patients and their service. We hope that it will also be useful for patients and carers who just want to know how best to understand all the plethora of confusing stories in the newspapers through to the journalists who write about health-care.

## People we want to thank

This book contains information taken from many clinical trials and many systematic reviews, and from many wonderful analyses and critiques about what makes good evidence. All of us are indebted to the millions of patients who agreed to participate in randomized trials and observational studies. We should also be grateful to the thousands of researchers who undertook those trials, and the hundreds of reviewers for pulling them all together.

We have been fortunate in some gifted researchers who have trained and worked with us and whose ideas, enthusiasm, and sheer hard work have contributed so much to our thinking and hence the work contained in this book. They are Dawn Carroll, Alex Jadad, Sally Collins, Martin Tramèr, Jayne Edwards, Anna Oldman, Lesley Smith, Jodie Barden, and Lorna Mason.

Special thanks go to a current member of our scientific team, Sheena Derry, who contributed an enormous amount to our thinking on adverse events. Some of our other regular collaborators also deserve our thanks, David Gavaghan, Helen Gaskell, John Reynolds, Eija Kalso, and Phil Wiffen.

Other people have helped us with our thinking over the years, particularly Dave Sackett (whom we miss now that he is back in Canada), Ceri Phillips, Michael Dunning, and Muir Gray. Many others have stimulated us by making us irritable, but perhaps it is more diplomatic not to name names.

We would like to acknowledge the unqualified support for our research that we have received from The BUPA Foundation, The Gwen Bush

Foundation, Pfizer, Astra Zeneca, Janssen Cilag, GSK, and Merck, Sharp and Dohme Ltd. They have all been very brave, because we only accept sponsorship if there is absolutely no control from the sponsoring body over what we write.

Catherine Barnes at OUP has been incredibly patient with us as we have amended our thinking. That we eventually got fingers to keyboard was due to the organizational ability and project management skills of Maureen McQuay.

Chris Glynn and Tim Jack, our clinical colleagues, are always useful sounding boards, and the nurses on the Pain Relief Unit helped us broaden our thinking. Maura Moore and Carole Newton provided much organizational support.

RAM, HJM 2006

# Contents

# Abbreviations

| | |
|---|---|
| ACR | American College of Rheumatology |
| ADE | adverse drug event |
| ADR | adverse drug reaction |
| AF | atrial fibrillation |
| AIS | Abbreviated Injury Scale |
| APACHE | acute physiology and chronic health evaluation |
| ARI | absolute risk increase |
| ARR | absolute risk reduction |
| ASD | autistic spectrum disorder |
| BMI | body mass index |
| BPH | benign prostatic hyperplasia |
| BSR | British Society of Rheumatology |
| CABG | coronary artery bypass grafting |
| CAMDEX | Cambridge Examination for Mental Disorders of the Elderly |
| CCT | controlled clinical trial |
| CDSS | clinical decision support systems |
| CEA | cost-effectiveness analysis |
| CER | control event rate or cost-effectiveness ratio |
| CHD | coronary heart disease |
| CHF | congestive heart failure |
| CHEC | Consensus on Health Economic Criteria |
| CI | confidence interval |
| CJD | Creutzfeldt–Jakob disease |
| COI | conflict of interest |
| COPD | chronic obstructive pulmonary disease |
| CRS | congenital rubella syndrome |
| DDD | defined daily dose |
| DMARD | disease-modifying anti-rheumatic drug |
| DSM | Diagnostic and statistical manual of mental disorder |
| EBM | evidence-based medicine |
| EER | experimental event rate |
| ESR | erythrocyte sedimentation rate |
| FDA | Food and Drug Administration (USA) |

| FEV$_1$ | forced expiratory volume in 1 second |
| --- | --- |
| FVC | forced vital capacity |
| GI | gastrointestinal |
| GORD | gastro-oesophageal reflux disease |
| H2A | histamine antagonist |
| HMO | health maintenance organization (US) |
| HRT | hormone replacement therapy |
| ICD | International Classification of Disease |
| ICER | incremental cost-effectiveness ratio |
| ICP | integrated care pathway |
| IM | intramuscular |
| IN | intranasal |
| INR | international normalized ratio |
| ITT | intention to treat (analysis) |
| ITU | intensive therapy unit |
| LDL | low-density lipoprotein |
| LoE | lack of efficacy |
| LOS | length of stay |
| LRTI | lower respiratory tract infection |
| LVH | left ventricular hypertrophy |
| MI | myocardial infarction |
| MMR | measles–mumps–rubella (vaccine) |
| MS | multiple sclerosis |
| NICE | National Institute for Clinical Excellence (UK) |
| NNH | number needed to harm |
| NNT | number needed to treat |
| NRT | nicotine replacement therapy |
| NSAID | nonsteroidal anti-inflammatory drug |
| OAD | obstructive airways disease |
| OPVS | Oxford Pain Validity Scale |
| OR | odds ratio |
| PBMA | programme budgeting and marginal analysis |
| PDD | pervasive developmental disorder |
| PEER | patient expected event rate |
| $p$O$_2$ | oxygen tension |
| POE | physician computer order-entry (system) |
| PPI | proton pump inhibitors |

| PSA | prostate-specific antigen |
| --- | --- |
| PUB | perforation, ulcer, or bleed |
| QALY | quality-adjusted life year |
| QHES | Quality of Health Economic Studies (instrument) |
| RA | rheumatoid arthritis |
| RCT | randomized controlled trial |
| RLS | restless legs syndrome |
| ROC | receiver operating characteristics (curve) |
| RR | relative risk |
| SC | subcutaneous |
| SCBU | special care baby unit |
| SSRI | selective serotonin reuptake inhibitor |
| TENS | transcutaneous electrical nerve stimulation |
| TIA | transient ischaemic attack |
| TNF | tumour necrosis factor |
| TOTPAR | total pain relief |
| UGIB | upper gastrointestinal bleed |
| UTI | urinary tract infection |
| UV | ultraviolet |
| WHO | World Health Organization |
| WOMAC | Western Ontario and McMaster Universities Arthritis Index |

# Introduction

This book was written as a simple guide for people who wish to make sense of evidence in the health-care setting and who want to avoid being misled by faulty evidence, but neither wish nor need to become pointy-headed academics. This book was not written as a comprehensive manual for those who want to do a systematic review or a meta-analysis, nor as a statistical or methodological textbook for students. Its origins lie in lectures for medical students, health-care professionals from a variety of tribes and settings, and journalists.

The reader will see references to Bandolier at various parts of the book. That's because the authors write *Bandolier*, an independent journal about evidence-based healthcare, published since February 1994 in print and on the web (*www.ebandolier.com*), and we use examples from *Bandolier* in this book.

Bandolier seeks information about evidence of effectiveness (or lack of it) in systematic reviews, meta-analyses, randomized trials, and from high-quality observational studies. This book is a summary of the tools that Bandolier uses to assess evidence, to be be able to distinguish good evidence from bad. We have an adage that we advocate tools not rules, because we hope to stimulate thought, debate, and innovation rather than to stifle.

There is a problem of language, though. As writers we inevitably use our own technical terms, which are meaningful to us, but not perhaps so meaningful to the reader. We do explain them in the text, but sometimes that explanation comes too late or too early. For that reason there is a glossary at the end of the book, to help if help is needed. We also occasionally repeat examples or thoughts. This is deliberate (well, usually).

These days everything is seemingly badged as 'evidence-based', irrespective of the amount or quality of evidence that is available. Too often someone will claim an evidence base when the evidence they have is a study of two men and a dog, in which the dog got better and the men weren't ill anyway. Being evidence-based is actually rather more than that. It should mean that there is a minimum amount of good-quality evidence, from valid studies, and free from bias.

Finding evidence to fit the bill is rather difficult. Consider the quotation by Richard Smith [1] of some words of David Eddy, an important original thinker about evidence, in 1991:

There are perhaps 30,000 biomedical journals in the world, and they have grown steadily by 7% a year since the seventeenth century. Yet about 15% of medical interventions are supported by solid scientific evidence...only 1% of the articles in medical journals are scientifically sound.

Bandolier's experience of reading lots of papers and systematic reviews over the past few decades is that, while the 1% may be difficult to pin down, this is not far from the right order of magnitude. For instance, some of our own work has identified that in some cases 1 in 10 trial reports contain serious errors (actually 2 in 13 [2]) and others have also found similar problems.

## Failure of peer review

Most of us think that the peer review process in journals should protect us—from mistakes, from inaccurate or inadequate conclusions, or even from fraud. It does not. One example will suffice, in part because it has a lively discussion about the history of failure of the peer review process.

Peer reviewers are usually busy people, who try to help editors, their professional colleagues, and authors of papers by giving freely of their time to judge manuscripts, and to improve them. Many of us who write papers are grateful to reviewers who have helped improve our papers. But just as often, unthinking, ignorant, or insulting remarks by reviewers drive us to fury. What about the reviewer from a journal at the leading edge of evidence who dismissed a negative systematic review of a procedure because 'they tried it once and it seemed to work'!

All too often accepting or rejecting submitted papers seems to be little less than the random play of chance. A study in neuroscience confirms just that [3]. Two journals that routinely sent manuscripts to two reviewers allowed access to the assessments of these manuscripts. One journal provided information on all manuscripts over a 6-month period (179), and the other provided information on 116 consecutive manuscripts. Both journals used a structured assessment, and assessors were asked to make the judgements: should the manuscript be accepted, revised, or rejected, and was the priority for publication low, medium, or high?

Agreement between reviewers was assessed using the kappa statistic. A value of 0 represents chance agreement, and a value of 1 perfect agreement. Scores of 0 to 0.2 are considered very poor, those between 0.2 and 0.4 poor, between 0.4 and 0.6 moderate, between 0.6 and 0.8 good, and between 0.8 and 1 excellent. Agreement was less than good, and was not convincingly better than chance for either journal for acceptance, revision, or rejection, or high, medium, or low priority.

## Problem of belief

It is all too easy to say that we 'know' a treatment works because we have seen the benefits for patients who have had the treatment. All too often, these beliefs can be exploded when good clinical studies that meet minimal rules of evidence are performed. An example is the use of hyperbaric oxygen for multiple sclerosis. A systematic review [4] showed that:
- four case series all showed benefit;
- one non-randomized comparative study showed benefit;
- of 12 randomized trials, not one showed anything other than trivial benefit.

The benefit seen in studies whose design leaves them open to bias was not seen in studies of more rigorous design. This happens frequently.

## Busy people

We are all busy people. In primary care in Europe, physicians have, on average, only a few minutes to spend with each patient (Figure 1) [5]. Nor is it so very different in hospitals, or with different professions, so there is precious little time to spare on evidence.

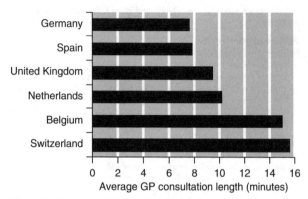

**Figure 1** Average consultation time for GPs in Europe.

We all have different backgrounds and experience. Some of us have spent many years doing research, exploring the bounds of our personal and corporate ignorance. Those who spend their lives doing research find it hard to take new findings on board, especially if there are methodological or statistical issues. Bandolier is reminded of a (clever) mathematician friend who gave a talk, full of symbols and equations. At best we saw through a glass darkly, and praised his ability to handle mathematics with such facility. His response was heartening that, when faced with new concepts and equations, it took him 3 years or so to become comfortable with them! What chance do we ordinary mortals have?

Most of us do not do research or have never done research. Not having done research at any deep level or for any prolonged time is the common experience, probably of about 99% of health-care professionals. Yet we are exhorted to include best research findings into our practice. Most of us just do not have the time to wade through long and complicated scientific papers, even if we had the skills to do so, so we just read the abstract to get the gist of what a paper says, and trust peer-review to eliminate the rubbish.

But most of us do want to know more, and that is exactly the target audience for this little book. For those who want to do more for themselves, this book might make a useful start, if only because it has a healthy dollop of scepticism, perhaps too often missing from those who preach the use of evidence.

### Being cautious

There are many traps and pitfalls to negotiate when assessing evidence, and it is all too easy to be misled by an apparently beautiful study that later turns out to be wrong, or by a meta-analysis with impeccable credentials that seems to be trying to pull the wool over our eyes. Although these are themes often found in the pages of *Bandolier*, a little reinforcement rarely comes amiss.

## Law of initial results

So often early promising results are followed by others that are less impressive. It is almost as if there is a law that states that first results are always spectacular, and subsequent ones are mediocre: the law of initial results. It now seems [6] that there may be some truth in this.

Three major general medical journals (*New England Journal of Medicine*, *Journal of the American Medical Association*, and *Lancet*) were searched for studies with more than 1000 citations published between 1990 and 2003. This is an extraordinarily high number of citations when you think that most papers are cited once if at all, and that a citation of more than a few hundred times is as rare as hens' teeth.

Of the 115 articles published, 49 were eligible for the study because they were reports of original clinical research (like tamoxifen for breast cancer prevention, or stent versus balloon angioplasty). Studies had sample sizes as low as 9 (nine) and as high as 87,000. There were two case series and four cohort studies, and 43 randomized trials. The randomized trials were very varied in size, though, from 146 to 29,133 subjects (median 1817 subjects; Figure 2). Fourteen of the 43 randomized trials (33%) had fewer than 1000 patients and 25 (58%) had fewer than 2500 patients.

Of the 49 studies, seven were contradicted by later research. These seven contradicted studies included one case series with nine patients, three cohort studies with 40,000–80,000 patients, and three randomized trials, with 200,875, and 2002 patients respectively. So only three of 43

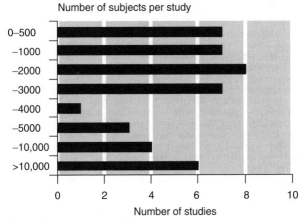

**Figure 2**  Size of highly cited RCTs.

randomized trials were contradicted (7%), compared with half the case series and three out of four cohort studies.

A further seven studies found effects stronger than subsequent research. One of these was a cohort study with 800 patients. The other six were randomized trials, four with fewer than 1000 patients and two with about 1500 patients.

Most of the observational studies had been contradicted, or subsequent research had shown substantially smaller effects, but most randomized studies had results that had not been challenged. Of the nine randomized trials that were challenged, six had fewer than 1000 patients, and all had fewer than 2003 patients. Of 23 randomized trials with 2002 patients or fewer, nine were contradicted or challenged. None of the 20 randomized studies with more than 2003 patients were challenged.

## Most published research false?

As we mentioned earlier, it has been suggested that only 1% of articles in scientific journals are scientifically sound [1]. Bandolier has often examined articles showing how we consumers of scientific literature can be misled, and how we often are. Another paper from Greece [7] is replete with Greek mathematical symbols and philosophy. It makes a number of important points.

1. The smaller the studies conducted in a scientific field, the less likely the research findings are to be true.
2. The smaller the effect sizes in a scientific field, the less likely the research findings are to be true.
3. The greater the number and the fewer the selection of tested relationships in a scientific field, the less likely the research findings are to be true.
4. The greater the flexibility in designs, definitions, outcomes, and analytical modes in a scientific field, the less likely the research findings are to be true.
5. The greater the financial and other interests and prejudices in a scientific field, the less likely the research findings are to be true.
6. The hotter a scientific field (the more scientific teams involved), the less likely the research findings are to be true.

Ioannides [7] then performs a pile of calculations and simulations but then demonstrates the likelihood of us getting at the truth from different typical study types (Table 1). This ranges from odds of 2:1 on (67% likely to be true) from a systematic review of good-quality randomized trials, to 1:3 against (25% likely to be true) from a systematic review of small inconclusive randomized trials, to even lower levels for other architectures.

There is much more in these fascinating papers, but from here on in it all gets more detailed and more complex without becoming necessarily much easier to understand. There is nothing here that contradicts what we already know, namely, that if we accept evidence of poor quality, without validity, or where there are few events or numbers of patients, we are likely, often highly likely, to be misled.

If we concentrate on evidence of high quality, which is valid, and with large numbers, that will hardly ever happen. As Ioannidis also comments, if

**Table 1** Likelihood of truth of research findings from various typical study architectures

| Example | Ratio of true to not true | Positive predictive value |
| --- | --- | --- |
| Confirmatory meta-analysis of good-quality RCTs | 2:1 | 0.85 |
| Adequately powered RCT with little bias and 1:1 pre-study odds | 1:1 | 0.83 |
| Meta-analysis of small, inconclusive studies | 1:3 | 0.41 |
| Underpowered, but poorly performed phase I/II RCT | 1:5 | 0.23 |
| Underpowered, but well performed phase I/II RCT | 1:5 | 0.17 |
| Adequately powered exploratory epidemiological study | 1:10 | 0.2 |
| Underpowered exploratory epidemiological study | 1:10 | 0.12 |
| Discovery-orientated exploratory research with massive testing | 1:1000 | 0.001 |

instead of chasing some ephemeral statistical significance we concentrate our efforts where there is good prior evidence, our chances of getting the true result are better—concentrating on all the evidence. Which may be why clinical trials on pharmaceuticals are so often significant statistically, and in the direction of supporting a drug. Yet, even in that very special circumstance, where so much treasure is expended, years of work with positive results can come to naught when the big trials are done and do not produce the expected answer.

That pretty much tells you what this book is about—avoiding the false.

## Humility

If a little knowledge is dangerous, where is the man who has so much as to be out of danger?

(T.H. Huxley, 1877)

To avoid any hubris, it is always a good idea to acknowledge both the limitations of one's own knowledge, and that the constraint of writing with a particular voice can occasionally lead to flirtation with oversimplification. The aim is to help people overcome their concerns, and to help any consumer of evidence to feel comfortable with thinking about it. Many professionals, and members of the public, have helped Bandolier over the years by suggesting ways we could do things better and being forthright about ways in which they would like data presented. A big thanks to all of them.

## References

1. Smith, R., quoting Professor David Eddy (1991). *British Medical Journal* **303**, 798–9.
2. Smith, L.A., Oldman, A.D., McQuay, H.J. and Moore, R.A. (2000). Teasing apart quality and validity in systematic reviews: an example from acupuncture trials in chronic neck and back pain. *Pain* **86**, 119–32.
3. Rothwell, P.M. and Martyn, C.N. (2000). Reproducibility of peer review in clinical neuroscience. Is agreement between reviewers any greater than would be expected by chance alone? *Brain* **123**, 1964–9.
4. Bennett, M. and Heard, R. (2001). Treatment of multiple sclerosis with hyperbaric oxygen therapy. *Undersea and Hyperbaric Medicine* **28**, 117–22.
5. Deveugele, M. *et al.* (2002). Consultation length in general practice: cross sectional study in six European countries *British Medical Journal* **325**, 472–5.
6. Ioannides, J.P.A. (2005). Contradicted and initially stronger effects in highly cited clinical research. *Journal of the American Medical Association* **294**, 218–28.
7. Ioannides, J.P.A. (2005). Why most published research findings are false. *PLoS Medicine* **2**, e124. (www.plosmedicine.org).
8. Huxley, T.H. (1877). On Elementary Instruction in Physiology. Published in Collected Essays, vol. 3 (1895).

# Basic understanding and tools

## 1.1   Evidence-based medicine

Evidence-based medicine is the conscientious, explicit and judicious use of current best evidence in making decisions about the care of individual patients.

This definition of evidence-based medicine (EBM) from a *BMJ* editorial [1] is probably the best there is. It points out that use of evidence is explicit, that the evidence should be current and the best available, and that it is all about making decisions for individual patients. Of course, evidence can also be used to make policy decisions in guidelines, for formularies, in health technology assessment, or for other reasons, but evidence is also really important for making decisions about individuals. Individuals are rarely if ever average, and recognizing that fact poses other challenges, both for evidence and for decision-making.

Perhaps the most challenging part of the quotation is that it wants us to use the best evidence, and the most up to date evidence. Of these, the hardest is to know when the evidence is the best. The trouble is that there are huge numbers of publications, perhaps several million each year. And many of these, perhaps more than 90%, have been criticized for some failing or other. We have information overload, when what we want is knowledge we can trust to use with wisdom (Figure 1.1.1). That often means using systematic reviews and meta-analyses, where good quality information is brought together. The process of systematic review distils information through quality filters and integrates different types of information to form knowledge, which can be used according to the unique biology of the patient, the values of society, and the conditions of the time.

EBM, then, is the process of systematically reviewing, appraising, and using clinical research findings to aid the delivery of optimum clinical care to patients. Increasingly, purchasers are looking to the strength of scientific

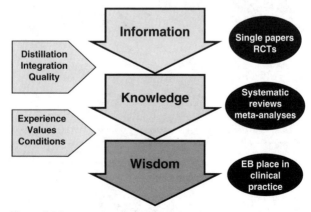

**Figure 1.1.1**   Information, knowledge, and wisdom.

evidence on clinical practice and cost-effectiveness when allocating resources. They are using this information to encourage everyone, from individual doctors and nurses in primary care through to huge hospitals, to adopt more clinically effective and cost-effective practices. This means that all of us have to have at least a passing knowledge of what constitutes good evidence, and this book aims to help busy professionals and interested lay people to get a handle on what constitutes good evidence.

Traditionally, when EBM forms part of the multifaceted process of assuring clinical effectiveness, the main elements are:

- production of evidence through research and scientific review;
- production and dissemination of evidence-based clinical guidelines;
- implementation of evidence-based, cost-effective practice through education and management of change;
- evaluation of compliance with agreed practice guidance and patient outcomes including clinical audit.

It can all get a bit formulaic, and many contend that the best use of EBM is to turn its spotlight on a specified problem, producing answerable questions by addressing:

- person or population in question;
- intervention given;
- comparison (if appropriate);
- outcomes considered.

Next, the problem is refined into explicit questions, which are then checked to see whether the evidence exists. But where can we find the information to help us make better decisions? The following are all common sources:

- personal experience;
- guesswork;
- reasoning and intuition;
- colleagues;
- file drawer (what we have in our filing cabinets);
- published evidence.

It is only by concentrating on the final category that ineffective, dangerous, or costly interventions can be reduced. For evidence to be useful we must:

- search for and locate it;
- appraise it;
- store and retrieve it;
- ensure it is updated;
- communicate and use it.

### Levels of evidence

Some of these topics will be looked at later in more detail. Usually, though, people like to have a framework for handling evidence, for pigeon-holing it, for knowing whether it is good or not. Academics have therefore tried to produce levels of evidence like these in Table 1.1.1, for trials of efficacy or harm, and for observational studies.

Suppose the meta-analysis is wrong and the non-experimental studies and opinion are right? How would you know? Much that goes under the heading of EBM is so formulaic that it can endorse things that are complete nonsense, and eliminate really useful evidence on spurious grounds. People who teach critical appraisal sometimes get upset when this is pointed out,

**Table 1.1.1** Levels of evidence

| Level | Therapy/prevention, aetiology/harm |
|---|---|
| 1a | Systematic review (with homogeneity) of RCTs |
| 1b | Individual RCT (with narrow confidence intervals) |
| 1c | All or none |
| 2a | Systematic review (with homogeneity) of cohort studies |
| 2b | Individual cohort study (including low quality RCT; e.g. < 80% follow-up) |
| 2c | Outcomes research; ecological studies |
| 3a | Systematic review (with homogeneity) of case-control studies |
| 3b | Individual case-control study |
| 4 | Case-series (and poor quality cohort and case-control studies) |
| 5 | Expert opinion without explicit critical appraisal, or based on physiology, bench research, or 'first principles' |

RCT, randomized controlled trial. From *www.cebm.net/levels_of_evidence.asp*.

but in truth they have an almost impossible job. Critical appraisal will be right most of the time, but usually it is insufficiently rigorous, and often that rigour can only come from people with an in-depth knowledge of the problem at hand.

Look at Figure 1.1.2, showing a slightly different paradigm from most critical appraisal. It begins familiarly enough, with concepts of finding evidence and assessing its quality. But then it asks more difficult questions, about credibility or validity, and then even more difficult ones about utility.

In reality EBM is a tad more difficult than following a few simple rules. Remember the old adage that for any complex question there is a simple answer—that's wrong!

### Where doctors get information

Where do doctors go to get their information? Lots of places—print, colleagues, meetings, lectures, Internet, and others. Part of the problem doctors face is the huge amount of stuff being produced. There are more and more randomized trials and systematic reviews, together with other papers on basic science and observational studies. It becomes impossible to keep track of this mass of information.

Doctors and others have to have a strategy that works for them, depending on where they are. Some places will be so computerized that nothing ever goes on to paper. Some will still be using a quill pen. Often the two will be side by side. A systematic review [2] tells us that, for the time being at least, printed papers seem to be king.

Several electronic databases were searched for papers examining information-seeking behaviour in doctors. Studies had to explicitly or implicitly define information sought as medical information, rather than some other form of information. Authors were contacted to seek information about other, unpublished, studies. If the instrument used in data collection was piloted before use, or otherwise independently examined, it was regarded as validated.

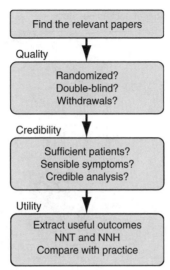

**Figure 1.1.2** A paradigm of EBM (NNT and NNH mean numbers needed to treat or harm, respectively, and are described later).

There were 19 papers published between 1978 and 2001, using questionnaires or interviews or both. Most involved doctors in primary care, mostly in the USA. Random sampling was used in eight studies. The median response rate was 80%.

Paper (books, papers, desk references) was the main source of information in 13 studies, colleagues were the main source in four, and one (published in 1996) found electronic sources to be the main source. There was no change over time.

Figure 1.1.3 shows the percentage of doctors using print sources. Most studies showed that print sources were used by over 50% of doctors. Figure 1.1.4 shows the percentage using colleagues. Most showed that colleagues were used by under 40%.

There was little recent information from outside the USA. In Britain and other countries with large socialized health-care systems, it seems a little odd that no one has bothered to find out how the main consumers of medical information get that information.

The authors of the review are in no doubt that convenience of access, reliability and high quality, quick use, applicability, and habit make information-seeking likely to occur and be successful. Lack of time, the huge amount of material, and forgetfulness hinder the process. This means that perhaps only one question in three or four gets followed up. Making it easier and better could improve this, and help doctors (and other professionals) use good evidence more.

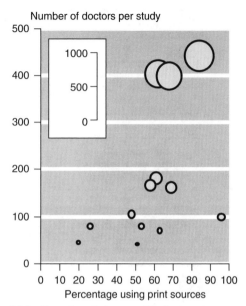

Number of doctors per study

**Figure 1.1.3** Doctors' use of print sources (this plot shows the percentage using print sources according to the number of doctors in each study, and the size of the symbol for each study is proportional to the number of doctors in it. The plot gives greater weight to larger studies).

## Barriers to EBM

A study conducted among 60 GPs in Sydney in mid-1999 [3] used methods and questions generally similar to those of a previous Wessex survey in the UK [4], but with additional questions. All 60 GPs returned their questionnaires.

Important barriers to the use of evidence-based medicine were four: unrealistic patient expectations; time; skills; and money (Figure 1.1.5).

The largest single barrier, noted by almost half these Australian GPs, is that patients demand treatment despite a lack of evidence of effectiveness, and one GP in five was concerned about unrealistic patient expectations driving treatment choice, rather than the evidence.

Time was a huge problem, whether for locating, reading, and appraising evidence, or for discussing the evidence with patients. One in four GPs was worried about the cost of purchasing resources for evidence-based practice, and lack of skills was important to a minority of GPs.

Clearly, top sources of EBM were evidence-based clinical practice guidelines and journals summarizing important research evidence, like *Evidence-based Medicine* and *Bandolier*, much the same as was found in Wessex some years earlier [4]. Systematic reviews, or original articles, including the Cochrane Library, were bottom of the list.

Number of doctors per study

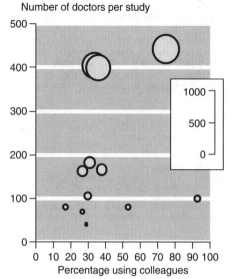

**Figure 1.1.4** Doctors' use of colleagues.

### Access and understanding

Internet access for 67%
Low understanding of EBM terms
Huge demand for more education

### Barriers to EBM

Unrealistic patient expectation and demand
Time, money, skills

### Resources to provide

Evidence-based practice guidelines
*Evidence-based Medicine*, *Bandolier*
Ongoing quality education

**Figure 1.1.5** Barriers to EBM.

## Commentary

Everyone wants to use the best evidence available. The message seems to be that, with limited time available, professionals have a hard time finding it, and being sure that it is the best. This obviously limits their ability to use it. There is much given in the way of guidance and guidelines, but even these can be such a burden as to be difficult to use, especially where guidelines and evidence disagree. This book should help in deciding how best to progress when that happens. But there are no simple answers, and few short cuts.

## References

1. Sackett, D.L. *et al.* (1996). Evidence-based medicine: what it is and what it isn't [editorial]. *British Medical Journal* **312**, 71–2.
2. Dawes, M. and Sampson, U. (2003). Knowledge management in clinical practice: a systematic review of information seeking behaviour in physicians. *International Journal of Medical Informatics* **71**, 9–15.
3. Young, J.M. and Ward, J.E. (2001). Evidence-based medicine in general practice: beliefs and barriers among Australian GPs. *Journal of Evaluation in Clinical Practice* **7**, 201–10.
4. McColl, A. *et al.* (1998). General practitioners' perceptions of the route to evidence-based medicine: a questionnaire survey. *British Medical Journal* **316**, 361–5.

# 1.2 Searching for evidence

The medical literature is vast, with tens of thousands of journals and millions of articles, and it is growing every day. It is estimated that there are over 30,000 biomedical journals, and tens if not hundreds of thousands of books. The journals publish three to six million papers every year. A 2005 estimate was that there were over 20,000 reports of clinical trials every year [1]. Then there is a whole tranche of publication that is called the 'grey' literature, not that it's boring, but not easily available, being in the form of reports, theses, or monographs.

Nobody has a library that takes every journal that might ever publish an article of interest and, even then, the task of finding that article by manual searching would be close to impossible. Fortunately, there are now a number of bibliographic databases available for electronic searching, which makes the task possible, and sometimes easy. We live in rapidly changing times, so that what is possible in 2005 could hardly have been dreamt of in 1995. More and better information is continually becoming available to enable any of us to access information that would previously been available only to the privileged few. Busy folk of the Cochrane Collaboration, for instance, have looked through dusty journal shelves to find almost 500,000 controlled clinical trials, and make their work available in the Cochrane Library.

To practice evidence-based medicine we need the 'best evidence', and the purists would say that we need to look at *all* relevant evidence to be sure that what we have is the 'best'. In practice this can never be possible—there is always a trade off between the comprehensiveness of a search and available time/expertise/resources. Whatever your own limits, a systematic approach is needed to identify the best evidence available to you.

Most of us are not going to do a systematic review from scratch every time we need to answer a question. What we want is a relatively simple way to know whether evidence exists, where it is, and what it is. For the most part, then we will work with a hierarchy of evidence—start by looking for systematic reviews or meta-analyses and avoiding reinventing wheels. If there are no systematic reviews, we might search for randomized trials or individual studies, and this section is about how busy people can most easily to do that.

## Basics of searching

The process of searching involves clearly identifying the question being asked, selecting a suitable database to search, choosing appropriate key words and combining them in a search strategy, running the search, reviewing the articles retrieved, and, if necessary, modifying the search strategy or searching a different database.

### The question

The first step in searching for evidence is to work out exactly what question you want answered. It is useful to think of four components, commonly known as PICO:

**P**opulation or Patient;
**I**ntervention (therapy, diagnostic test, exposure, risk factor);
**C**omparison to the intervention;
**O**utcome(s) of interest.

For example, we might ask: *Is acupuncture effective in chronic back pain?* As stated, this is a very broad question. Think about it a bit more deeply for a moment.

- The **population** is patients with chronic back pain: do you want to include all patients with chronic back pain, or restrict the population to, for example, those with pain resulting from osteoarthritis, or after back surgery?
- The **intervention** is acupuncture: do you want to include studies involving only one treatment, or only those providing a course of, say, a minimum of four treatments? Do you have any preconceptions about different 'types' of acupuncture?
- The **comparison** might be no treatment, or analgesics, but you might want only to consider studies in which the patient was blinded to the treatment received, in which case the comparison would need to be sham acupuncture.
- The **outcome** might be a measure of pain or mobility or quality of life, but you may also be worried about rare but serious adverse events.

Most clinicians want an answer that helps them to treat the patient sitting in front of them, but it is important to remember not to be too specific about the defined population when formulating a question. Your patient may be a 65-year-old Afro-Caribbean woman, but searches for relevant trials in only older Afro-Caribbean women may retrieve very few, if any, articles. You need to decide whether trials conducted in Caucasians, or men, or younger or older patients are still relevant.

### Databases

The largest, and probably best known, general biomedical database is MEDLINE, which indexes over 4800 journals, has over 12 million records dating back to 1966, and is produced by the US National Library of Medicine. The other large general database is EMBASE, which indexes a similar number of journals, has records back to 1980, and is produced by Elsevier Science. Although the databases index a similar number of journals, these are overlapping sets, with some journals indexed by both. EMBASE has more pharmacology-related and European journals than MEDLINE. There are other more specialized databases that concentrate on specific areas of medicine. For example, PsychINFO contains psychological studies, CINHAL contains nursing and allied health studies, and Allied and Complementary Medicine Database contains studies of complementary and alternative medicine. There are also databases that provide evidence-based reviews, such as the Cochrane Database of Systematic Reviews (in the Cochrane Library) and ACP Journal Club.

Whichever database(s) you choose to search, it is a good idea to invest a little time finding out how it conducts its searches, as they do differ in the format required for entry of search terms and the way in which they search the records. They all have good user guides.

### Search strategy

It is unlikely that any electronic search is capable of finding all the papers you want. This may be because the papers are not in databases, or there are errors, but even the best search strategies are unlikely to get the lot. Even people who work on this full time on academic projects cannot do much better than a sensitivity of 97–99% [2].

Having decided what question is being asked and which databases you will use, the next step is to choose key words or search terms. The search does not need to include key words for all of the components of the question. In our example we might choose: osteoarthritis and pain and acupuncture.

- When selecting key words it is important to think about possible different spellings of a word, e.g. hemoglobin/haemoglobin. You will need to search for **hemoglobin** or **haemoglobin**, or use a wildcard symbol. The wildcard symbol replaces one letter or none, and in this example would be **h?emoglobin**.

- You may want to retrieve variants of a single word, e.g. bleed, bleeds, bleeding, by using the truncation symbol, which identifies all words with the same stem. In this case it would be **bleed\***.

- You may also need to think about different words to describe the same thing (synonyms). For example, if your outcome of interest is **death** you may also need to search for **mortality** and **survival**.

Bibliographic databases contain records of individual published articles, with the content allocated to distinct fields, e.g. title, author, abstract. When the article is indexed it is also allocated a number of terms, using controlled vocabulary (Unified Medical Language System), that describe the article in terms of the population, intervention, comparator, and outcomes. These are called MESH (Medical Subject Headings) descriptors in MED-LINE, and SU (Subjects) descriptors in EMBASE. Other terms are allocated to describe characteristics such as the design of the study, the age range of the participants, and whether they were male or female, human or animal. You can search in all the fields (default), or in selected fields, by adding a field tag, e.g. [ti] for title. You can also search using free text words, or controlled vocabulary.

Key words are combined using Boolean operators. The most commonly used operators are AND, OR, and NOT (Figure 1.2.1). Combining two key words with AND will retrieve records that contain both words, combining them with OR will retrieve records that contain either word (or both), and combining them with NOT will retrieve records that contain the first, but not the second term. The operator WITH retrieves records in which the two words appear in the same record, and NEAR retrieves records in which the two words appear in the same sentence, or within a specified number of words.

The search 'string' is read from left to right, and can contain brackets, obeying the laws of algebra. For instance, if we wanted to know about paracetamol in osteoarthritis we could search for 'paracetamol AND osteoarthritis'. But paracetamol is known as acetaminophen in some parts of the world, so we should include that, too. The use of brackets makes this simple.

(acetaminophen OR paracetamol) AND osteoarthritis

There is no right or wrong way to build a search strategy. Using the operators AND and NOT has the effect of limiting the number of articles retrieved, while using OR will increase the number of articles retrieved. Be careful when using NOT as it is easy to eliminate useful studies, especially if double negatives are involved. In the example of acupuncture for back pain due to osteoarthritis, we might want to eliminate studies in patients with

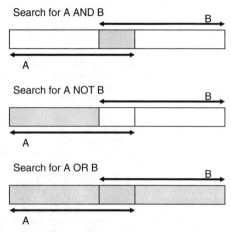

**Figure 1.2.1** Boolean operators AND, OR, NOT.

osteoarthritis of the knee, so include **NOT knee** in the search string. This would also eliminate articles that included patients with osteoarthritis of either the back or knee, and also studies with osteoarthritis of the knee as an exclusion criterion.

Most people start with a broad search strategy, retrieving probably all relevant articles, but also a high proportion of non-relevant ones (high **sensitivity** search). By reviewing the articles retrieved you can then refine the search to eliminate more of the non-relevant articles, increasing the **specificity** of the search. The danger is that, in eliminating the non-relevant articles, relevant ones are also lost, so it is useful to check as you go, and inevitably a compromise will need to be made between sensitivity (finding all the relevant articles) and specificity (eliminating the non-relevant articles).

### Using PubMED

MEDLINE is available free using the PubMED website (*www.pubmed.gov*), is user-friendly, and the usual starting point for most people. PubMED searches using **automatic term mapping**, which essentially means that it searches for the term entered (and its synonyms) as a MESH term in addition to a text word, unless instructed otherwise. It does a lot of the work for you, and takes much hassle out of simple searches. The Boolean operators AND, OR, and NOT are recognized and need to be in capital letters. NEAR and NEXT are not recognized, but PubMED uses automatic term mapping to recognize phrases, or quotation marks can be used.

"febrile convulsion", "home visit"

We can enter our search string **osteoarthritis AND pain AND acupuncture** into the query box on the general search page, then click on the Go button. The results of the search are displayed in Figure 1.2.2. By

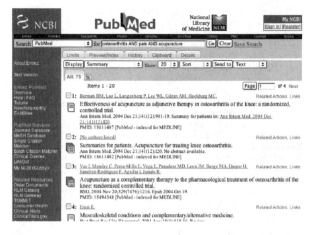

**Figure 1.2.2**

default, results are displayed as citations (author, title, source). To see the abstract, click on either the author or the page icon to the left of the title. From this page it may be possible to link out to the journal or PubMED Central to obtain the full text article, although this sometimes requires a subscription or payment.

There are five tabs beneath the query box. Clicking on the **Limits** tag gives us the option to limit the search to specific fields, publication types, etc. We might choose to limit our search to randomized controlled trials in human adults. Select the appropriate options and click Go. The number of retrieved records is considerably reduced, and should be more relevant (Figure 1.2.3). You can see the exact search string that PubMED has used by clicking on the **Details** tab.

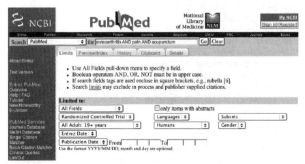

**Figure 1.2.3**

The search strategy and results of each search are saved (up to a limit of 100 searches) and can be seen by clicking on the **History** tab. They are numbered consecutively, and can be combined or modified using these numbers, e.g. #1 AND #3, or #2 AND Smith AN). To re-run a search, click on the number under Result on the right hand side.

Articles of interest can be saved to the clipboard for future use. Tick the box to the left to the article(s), then from the **Send to** menu select **Clipboard**, then click on the **Send to** button. Up to 500 citations can be stored on the clipboard. To see what you have saved to the clipboard, click on the **Clipboard** tab.

To print saved citations, first select the output you want (e.g. citation or abstract) from the **Display** menu, and click on the button, then select **Text** from the Send to menu, and click on the button. This will open a text file containing your saved citations, which can then be printed. To save citations for transfer to a reference management application, select **MEDLINE** from the Display menu, and **File** from the Send to menu. Save the file, which can then be imported into your reference management software (like ProCite, or EndNote).

### Searching by field

You can search for a particular term in a particular field by adding the correct **field tag**, enclosed in square brackets, to the term. A list of field tags is available in the Help section.

Acupuncture[ti], Walters[au], BMJ[so]

For authors, entering the name as surname, space, initial(s) (up to two), will automatically force the search in the author field, without using the tag.

Walters AB

### Searching with MESH terms

The National Library of Medicine uses a controlled vocabulary thesaurus known as MESH (Medical Subject Headings) to index articles for MEDLINE. Experienced indexers assign these headings according to a paper's importance to the subject. The aim is to facilitate retrieval of information relating to a particular subject or concept despite use of different terminology. Sets of terms naming descriptors are arranged in 'trees' in alphabetic and hierarchical structure. At higher levels the headings are broad and general (e.g. disease category), becoming increasingly specific at lower levels (pain, back pain, low back pain).

On the general search page, select Search MESH, and type your term into the query box. A list of potentially relevant terms will be displayed together with a definition of each. Select the one you want, and follow the instructions to either search for all records in PubMed with that term, or Send to Search Box to refine the search further and/or combine it with other terms. As a default, PubMed will 'explode' the MESH term selected, to include terms found below this term in the MESH tree. Phrase searching with quotation marks turns off the MESH explosion. Articles in PreMEDLINE have no MESH terms assigned, so will not be identified by searching the MESH fields.

### Clinical queries

Under PubMED services in the blue strip on the left-hand side of the PubMED screen, is a heading **Clinical Queries**. This feature is intended for use by clinicians, and has three specialized types of searches: clinical study category; systematic review; and medical genetics.

The first uses built-in **methodological filters** to identify articles falling into four categories based on research methods: aetiology ('etiology' in PubMed, because it is US); diagnosis; therapy; and prognosis. You can also choose whether to conduct a broad (sensitive) or narrow (specific) search. Simply enter your search terms, select the category and breadth of search required and click on Go (Figure 1.2.4). The results are displayed, and the usual tabs are available for modifying the search, saving, etc. To see the search strategy for the filter used, click on Details (Figure 1.2.5).

The second type of search uses methodological filters to identify studies that are **systematic reviews** or similar articles (meta-analyses, reviews of clinical trials, evidence-based medicine, consensus development conferences, and guidelines).

### Using methodological filters

Controlled clinical trials (randomized or not) are probably the only study types that can reliably be identified using only MESH terms. This is because the Cochrane Collaboration and the National Library of Medicine have put

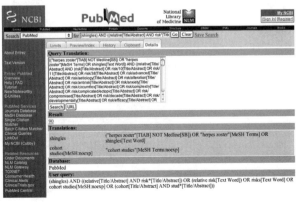

**Figure 1.2.4**

**Figure 1.2.5**

a great deal of effort into identifying and correctly indexing all controlled trials. Indexing of other study types, including all epidemiological studies, is less reliable, particularly in earlier records.

## Using the Cochrane Library

The Cochrane Library is available free to NHS staff, patients, and the public in England through the NLH, at *www.library.nhs.uk/*. The library is updated four times a year, and contains a number of databases, including:
- Cochrane Database of Systematic Reviews (CDSR)—systematic reviews of the effects of healthcare, carried out by the Cochrane Collaboration. Both completed reviews and protocols for reviews in progress are included, and completed reviews are regularly updated.
- Database of Abstracts of Reviews of Effects (DARE)—structured abstracts of critically appraised systematic reviews published elsewhere.
- Cochrane Central Register of Controlled Trials (CENTRAL)—this is the largest register of reports of controlled trials in the world, compiled by electronic searching of bibliographic databases and hand searching of journals.

The query box is in the top right-hand corner of the home page. Boolean operators are recognized and do not have to be in capitals. Two terms entered without an operator are searched as if they were joined by 'and'. To search as a phrase enclose the word in quotation marks (e.g. "back pain"). We can type in our search strategy and using the default of **Search all Text**, click on Go (Figure 1.2.6).

The results are displayed showing the number of records retrieved in each database, and listing those found in Cochrane Reviews. Select another database to see the records there (Figure 1.2.7). The results can be

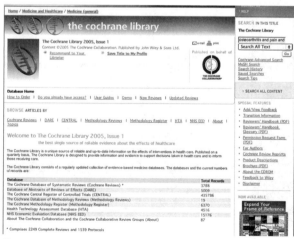

**Figure 1.2.6**

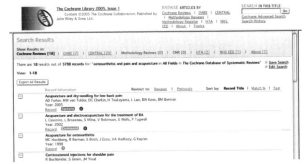

**Figure 1.2.7**

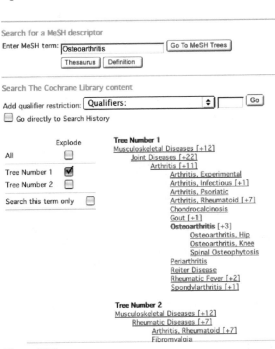

**Figure 1.2.8**

**Table 1.2.1** Internet sites for finding papers

| Website | Address |
|---|---|
| Bandolier | www.ebandolier.com |
| PubMed | www.ncbi.nlm.nih.gov/entrez |
| US National Library of Medicine | www.nlm.nih.gov/entrez |
| UK National Library of Health | www.library.nhs.uk |
| Cochrane Library | www.thecochranelibrary.com |
| Embase | www.embase.com |
| Psychinfo | www.psychinfo.com |
| CINHAL | www.cinhal.com |
| ACP Journal Club | www.acponline.org / Journals / EBM/EBMmenu.html |
| Medscape | www.medscape.com |
| Allied & Complementary Medicine Database | www.bl.uk/collections/health/amed.html |
| Netting the evidence | www.shef.ac.uk/scharr/ir/netting |

restricted to reviews or protocols as required, complete records can be accessed, searches can be saved, and citations exported by clicking on the relevant buttons and following simple instructions where appropriate.

Searching all text will identify articles that contain your search term(s) anywhere in the record, and can give large numbers of irrelevant articles. The **Cochrane Advanced Search** allows you to refine the search using specific fields for different terms. The **MESH Search** allows you to identify the relevant MESH term and execute the search. The default search is set to include all terms below the selected term in the MESH tree(s) (explode). To search ONLY the selected term, or to explode a particular MESH tree, tick the relevant box(es). Searching for the osteoarthritis term only would not retrieve reviews indexed as spinal osteophytosis (Figure 1.2.8).

### Other places to visit

Website addresses useful for finding papers are given in Table 1.2.1. **Netting the Evidence** contains links to a wide variety of on-line resources that might help in finding the best evidence. It includes sections on Searching, Journals, and Databases. The content of most of the journals and databases is evidence-based reviews, summaries, and guidelines.

### And finally

Readers will understand that while all the above was correct at the time it was written, it may not be current when the book is published and read. General principles should not change, though design of interfaces may change.

### References

1. Sackett, D. (2005). Participants in research. *British Medical Journal* **330**, 1164.
2. Haynes, R.B. *et al.* (2005). Optimal search strategies for retrieving scientifically strong studies of treatment from Medline: analytical survey. *British Medical Journal* **330**, 1179–82.

# 1.3  The importance of size

The sock-drawer problem seemed to be a good place to start when thinking about size (or numbers), especially on cold, dark, winter mornings. When we think about size (or numbers) in the sock drawer or any other context, the numbers we need to answer a question depend on the precise question asked. Socks can help us get our brains around it (and help us to look clever at dinner parties).

### The scenario

We have 20 pairs of socks: 10 pairs of red socks (20 red socks in total) and 10 pairs of white socks (20 white socks in total). The problem is that they are all mixed up in my sock drawer, and it is dark, so I can't see the colour of the socks I am taking out of the drawer. We can ask a number of subtly different questions.

Q1:  How many socks do I have to take out to be sure that I have a pair of socks?

A1:  Two socks, as long as I don't care what colour they are. I may have two red socks, two white socks, or one white and one red. Whichever I have my two socks, and by many definitions that constitutes a pair.

Q2:  How many socks do I have to take out to be sure that I have a pair of socks of the same colour?

A2:  Three socks, so long as I don't care what colour they are. I may have three red socks, three white socks, two white and one red, or one white and two red. Whichever I have, I have two socks of the same colour in my three sock sample.

Q3:  How many socks do I have to take out to be sure that I have a pair of red socks?

A3:  Twenty-two socks, because it could be that just by chance I pull out all 20 white socks first, and then have to pull out two of the remaining 20 red socks.

But that is unlikely. So how many socks do I need to pull out to be 95% sure (or 90%, or 75%, or 50%) of having a pair of red socks in the sample of socks I take from the drawer? That depends. It depends on how confident I want to be. If I want to be 100% sure, it is 22 socks. If I am prepared to take more of a chance, then I can sample fewer socks. The point is that the number of socks I need to pull out rises sharply with the confidence I need to put in the answer.

These answers to all these questions will depend on the proportion of red and white socks in the drawer. The numbers will change as the proportion of red socks in the drawer changes.

### Clinical trials

A clinical trial is a bit like two sock drawers (or more), with different proportions of socks in each, where we try to find out the proportion of red socks by randomly choosing socks from each drawer until we have enough to answer the question.

But what is the question? You have several choices here, including these:
- Are there more red socks in drawer 1 than in drawer 2?
- How big is the difference in the proportion of red socks between drawer 1 and drawer 2?
- What proportion of red socks is in drawer 1?

Think about ibuprofen used as an analgesic. In clinical trial terms these sock drawer questions are roughly like asking whether ibuprofen is a better analgesic than placebo, by how much is it better, and what proportion of people with pain have their pain relieved by ibuprofen? There are different answers to different questions, and the numbers of socks or patients needed to answer them differ.

### Random chance, quality, and size

These are all related topics. This section therefore examines aspects of all of them. First it looks at the effects of random chance that we can get just by rolling dice. Then it examines how likely our results are to change, depending on the amount of information we have available, and finally it reverts to the answers to the sock drawer, or ibuprofen question.

#### Rolling dice

'There is much luck in the world, but it is luck. We are none of us safe.' So said E.M. Forster nearly 100 years ago. It is astonishing how many people appreciate the importance of chance, in, say, winning a lottery or avoiding a car accident, but not in clinical trials. Perhaps it is all down to the way statistics are taught. We should forget probabilities and p-values, and acquaint ourselves with more relevant information, notably how much data do we need to be sure that an observation is not likely to occur just by chance.

Why are people impressed with p-values? The cherished value of 0.05 merely says that a result is likely to have occurred by chance no more than 1 time in 20. Most of us have played Monopoly or other games involved with throwing dice. We will have experienced that throwing two sixes with two dice happens relatively often, yet the chance of that is about 1 time in 36.

Look at it another way. If you were about to cross a bridge, and were told that there was a 1 in 20 chance of it falling down when you were on it, would you take the chance? What about 1 in 100, or 1 in 1000? That p-value of 0.05 also tells you that 1 time in 20 the bridge is likely to fall down.

The dice analogy is pertinent, because there are now (at least) two papers that look at random chance and clinical trials, reminding us how often and how much chance can affect results. An older study actually used dice to mimic clinical trials in stroke prevention [1], while a more recent study [2] used computer simulations of cancer therapy.

#### DICE 1

In this study [1] participants in a practical class on statistics at a stroke course were given dice and asked to roll them a specified number of times to represent the treatment group of a randomized trial of a 'new' treatment for stroke. If a six was thrown, this was recorded as a death, with any other number a survival. The procedure was repeated for a control group of similar size. Group size ranged from 5 to 100 patients.

The paper gives the results of all 44 trials for 2256 'patients'. While the paper does many clever things, it is perhaps more instructive to look at the results of the 44 trials. Since each arm of the trial looks for the throwing of one out of six possibilities for standard dice, we might expect that the rate of events was 16.7% (100/6) in each, with an odds ratio or relative risk of 1.

Figure 1.3.1 shows a L'Abbé plot of the 44 trials. In a L'Abbé plot, each trial is represented by a symbol whose size is proportional to the size of the trial; if there is no difference between treatments the symbols should fall along the line of equality. The expected result in this case is a grouping in the bottom left, on the line of equality, at about 17%. Actually, it is a bit more dispersed than that, with some trials far from the line of equality.

The odds ratios for individual trials are shown in Figure 1.3.2. Two trials (with 20 and 40 'patients' in total) had odds ratios statistically different from 1. That's one time in every 22 trials, and is what we expect by chance.

The variability in individual trial arms is shown in Figure 1.3.3, where the results are shown for all 88 trial arms. The vertical line shows the overall result (16.7%). Larger samples come close to this, but small samples show values as low as zero, and as high as 60%.

The overall result, pooling data from all 44 trials, showed that events ('deaths') occurred in 16.0% of treatments and 17.6% of controls (overall mean 16.7%). The relative risk was 0.8 (0.5 to 1.1). The NNT was 62, with a 95% confidence interval that went from one benefit for every 21 treatments to one harm for every 67 treatments (Table 1.3.1).

Many of the experimental DICE trials were quite small, with as few as five per group. The smaller trials, with 40 per group or less, actually came

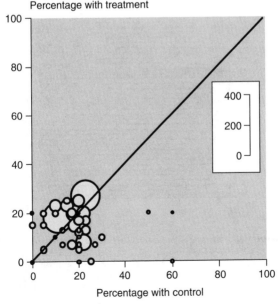

Percentage with treatment

**Figure 1.3.1**    L'Abbé plot of DICE 1 trials.

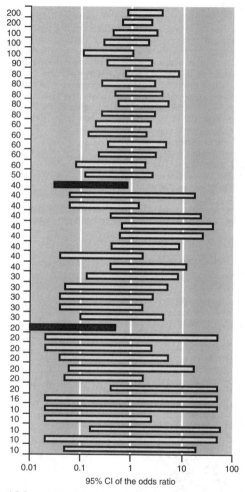

**Figure 1.3.2** Odds ratios for individual DICE studies, by number in 'trial'. Filled bars were statistically significant.

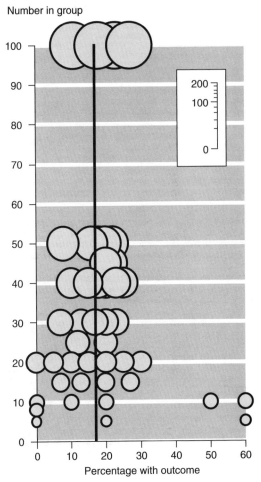

**Figure 1.3.3** Percentage of events in each trial arm of DICE 'trials'.

**Table 1.3.1** Meta-analysis of DICE trials, with sensitivity analysis by size of trial

|  | Number of | | Outcome (%) with | | Relative | NNT |
|---|---|---|---|---|---|---|
|  | Trials | Patients | Treatment | Control | risk (95% CI) | (95% CI) |
| All trials | 44 | 2256 | 16.0 | 17.6 | 0.8 (0.5 to 1.1) | 62 (21 to −67) |
| Larger trials (> 40 per group) | 11 | 1190 | 19.5 | 17.8 | 1.1 (0.9 to 1.4) | −60 (35 to −16) |
| Smaller trials (< 40 per group) | 33 | 1066 | 12.0 | 17.3 | 0.7 (0.53 to 0.94) | 19 (11 to 98) |

up with a statistically significant result (Table 1.3.1). The NNT here was 19 (11 to 98).

*DICE 2*

Information on the time between randomization and death in a control group of 580 patients in a colorectal cancer trial was used to simulate 100 theoretical clinical trials. Each time the same 580 patients were randomly allocated to a theoretical treatment or control group, and survival curves calculated [2].

Four of the trials generated artificially had statistically significant results. One was significant at the $p = 0.003$ level (1 in 333) and showed a large theoretical decrease in mortality of 40%.

Subgroup analysis was done for this trial by randomly allocating patients to type A or type B, and doing this 100 times. Over half (55%) of the subgroup analyses showed statistical significance between subgroups. The extremes of results were on the one hand no difference between subgroups, and on the other a result with a difference of very high statistical significance (0.00005, or 1 in 20,000). In another trial that had bare statistical significance, four of 100 simulated subgroups had statistical significance at the 1 in 100 level.

*What do these trials tell us?*

They emphasize that the random play of chance is a factor we cannot ignore, and that small trials are more prone to chance effects than larger ones. And it is not just an effect seen in single trials. Even when we pool data from small trials just from rolling dice, as in DICE 1, a meta-analysis can come up with a statistically significant effect when there was none.

High levels of statistical significance can be generated just by the random play of chance. DICE 2 found levels of statistical significance of 1 in 333 for at least one simulated trial, and 1 in 20,000 for a subgroup analysis of that trial.

Not only do we need well-conducted trials of robust design and reporting, we also need large amounts of information if the size of a clinical effect is to be accurately assessed. The rule of thumb is that where the difference between control and treatment is small we need very large amounts of information. Only when the difference is large (an absolute risk increase or decrease of 50%, affecting every second patient) can we be reasonably happy with information from 500 patients or fewer.

When we see differences in results between trials, or between responses to placebo, the rush is often to try and explain away the difference as due to some facet of trial design or patient characteristic. Almost never does anyone ask how likely the difference is to occur just by the random play of chance.

## Quality and size

Study architecture and size are often linked. Three Danish researchers looked for large clinical trials with at least 1000 patients together with meta-analyses of small trials [3]. They were asking the sensible question about how possible discrepancies between large trials and meta-analyses of small trials could be affected by methodological quality.

They found 14 meta-analyses with corresponding large RCTs, pulled all the original papers, subjected those to quality review, and examined outcomes in terms of odds ratios. They then used the ratio of the odds ratio in the large randomized trial to that from the meta-analysis of small trials to produce a 'ratio of odds ratios' as the final outcome. When the ratio of odds ratios was significantly less than 1, that indicated that small trials with particular quality criteria exaggerated the effect of an intervention compared with the large trial.

The quality criteria they tested for were generation of the allocation sequence (randomization), allocation concealment, double-blinding, and withdrawals or drop-outs. The relevant criteria are shown in Table 1.3.2.

The researchers used 23 large trials and 167 small trials with 136,000 patients. Compared with large trials, small trials with inadequate generation or allocation concealment of the randomization sequence, or those that were not adequately double-blinded overestimated the effect of treatment (Table 1.3.3). When methodological quality was compared in large and small trials, inadequate generation of the randomization sequence and inadequate double-blinding caused overestimation of the treatment effect

**Table 1.3.2** Quality criteria tested

| Quality feature | Adequate | Inadequate |
| --- | --- | --- |
| Generation of the allocation sequence | Computer-generated random number or similar | Not described |
| Allocation concealment | Central independent unit, sealed envelope, or similar | Not described, or open table of random numbers |
| Double blinding | Identical placebo or similar | Not described or tablets versus injection not double dummy |
| Withdrawals or drop-outs | Number and reasons for drop-outs | Not described |

**Table 1.3.3** Comparison of large trials with small trials with different quality criteria

| Common comparator | Comparison | Ratio of odds ratios (95% CI) |
| --- | --- | --- |
| Large trials | Small trials with inadequate generation of allocation sequence | **0.46 (0.25 to 0.83)** |
| Large trials | Small trials with adequate generation of allocation sequence | 0.90 (0.47 to 1.76) |
| Large trials | Small trials with inadequate allocation concealment | **0.49 (0.27 to 0.86)** |
| Large trials | Small trials with adequate allocation concealment | 1.01 (0.48 to 2.11) |
| Large trials | Small trials with inadequate or no double blinding | **0.52 (0.28 to 0.96)** |
| Large trials | Small trials with adequate double blinding | 0.84 (0.43 to 1.66) |
| Large trials | Small trials with inadequate follow-up | 0.72 (0.30 to 1.71) |
| Large trials | Small trials with adequate follow-up | 0.58 (0.32 to 1.02) |

When the ratio of the odds ratios is less than 1, it indicates that the feature (inadequate blinding, for example) exaggerates the intervention effect. Shaded and bold indicates statistical significance.

(Table 1.3.4), and much the same was found for a similar analysis of small trials alone.

In these tables, small trials with a characteristic have been compared with large trials, and odds ratios compared. If the ratio is below 1 (that is, the 95% confidence interval does not include 1), then a feature exaggerates the treatment effect.

Quality scoring using the Oxford system [4], perhaps one of the most commonly used scoring systems in systematic reviews (see later), produced sensible results. Small trials with lower quality scores overestimated

**Table 1.3.4** Comparison of adequate versus inadequate quality criteria in large and small trials

| Common comparator | Comparison | Ratio of odds ratios (95% CI) |
| --- | --- | --- |
| Adequate | Inadequate generation of allocation sequence | **0.49 (0.30 to 0.81)** |
| Adequate | Inadequate allocation concealment | 0.60 (0.31 to 1.15) |
| Adequate | Inadequate or no double blinding | **0.56 (0.33 to 0.98)** |
| Adequate | Inadequate follow-up | 1.50 (0.80 to 2.78) |

When the ratio of the odds ratios is less than 1, it indicates that the feature (inadequate blinding, for example) exaggerates the intervention effect. Shaded and bold indicates statistical significance.

treatment effects compared with large trials. Small trials with higher quality scores did not. In both large and small trials, treatment effects were exaggerated with low versus high quality scores.

At first look this is all complicated pointy-head stuff, but actually it's no more than simple common sense. If trials are not done properly, they might be wrong. If trials are small, they might be wrong. To be sure of a result we need large data sets of high quality, whether from single trials or meta-analyses. The corollary is that, if we have small amounts of information, or information of poor quality, the chance of that result being incorrect is substantial, and then we need to be cautious and conservative.

### Variability and size

Clinical trials should have a power calculation performed at the design stage. This will estimate how many patients are needed so that, say, 90% of studies with $X$ patients would show a difference of $Y$% between two treatments. When the value of $Y$ is very large, the value of $X$ can be small. More often the value of $Y$ is modest, or small. In those circumstances, $X$ needs to be larger, and more patients will be needed in trials for them to have a hope of showing a difference.

Yet clinical trials are often ridiculously small. *Bandolier*'s record is a randomized study on three patients in a parallel group design. But when are trials so tiny that they can be ignored? Many take a pragmatic view that trials with fewer than 10 patients per treatment arm should be ignored, and not included in a systematic review, though others may disagree, and context may be important. In a rare disease or a rare condition, small trials may be vital and necessary. In common diseases or conditions there is really no excuse for not making the trial of sensible size.

### Random play of chance

The degree of variability between trials of adequate power is still large, because trials are powered to detect that there is a *difference* between treatments, rather than *how big* that difference is. The random play of chance can remain a significant factor despite adequate power to detect a difference.

Figure 1.3.4 shows the randomized, double-blind studies comparing ibuprofen 400 mg with placebo in acute postoperative pain [5]. The trials had the same patient population, with identical initial pain intensity and with identical outcomes measured in the same way for the same time using standard measuring techniques. There were big differences in the outcomes of individual studies.

Figure 1.3.5 shows the results of 10,000 studies in a computer model based on information from about 5000 individual patients [6]. Anywhere in the grey area is where a study could occur just because of the random play of chance. And for those who may think that this reflects on pain as a subjective outcome, the same variability can be seen in other trial settings, with objective outcomes.

### Minimum number of events

If random chance is so important, how can we know when there is sufficient information for us not to be misled? There are two simple things to bear in mind. The first is that we have to recognize the difference between number of events (successful or unsuccessful outcome of a trial) and number of

Adequate pain relief with ibuprofen 400 mg (%)

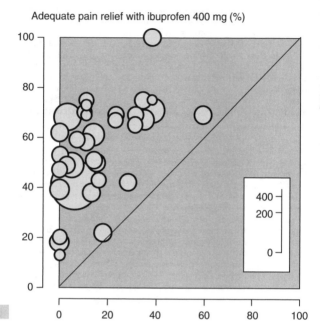

Adequate pain relief with placebo (%)

**Figure 1.3.4** Trials of ibuprofen in acute pain that are randomized, double-blind, and with the same outcomes over the same time in patients with the same initial pain intensity.

people. A sample of 10,000 people where there are only two events is not more impressive than a group of 40 patients in whom 20 events occur. We have to be mindful of the number of events as well as the number of patients in a sample. Of course, it depends on whether you are looking at efficacy events or adverse events, when 2 in 20,000 would be more useful.

If no events occur in, say, 5000 patients, then the best we can say is that we can be 95% confident that the event does not occur more frequently than once every 5000/3, or 1667 patients [7]. This inverse rule of 3 is useful when we think that new treatments are often launched following experience in only a few thousand patients.

We can investigate the effect of numbers on our confidence by the simple expedient of feeding different numbers with the same percentage into a standard method of calculating the 95% confidence interval of proportions. If we use 30% and feed in 3 of 10, 30 of 100, 300 of 1000, and so on, the results can be seen graphically in Figure 1.3.6. Quite clearly our estimate of the proportion is quite tight when we have 300 events and

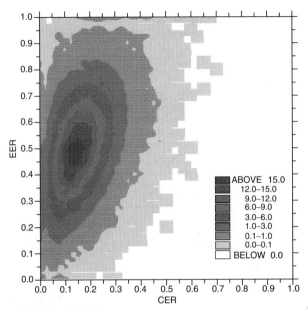

**Figure 1.3.5** Computer model of trials of ibuprofen in acute pain. Intensity of shading matches probability of outcome of a single trial. CER (control event rate) is equivalent to placebo and EER (experimental event rate) to ibuprofen in clinical trials.

total numbers of 1000. But when the total is below 500, and especially below 100 when there are fewer than 30 events, we can have virtually no confidence in the result.

Real-life examples can be compared with the theoretical picture generated in Figure 1.3.6. The first (Figure 1.3.7) shows the percentage of patients with at least 50% pain relief with placebo in 56 meta-analyses in acute pain in which the overall mean was about 18%, with about 12,000 patients given placebo. All the trials were randomized, all double-blind, and all used the same outcome, measured in the same way, over the same period of time, in similar pain models and patients. Only those meta-analyses with at least 1000 patients given placebo correctly measured the event rate with placebo. Where the numbers given placebo were small, the estimate varied widely from 0 to 60%.

The next example is sperm counts. A review a decade ago [8] started us worrying about falling sperm counts, probably wrongly. If we take the data on sperm counts from that paper and calculate a weighted mean value (overall average in which studies contribute according to the number of men in them) in thousands of men, the mean is about 77 million sperm per mL. Large studies with many men confirm this, but small studies produce

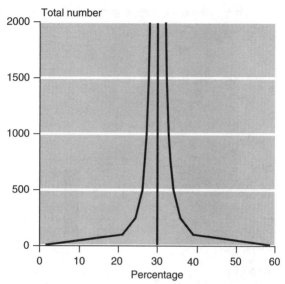

**Figure 1.3.6** Confidence intervals around the proportion of 30% as number of observations increase. The vertical line represents the overall proportion and the other lines the upper and lower limit of the 95% confidence interval.

results that are all over the place (Figure 1.3.8). Small samples (some as few as seven men, which don't even show on the graph) produced widely differing results. For sperm counts, size really is everything.

The final example is the relative risk of perforation, ulcer, or bleed (PUB) in people taking NSAIDs compared with people not taking NSAIDs (Figure 1.3.9), taken from an analysis of good-quality epidemiological studies published in the 1990s [9]. The overall relative risk was 4. Studies with 1000 PUBs or more measured this accurately. Those with fewer did not. Below 200 PUBs the relative risks varied from no increased risk to an eightfold increased risk.

The lessons from these examples (and there are many others that one could use) are that we need reasonably large data sets to be confident of a result, and that conclusions drawn from limited amounts of information might mislead.

### How much information is enough?

While it is relatively easy to demonstrate that inadequate amounts of information can result in erroneous conclusions, the alternative question—how much information do we need to avoid erroneous conclusions—is more difficult to answer. It depends on a number of things. Two important issues are the size of the effect you are looking at (absolute differences between treatment and control), and how sure you want to be.

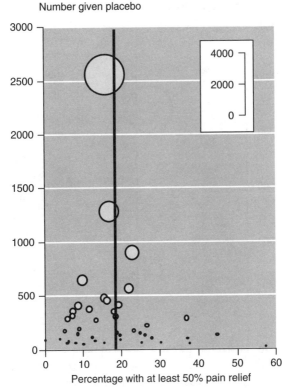

**Figure 1.3.7** Percentage of patients with at least 50% pain relief with placebo in 56 meta-analyses in acute pain. Size of symbol is proportional to number of patients given placebo. Vertical line is the overall average.

A worked example using simulations of acute pain trials [6] gives us some idea. Using the control event rate of 16% as in DICE 1 (because it happens to be what is found with placebo), it looked at experimental event rates (percentage or proportion benefiting with treatment) of 40%, 50%, and 60% (or 0.4, 0.5, 0.6 as proportions), equivalent to NNTs of 4.2, 2.9, and 2.3. The numbers in treatment and placebo group were each simulated from 25 patients per group (trial size 50) to 500 patients per group (trial size 1000). For each condition 10,000 trials were simulated and the percentage where the NNT was within ±0.5 of the true NNT counted.

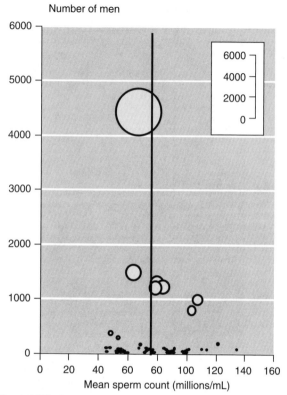

**Figure 1.3.8** Sperm counts and size of study. Size of symbol is proportional to number of men. Vertical line is the overall average.

### Statistical significance

Table 1.3.5 shows the number of patients needed for statistical significance for a variety of experimental event rates, and a variety of levels of confidence. When we want to be 95% confident that ibuprofen with an event rate of about 0.5 (50%) is better than placebo with an event rate in this example of 0.16 (16%), we need 41 patients in each treatment arm (41 for ibuprofen, 41 for placebo) making a total of about 80 patients. This is the median number found in actual clinical trials (Figure 1.3.4). If we can afford to be less confident, or if we have an analgesic expected to be much better than ibuprofen, we can do with fewer patients. But if our analgesic is less efficacious than ibuprofen, we need many more patients.

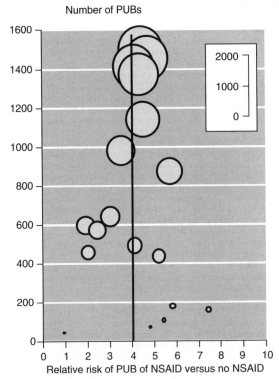

**Figure 1.3.9** Relative risk of perforation, ulcer, or bleed (PUB) in people taking NSAID compared with people not taking NSAID. Size of symbol is proportional to number of PUBs. Relative risks have been plotted from zero for convenience. Vertical line is the overall average.

**Table 1.3.5** Number of patients required in each group for a statistically significant result that experimental is better than control

| Probability | Group size needed for experimental event rate | | | | | |
| | 0.30 | 0.40 | 0.50 | 0.60 | 0.70 | 0.80 |
|---|---|---|---|---|---|---|
| 0.50 | 83 | 26 | 17 | 13 | 10 | 7 |
| 0.75 | 137 | 40 | 27 | 21 | 14 | 10 |
| 0.90 | 200 | 57 | 34 | 29 | 20 | 13 |
| 0.95 | 244 | 68 | 41 | 33 | 23 | 16 |

Group sizes required to obtain a probability of 0.5, 0.75, 0.9, and 0.95 of obtaining a statistically significant result from the chi-squared test with a CER of 0.16 and EERs from 0.3 to 0.8.

*Clinical significance*

Suppose instead that we want to be clinically confident of the result. First, we need a definition of clinical confidence. For the sake of argument, let's say that we want to be 95% sure that the true number needed to treat is within plus or minus 0.5 of the observed NNT. So if the NNT is 3, we want to know that the true NNT is within 2.5 to 3.5.

In that case we need many more patients (Table 1.3.6). Now we need not 41 patients per group, but rather 470 per group or nearly 1000 in all. This is equivalent to more than 10 average sized randomised controlled trials designed to achieve statistical rather than clinical significance. Again if we can afford to be less confident, or if the treatment has a bigger effect, we can do with fewer patients. But if we have a treatment that is less effective than ibuprofen, suddenly we need many, many patients.

To expand on this point, Table 1.3.7 looks at a range of group sizes and a range of experimental event rates between 0.4 and 0.6, and calculates the proportion of trials that, by the random play of chance alone, would have an NNT within ±0.5 of the true NNT. With 1000 patients in a trial where the NNT was 2.3, we could be 100% sure that the NNT measured was within ±0.5 of the true NNT; all trials of this size would produce values between 1.8 and 2.8. In a trial of 50 patients where the NNT was 4.2, only one in four trials would produce an NNT within ±0.5; the true value is between 3.7 and 4.7, and three-quarters of trials (or meta-analyses) of this size would produce NNTs below 3.7 or over 4.7.

The study also shows that, to be certain of the size of the effect (the NNT, say), we need ten times more information than when we just need to know that there is statistical significance.

## Does this thinking work in practice?

We can test whether this works in practice by looking at four large data sets with meta-analyses in acute pain. For four drugs and doses, ibuprofen 400 mg, aspirin 600/650 mg, paracetamol 975/1000 mg, and ibuprofen 200 mg we have a sufficient number of trials to perform cumulative meta-analyses. In a cumulative meta-analysis we take the first trial to be published and calculate the NNT, then the first plus the second, then the first, plus second and third, and so on. Over time, more and yet more information becomes available, and we can compare results at any one time

**Table 1.3.6** Number of patients required in each group for a clinically relevant number needed to treat

| Probability | Group size needed for experimental event rate | | | | | |
| | 0.30 | 0.40 | 0.50 | 0.60 | 0.70 | 0.80 |
| --- | --- | --- | --- | --- | --- | --- |
| 0.50 | >500 | 200 | 50 | 20 | 10 | <10 |
| 0.75 | >500 | >500 | 150 | 60 | 25 | 10 |
| 0.90 | >500 | >500 | 320 | 110 | 50 | 20 |
| 0.95 | >500 | >500 | 470 | 180 | 80 | 40 |

Group sizes required to obtain a probability of 0.5, 0.75, 0.9, and 0.95 of obtaining a clinically relevant NNT (NNT within ±0.5 of true value) with a CER of 0.16 and EERs from 0.3 to 0.8.

**Table 1.3.7**   Effect of size and size of effect on confidence in measured treatment effect

| E E R | 40 | 50 | 60 |
|---|---|---|---|
| C E R | 16 | 16 | 16 |
| N N T | 4.2 | 2.9 | 2.3 |

| Group size | Percentage of results within ± 0.5 of NNT | | |
|---|---|---|---|
| 25 | 26 | 37 | 57 |
| 50 | 28 | 51 | 73 |
| 100 | 38 | 61 | 88 |
| 200 | 55 | 81 | 96 |
| 300 | 63 | 89 | 99 |
| 400 | 71 | 93 | 99 |
| 500 | 74 | 95 | 99 |

| At least | |
|---|---|
| 50% | within ± 0.5 |
| 80% | within ± 0.5 |
| 95% | within ± 0.5 |

and when all the information is available. Remember that these trials are all randomized and double-blind, measuring the same outcome over the same period in the same way and with similar patients in similar clinical situations, so they are as close to identical as it is possible to be.

Figure 1.3.10 shows the data for ibuprofen 400 mg. The overall NNT was 2.5 and the horizontal lines are ±0.5 NNT from this, giving the confidence range we want of 2.0 to 3.0. The confidence interval was wide initially, but as the numbers of patients increased the confidence interval narrowed rapidly and, by the time about 1000 patients' worth of information was available, the confidence interval was within the boundary of ±0.5 of an NNT. This is just what we expected where the experimental event rate was about 0.55.

We have a similar pattern for aspirin 600/650 mg (Figure 1.3.11). Here, though, the NNT was 4.5 and the experimental event rate about 0.4. Again the confidence interval narrowed as more information became available, but only with almost 5000 patients was the interval within ±0.5 of an NNT unit. Again, this is about what we would have expected with this lower event rate.

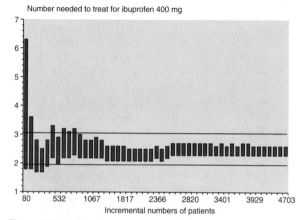

**Figure 1.3.10** Cumulative meta-analysis for ibuprofen 400 mg (bars show the 95% confidence interval of the NNT).

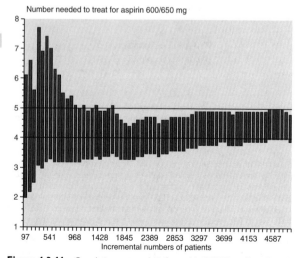

**Figure 1.3.11** Cumulative meta-analysis for aspirin 600/650 mg (bars show the 95% confidence interval of the NNT).

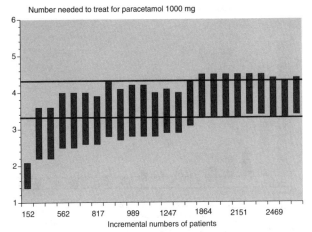

Number needed to treat for paracetamol 1000 mg

Incremental numbers of patients

**Figure 1.3.12** Cumulative meta-analysis for paracetamol 1000 mg (bars show the 95% confidence interval of the NNT).

For paracetamol 1000 mg the picture is somewhat different (Figure 1.3.12). The overall NNT is about 3.7, but early trials were wildly inaccurate, and overestimated the treatment efficacy (a lower NNT). Only as more information became available did the confidence interval come into line with that obtained from all the clinical trial information eventually available.

For ibuprofen 200 mg, we see a similar picture as for paracetamol, but in the opposite direction (Figure 1.3.13). Early trials wildly underestimated drug efficacy, and only as more information accumulated did the result begin to give the same picture as for all clinical trial information.

## Cumulative meta-analysis

Cumulative meta-analysis is a useful technique for visually examining the results of all the trials as they are published, and has value as a quality control check for those doing systematic reviews. It has also been used to examine the effects of size [9].

It is obvious that, if we have a very small amount of information, from few patients, the effects of random chance can be significant. As the amount of information or number of patients increases, then the effects of chance will diminish. In some circumstances, like acute pain trials, we can define how much information is needed for us to be confident, not only that a treatment works, but also how big is the effect of that treatment [6].

Confirmation that our estimate of the effect of treatment can be heavily dependent on size comes from a study from the USA and Greece [9]. Researchers looked at 60 meta-analyses of randomized trials where there were at least five trials published in more than three different calendar

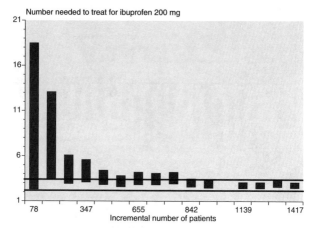

**Figure 1.3.13** Cumulative meta-analysis for ibuprofen 200 mg.

years. The trials were in either pregnancy and perinatal medicine or in myocardial infarction.

For each meta-analysis, trials were chronologically ordered by publication year and cumulative meta-analysis performed to arrive at a pooled odds ratio at the end of each calendar year. The relative change in treatment effect was calculated for each successive additional calendar year by dividing the odds ratio of the new assessment with more patients by the odds ratio of the previous assessment with fewer patients. This gives a 'relative odds ratio', in which a number greater than 1 indicates more treatment effect, and one less than 1 indicates less treatment effect. The relative odds ratio can be plotted against the number of patients included. The expected result is a horizontal funnel, with less change with more patients, and the relative odds ratio settling down to 1.

The two graphs produced for pregnancy/perinatal medicine and myocardial infarction show exactly this expected pattern. Below 100 patients, the relative odds ratios vary between 0.2 and 6. By the time 1000 patients are included the ratios are between 0.5 and 2. By the time we have about 5000 patients they settle down to close to 1. The 95% prediction interval for the relative change in the odds ratio for different numbers for both examples is shown in Table 1.3.8.

When evidence was based on only a few patients there was substantial uncertainty about how much the pooled treatment effect would change in the future. With only 100 patients randomized, additional information from more trials could multiply or divide by three the odds ratios we have at that point.

## Commentary

The lesson is simple. We need large amounts of information to obtain credible estimates of the true clinical efficacy of a treatment. Single small

**Table 1.3.8** Effect of size on prediction of relative change in odds ratios with additional patients randomized

| Number of patients | Fixed effect prediction interval for relative change in odds ratio | |
|---|---|---|
| | Pregnancy/perinatal | Myocardial infarction |
| 100 | 0.32–2.78 | 0.18–5.51 |
| 500 | 0.59–1.71 | 0.60–1.67 |
| 1000 | 0.67–1.49 | 0.74–1.35 |
| 2000 | 0.74–1.35 | 0.83–1.21 |
| 15,000 | 0.85–1.14 | 0.96–1.05 |

trials, even if performed impeccably, can give the wrong result because of the random play of chance. They can mislead. Together, quality and size represent the keys to understanding clinical, as opposed to statistical, results. If we base practice on statistical results alone, we head for trouble. The need for size is the single biggest justification for using information from systematic reviews, rather than relying on individual small efficacy trials.

Early in the reign of Augustus, Dionysius of Halicarnasus commented 'history is philosophy from examples' (RARS Rhetorica Ch 11, Section 4). We think of evidence in much the same way, in seeking examples from the archaeology of medicine to learn what constitutes good science and what bad, perhaps leavened here and there with a bit of real philosophy and science. Theory tells us that randomization is good, and examples from reviews frequently confirm it. Yet we are condemned to re-learn the lessons because so many systematic reviews include trials whose architecture potentially misleads.

Cynics might say that much decision-making in health-care is done on small amounts of inadequate information. They may be right, but knowing that that information may be misleading is still helpful. We know that we need to examine what we do in practice to check that it conforms with what we thought we started out with. Suspending belief is not an option.

The simple fact is that none of this is particularly new. The idea that larger studies are more reliable has been known for some time [10], and suggestions have been put forward about defining the amount of information required before a result can be known with accuracy [6, 11].

Suggested answers to the sock problem included turning the light on, having only red socks, keeping them in different drawers, and washing them together so that they all go pink. With clinical trials it is a bit different, but the one that we can use is that of turning the light on. For any problem we need to be clear what the question is, and apply what is known about the amount of information needed to answer it.

We should also be crystal clear that small studies, even if impeccably performed and reported, can give the wrong answer just because of the random play of chance. That can be true of small, randomized studies with few patients and few events, and of observational studies that may be large in numbers of patients but still have few events.

## References

1. Counsell, C.E. et al. (1994). The miracle of DICE therapy for acute stroke: fact or fictional product of subgroup analysis? *British Medical Journal* **309**, 1677–81.
2. Clarke, M. and Halsey, J. (2001). DICE2: a further investigation of the effects of chance in life, death and subgroup analyses. *International Journal of Clinical Practice* **55**, 240–2.
3. Kjaergard, L.L. et al. (2001). Reported methodologic quality and discrepancies between large and small randomised trials in meta-analyses. *Annals of Internal Medicine* **135**, 982–9.
4. Jadad, A.R. et al. (1996). Assessing the quality of reports of randomized clinical trials: is blinding necessary? *Controlled Clinical Trials* **17**, 1–12.
5. Collins, S.L. et al. (2002). Single dose oral ibuprofen and diclofenac for post-operative pain (Cochrane Review). In The Cochrane Library, Issue 4, 2002. Oxford: Update Software.
6. Moore, R.A. et al. (1998). Size is everything—large amounts of information are needed to overcome random effects in estimating direction and magnitude of treatment effects. *Pain* **78**, 209–16.
7. Hanley, J.A. and Lippman-Hand, A. (1983). If nothing goes wrong, is everything alright? *Journal of the American Medical Association* **249**, 1743–5.
8. Carlsen, E. et al. (1992). Evidence for decreasing quality of semen during past 50 years. *British Medical Journal* **305**, 609–13.
9. Ioannidis, J.P.A. and Lau, J. (2001). Evolution of treatment effects over time: empirical insight from recursive cumulative metaanalyses. *Proceedings of the National Academy of Sciences USA* **98**, 831–6.
10. Flather, M.D. et al. (1997). Strengths and limitations of meta-analysis: larger studies may be more reliable. *Controlled Clinical Trials* **18**, 568–79.
11. Pogue, J.M. and Yusuf, S. (1997). Cumulating evidence from randomized trials: utilizing sequential monitoring boundaries for cumulative meta-analysis. *Controlled Clinical Trials* **18**, 580–93.

# 1.4 Simple statistics

This book is not about statistics. Inevitably, though, we have to have a minimum understanding of a few statistical terms to get to grips with any numerical results we need to deal with. There really are not all that many, and some are explained later. Two concepts of general importance though are the $p$-value and confidence intervals.

### $p$-Value

A $p$-value is the probability (ranging from zero to one) that the results observed in a study could have occurred by chance. $p$-Values are written as decimal fractions of 1, such as 0.1, 0.05, or 0.01, or possibly as percentages, when the same $p$-values would be written as 10%, 5%, or 1%.

We often want to know whether there is a difference between two things, such as a new treatment and placebo, or whether there has been a change in something, or whether there is an association between two things. We start from the premise that there is no real difference (the null hypothesis), the opposite of what might be the research hypothesis that there is a difference. Statistical tests are performed, and they produce a $p$-value (as well as lots of other useful stuff).

A result for the $p$-value of 1 confirms that there is no difference, whereas a $p$-value of 0 says that there is a difference. If the $p$-value is small we can say that the research hypothesis is true, and the null hypothesis is false. It may help to have some $p$-values, and the probabilities they mean. Table 1.4.1 gives a list of them, from those things that are likely to occur by chance, to those that are very unlikely.

Statistically significant results are those that are unlikely to have occurred by chance. Non-significant results are those in which a chance occurrence has not been ruled out, and the result obtained could have occurred just because of the random play of chance. It all depends on the risk we are prepared to accept of a result being obtained by chance alone.

By convention we accept a $p$-value of 0.05 or below as being statistically significant. This convention has no solid basis, other than being the number chosen many years ago. When many comparisons are being made, statistical significance at this level can occur just by chance 1 time in 20,

**Table 1.4.1**  $p$-Values and chance

| $p$-Value | Probability of obtaining a result by chance |
|-----------|---------------------------------------------|
| 0.5 | 1 in 2 |
| 0.2 | 1 in 5 |
| 0.1 | 1 in 10 |
| 0.05 | 1 in 20 |
| 0.025 | 1 in 40 |
| 0.01 | 1 in 100 |
| 0.001 | 1 in 1000 |
| 0.0001 | 1 in 10,000 |

which is not very unlikely. A more stringent rule is to use a $p$-value of 0.01 (1%; 1 in 100) or below as statistically significant, though some folk get hot under the collar when you do it.

However, it is a useful general rule to be unimpressed when some not very likely difference in a small sample is hailed as important with a barely significant $p$-value of 0.049 (although there will be occasions when even that will have its wow factor). It is far better to be impressed by very small $p$-values in much larger samples, when the result is much more likely to be true.

Think for a moment that you have to drive across a bridge over a fast-flowing river, with your family in the car. If you were told that there was a 1 in 20 chance that the bridge would collapse into the river when you drove over it, would you take it? Or a 1 in 100, or a 1 in 1000 chance? Of course the question begs what alternative you have in not driving over the bridge, where you are going, and the tank behind you.

## Confidence interval

Confidence intervals provide different information from that arising from hypothesis tests, which is what we call the sort of statistical tests that generate $p$-values around our research or null hypothesis. Confidence intervals provide a range about the observed effect size, whether that effect size is a statistical output like and odds ratio or relative risk, or a number needed to treat, a difference between two things, or a proportion.

This range is constructed in such a way that we know how likely it is to capture the true, but unknown, effect size. The formal definition of a confidence interval is:

A range of values for a variable of interest constructed so that this range has a specified probability of including the true value of the variable. The specified probability is called the confidence level, and the end points of the confidence interval are called the confidence limits.

Conventionally we create confidence intervals at the 95% level. This means that 95% of the time properly constructed confidence intervals should contain the true value of the variable of interest. The confidence interval provides a range for our estimate of the true treatment effect that is plausible given the size of the difference (or population) actually observed.

A caveat is that the confidence interval relates to the population sampled. If we have a small sample of part of a population, or a very small sample of the whole population, then the confidence interval that is generated is not necessarily that for the whole population. This is not always remembered when people deal with small samples.

We can use confidence intervals to look at statistical significance, just like $p$-values. Table 1.4.2 gives some simple rules for determining statistical significance with different measures. If the 95% confidence interval includes 1, infinity, or zero, this is non-significance at the 5% level (so $p$ is greater than 0.05), and there is more than a 1 in 20 likelihood that the result was due to random chance.

Confidence intervals provide additional information. The upper and lower bounds of the interval provide information on how big or small the true effect might plausibly be, and the width of the confidence interval also conveys some useful information. If the confidence interval is narrow, capturing only a small range of effect sizes, we can be quite confident

**Table 1.4.2**   Using confidence intervals to look for statistical significance

| Measure | Statistical significance using confidence intervals | Reason |
|---|---|---|
| Odds ratio | Statistical significance when confidence interval does not include 1 | Odds ratio of 1 shows no difference between two samples |
| Hazard ratio | Statistical significance when confidence interval does not include 1 | Hazard ratio of 1 shows no difference between two samples |
| Relative risk | Statistical significance when confidence interval does not include 1 | Relative risk of 1 shows no difference between two samples |
| Number needed to treat | Statistical significance when confidence interval does not include infinity | Number needed to treat becomes infinity when there is no difference |
| Difference between two populations | Statistical significance when confidence interval does not include zero | Zero would indicate that there was no difference in a proportion between two populations |

The derivation of each of these measures requires a comparison between two alternatives. These may be active treatment and placebo, or two different active treatments.

that any effects far from this range have been ruled out by the study. This situation usually arises when the study population, or number of events, is quite large and hence the estimate of the true effect is quite precise.

If the confidence interval is quite wide, capturing a diverse range of effect sizes, we can infer that the study was probably quite small. Thus, any estimates of effect size will be quite imprecise. Small studies, of course, run the risk of surveying a population that is different from the overall population, and so can mislead us.

### Some other terms to remember

Populations can have a normal distribution, like height or serum sodium, for instance, in which many of the population are close to the average, with small numbers at either extreme (very tall or short people, or people with high or low serum sodium). Other distributions are different. Most people have reasonably low but measurable serum prolactin levels, but lactating women, people on some drugs, people under stress, or those with pituitary tumours have high, sometimes extraordinarily high values. This is a skewed distribution. Many types of distribution are skewed, so let's remind ourselves of ways we describe values from different distributions.

#### Mean

The average value, calculated by adding all the observations and dividing by the number of observations.

#### Median

Middle value of a list. If you have numbers 2, 3, 4, 5, 6, 7, and 8, the median is 5. Medians are often used when data are skewed, meaning that the distribution is uneven. In that case, a few very high numbers could, for instance, change the mean, but they would not change the median.

Other definitions include the smallest number such that at least half the numbers in the list are no greater than it. If the list has an odd number of entries, the median is the middle entry in the list after sorting the list into increasing order. If the list has an even number of entries, the median is equal to the sum of the two middle (after sorting) numbers divided by two. The median can be estimated from a histogram by finding the smallest number such that the area under the histogram to the left of that number is 50%. But all mean the same thing in the end.

### Mode

For lists, the mode is the most common (frequent) value.

## Commentary

That's about it for statistics, because this book isn't about statistics. It is interested in where evidence, even with good statistical analysis, is just plain wrong, and when we can trust evidence. Statistical significance alone is not enough to allow us to trust a result.

# Section 2

# Clinical trials

# 2.1 Clinical trial fundamentals

While there are some fundamental properties necessary to produce a good clinical trial, what makes a clinical trial good depends on a number of factors, and there are no absolute hard and fast rules that can cover every clinical eventuality. And there are different reasons for doing clinical trials—for instance, proving whether one treatment is better than another requires a different approach from telling whether two treatments have the same effect. But we can make some important observations about what to look for in a good clinical trial, and we do know that if clinical trials of efficacy are not done properly any results they produce will be worthless.

## Randomization

We randomize trials to exclude selection bias. Trials are usually performed where there is uncertainty as to whether a treatment works (is better than no treatment or placebo), or whether one treatment is better than another. We start from a position of intellectual equipoise, that there is no proven difference between treatments. But trials are often done by believers, and belief, even subconscious belief, might influence our choice of treatment for particular patients if we could choose. To avoid this, and to ensure that the patients allocated to each intervention are identical, we make the treatment choice randomly. This might be by tossing a coin, or more often by computer-generated randomization. If we do not randomize we can end up with treatment groups that are not the same, thus invalidating the trial, or with a trial that no-one will believe because trials that are not randomized are often shown to be wrong (Chapter 2.4). Randomization is essential in almost all cases.

Another important aspect of randomization is concealment—hiding the result of random allocation from everyone involved in the trial. Concealment might be achieved by putting the treatment choice in a sealed envelope, for instance. That way no one can know in advance which treatment the next patient will have, and this again prevents patients being consciously or unconsciously selected for a particular treatment. Faulty methods of randomization include assignment by date of birth, or hospital number, because they are not random (and treatment allocation may or may not be concealed).

Randomization is important because we know that non-randomized or inadequately randomized studies tend to give overly optimistic results compared with those that are properly randomized. Look at the example in Table 2.1.1, examining clinical trials of transcutaneous electrical nerve stimulation (TENS) in acute pain [1]. Almost all of the trials that were not properly randomized gave results that told us that TENS was beneficial. By contrast, almost all of the trials that were randomized told us that TENS had no effect. This wasn't just a slight change in emphasis, but a completely different result!

If a trial says it is properly randomized, how can we tell that it has been? The obvious thing is to look for a table describing the randomized groups of patients at the start of the trial. If randomization has been done properly, the two groups should be very similar or identical to one another. So you would expect to see that average age, and age range, are about the

**Table 2.1.1** Effect of adequacy of randomization on outcomes of clinical trials of transcutaneous electrical nerve stimulation in acute pain

| | Trial conclusion | |
| --- | --- | --- |
| **Adequacy of randomization** | **Beneficial** | **Not beneficial** |
| Properly randomized | 2 | 15 |
| Inadequately randomized or not randomized | 17 | 2 |

same, with the same proportions of men and women, or patients with different severities of disease, or co-morbidities, or already being treated with certain therapies for those co-morbidities. If trials are small (a few tens of patients), randomization can fail because of the random play of chance. In reasonably sized trials with many tens or hundreds of patients, a major discrepancy in patient characteristics implies that researchers have been very unlucky, or that there was a systematic failure in randomization. Whether it is bad luck or failure to randomize properly, important differences between groups at the start of a trial are a good reason to be cautious about the result. In any event, it is worth checking any paper that describes itself as randomized, because some that do are not.

### Blinding

We conduct trials blind to minimize observer bias. Double-blind means that neither the patient nor the health-care professional knows which treatment has been given. Single-blind means that the patient doesn't know but the health-care professional does, or sometimes that the patient does but the health-care professional making outcome assessments doesn't. It's belief again because, even if the trial is randomized, if we know that Mrs Jones has treatment A and Mr Smith treatment B, our observations may be biased by our belief that Mr Smith overstates his complaint and Mrs Jones understates hers. Only if we have no idea which treatment they received will we be free from a bias that is known to deliver incorrect results.

A good example of this is acupuncture for back pain [2]. Here the overall result was statistically in favour of acupuncture over the control, in this case a form of sham acupuncture, with acupuncture and control techniques checked by a panel of acupuncture experts. Yet, as Figure 2.1.1 shows, those trials that were blind, where observers did not know what treatment patients had, showed negligible difference. Any difference came from trials in which the observers knew whether the patients had real acupuncture or sham acupuncture. Our conclusion might be that the best trials showed no effect, yet this meta-analysis has been used to demonstrate both that acupuncture is effective and that it should be used to treat patients with back pain.

Blinding is the ideal, and it *can* be done, even for non-drug trials. An arthroscopy trial is a good example, in which patients in the placebo group received skin incisions and underwent a simulated debridement without insertion of the arthroscope; patients and assessors of outcome were blinded to the treatment-group assignment [3]. As a simple rule, if a trial

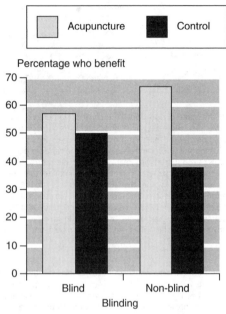

**Figure 2.1.1** Effect of adequacy of blinding on trials of acupuncture for back pain.

is not blinded then it will need to be much larger to be credible to minimize the risk of observer bias. The more objective the outcome the better if the trial is not to be blinded, because more objective outcomes limit the potential impact of observer bias.

How do you know a trial has been properly blinded? The obvious thing is to look at the description of treatments used. If, for instance, they describe treatments as identical numbers of tablets, identical in appearance and taste, given at the same intervals during the day, that pretty much describes adequate double-blinding, where neither patient nor professional should know who gets what. If there are different treatment regimens, then double-dummy techniques can be used. This might involve two sets of therapies, active A plus placebo B, or placebo A plus active B, and that can work for tablets or combinations of tablets and injection.

Sometimes blinding needs to be complicated. Homeopathy is often said to require individualization for patients, a technique that is hard to blind. One method used an individualized homeopathic remedy as prescribed by a practitioner or placebo dispensed from a notary public, who held the randomization schedule and mailed out the treatments. Reporting was to a study secretariat unconnected with the patients [4]. This was described as triple-blind.

So blinding is possible even for surgery as the arthroscopy trial [3] shows. Even so, it is worth checking the methods section of any paper that describes itself as double-blind, because some trials that so describe themselves really are not double-blind.

### Placebo

Clinical trials sometimes, but not always, and in some cases never, compare treatment directly with placebo. The reason for using a placebo is that there are many circumstances where people get better by themselves, without intervention, or despite it. It is said that the common cold takes 7 days to get better if you do nothing, but only 1 week if you treat it. In the example of back pain above, about 50–60% of patients had a 'cure' when no active treatment was used, mostly in short-term trials. That is exactly what we expect with back pain. If we did not have a placebo control, we might have thought that acupuncture was as miraculous as some enthusiasts claim. In other circumstances, like oncology, placebo on its own is almost never used, and instead we use add-on trials, where new treatment or placebo are compared added on to treatments known to be effective.

Placebo deserves a section all on its own, to think about both how it is best used in clinical trials, and whether there is such a thing as the 'placebo effect', where giving placebo has added benefit from doing nothing.

### Superiority trials

Most clinical trials are superiority trials, where an intervention is tested either against an inactive therapy (placebo, say) or an active therapy. The aim of the trial is to show that the intervention is superior to the comparator. Historically, the gold standard for drug approval by regulatory authorities has been convincing evidence of efficacy in double-blind, placebo-controlled, clinical trials. Because a placebo-controlled superiority trial provides the most straightforward opportunity for demonstrating efficacy, it is the most widely used regulatory benchmark in the drug approval process. In a superiority trial comparing a test drug with an active control, the difference between the two drugs is smaller than the expected difference between drug and placebo, resulting in the need for larger sample size.

The format of a superiority trial can be expressed by two hypotheses: the null hypothesis stating that there is no difference between the test drug and control in terms of some outcome variable and the alternate hypothesis stating that there is a difference. For the purposes of regulatory approval, effectiveness is shown when the difference between observed treatment effect of the test drug compared with that of the control exceeds some prespecified threshold considered to be clinically relevant.

Superiority trials often have a parallel group design in which two or more separate groups of patients are assigned randomly to one of two or more different treatments. They can, in some circumstances, have a cross-over design. Here there is random allocation to one of two or more treatments but, after a specified time, usually after a shorter intervening period with limited or no treatment (called a wash-out period), the patients are given the alternate treatment.

### Equivalence trials

Studies of an A versus B design, where two similar interventions are compared to show they are equivalent, are notoriously difficult to interpret, but we have guidance as to what to expect from equivalence trials and useful guides about what features of equivalence trials are important in determining their validity [5]. The intellectual problem with equivalence (A versus B) trials is that the same result for A and B is consistent with three conclusions.

- A and B are equally effective.
- A and B are equally ineffective.
- The trial was inadequate to detect differences between A and B.

To combat the problems posed by the latter two conclusions, McAlister and Sackett [5] suggest several criteria in addition to those used for superiority trials (A and/or B versus placebo). These are shown in Table 2.1.2 and compared with superiority trials for those aspects we need to think about. This table provides a useful checklist when we are presented with an equivalence trial, and we want to know how good it is.

- *Control shown previously to be effective?* Ideally documented in a systematic review of placebo-controlled trials with benefits exceeding a clinically important effect. Without this information, both active treatments may be equally ineffective.
- *Patients and outcomes similar to original trials?* Obvious, this one. If they are not similar, then any conclusion about equivalence is doomed. Beware, though, of trials designed to show equivalent efficacy being used to demonstrate differences in harm or toxicity, for which they were not designed, and for which they lack sufficient statistical power.
- *Regimens applied in identical fashion?* The most common example is that of choosing the best dose of A versus an ineffective dose of B (no names, no pack drill, but no prizes for picking out numerous examples especially from pharmaceutical company-sponsored trials showing 'our drug is better than yours'). Should be OK if licensed doses are chosen.

Other pitfalls to look out for are low compliance or frequent treatment changes, incomplete follow-up, disproportionate use of co-interventions, and lack of blinding.

### Appropriate statistical analysis?

Equivalence trials are designed to rule out meaningful differences between two treatments. Often the statistical tests used are one-sided tests of difference. Lack of significant superiority is not necessarily the same as defining an appropriate level of equivalence and testing for it.

Intention to treat analysis confers the risk of making a false-negative conclusion that treatments have the same efficacy when they do not. In equivalence trials the conservative approach may be to compare patients actually on treatment (per protocol analysis). Both analyses should probably be used.

### Prespecified equivalence margin?

How different is different? Equivalence trials should have a prior definition of how big a difference is a difference, and justify it. Even more than that, they have to convince you that the lack of that difference means that treatments would, in fact, be equivalent.

**Table 2.1.2** Criteria for validity in superiority and active-control equivalence trials

| Superiority trials | Active-control equivalence trials |
| --- | --- |
| Randomized allocation | Randomized allocation |
| Randomization concealed | Randomization concealed |
| All patients randomized accounted for | All patients randomized accounted for |
| Intention to treat analysis | Intention to treat analysis and on-treatment analysis (per protocol) |
| Clinicians and patients blinded to treatment received | Clinicians and patients blinded to treatment received |
| Groups treated equally | Groups treated equally |
| Groups identical at baseline | Groups identical at baseline |
| Clinically important outcomes | Clinically important outcomes<br>**Active control previously shown to be effective**<br>**Patients and outcomes similar to trials previously showing efficacy**<br>**Both regimens applied in an optimal fashion**<br>**Appropriate null hypothesis tested**<br>**Equivalence margin pre-specified** |
| Trial of sufficient size | Trial of sufficient size |

### Size?

Most equivalence trials are not large enough to detect even a 50% difference between treatments, and a 1994 review [6] found that 84% of equivalence trials were too small to detect a 25% difference. Size is everything when we want to show no difference and, the smaller the difference that is important, the larger the trial has to be. A more detailed look at size and the power of numbers comes later.

### Non-inferiority trials

Non-inferiority is a relatively new term that has not been universally adopted, and in the past non-inferiority and equivalence trials, which have an important distinction, have both been referred to as equivalence trials. To make the confusion even worse, both of these terms are somewhat misleading.

It is fundamentally impossible to prove that two treatments have exactly equivalent effects. Equivalence trials, therefore, aim to show that the effects differ by no more than a specific amount. In an equivalence trial, if the effects of the two treatments differ by more than the equivalence margin in either direction, then equivalence does not hold.

Non-inferiority trials, on the other hand, aim to show that an experimental treatment is not worse than an active control by more than the equivalence margin. An improvement of any size fits within the definition of non-inferiority. Bioequivalence trials (two forms of the same medicine, for instance) are true equivalence trials, but it is difficult to imagine any trial comparing the clinical effects of an experimental treatment and active control that would not more appropriately be termed a non-inferiority trial.

These trials have a number of inherent weaknesses that superiority trials do not: no internal demonstration of assay sensitivity; no single conservative analysis approach; lack of protection from bias by blinding; and difficulty in specifying the non-inferiority margin. Non-inferiority trials may sometimes be necessary when a placebo group cannot ethically be included, but it should be recognized that the results of such trials are not as credible as those from a superiority trial.

## When can we say that drugs have a 'class effect'?

Class (noun): 'any set of people or things grouped together or differentiated from others'. An increasingly asked question is whether a set of drugs forms a class, and whether there is a 'class effect'. Class effect is usually taken to mean similar therapeutic effects and similar adverse effects, both in nature and extent. If such a 'class effect' exists, then it makes decision-making easy: you choose the cheapest. An example is the statins: do statin drugs show a class effect? Of course, they do, in that they all reduce cholesterol, though the amount of reduction for particular doses might be different one from another.

Criteria for drugs to be grouped together as a class involve some or all of the following [7]:

- drugs with similar chemical structure;
- drugs with similar mechanism of action;
- drugs with similar pharmacological effects.

Declaring a class effect requires a bit of thought, though. How much thought, and of what type, has been considered in one of that brilliant *Journal of the American Medical Association* series on users' guides to the medical literature [7]. No one should declare a class effect and choose the cheapest without reference to the rules of evidence set out in this paper.

### Levels of evidence for efficacy for class effects

These are shown in Table 2.1.3 though, if it comes down to levels 3 and 4 evidence for efficacy, the ground is pretty shaky. Level 1 evidence is what we always want and almost always never get, the large randomized head to head comparison. By the time there are enough compounds around to form a class, there is almost no organization interested in funding expensive, new, trials to test whether A is truly better than B.

Most of the time we will be dealing with randomized trials of A versus placebo or standard treatment and B versus placebo or standard treatment. This will be level 2 evidence based on clinically important outcomes (a healing event) or validated surrogate outcomes (reduction of cholesterol with a statin). So establishing a class effect will likely involve quality systematic review or meta-analysis of quality randomized trials.

What constitutes quality in general is captured in Table 2.1.3, though there will be some situation-dependent factors. The one thing missing from consideration in Table 2.1.3 is size. There probably needs to be some prior

**Table 2.1.3** Levels of evidence for efficacy for class effect

| Level | Comparison | Patients | Outcomes | Criteria for validity |
|---|---|---|---|---|
| 1 | RCT direct comparison | Identical | Clinically important | Randomization concealment Complete follow-up Double-blinding Outcome assessment must be sound |
| 2 | RCT direct comparison | Identical | Valid surrogate | Level 1 plus Validity of surrogate outcome |
| 2 | Indirect comparison with placebo from RCTs | Similar or different in disease severity or risk | Clinically important or valid surrogate | Level 1 plus Differences in methodological quality End points Compliance Baseline risk |
| 3 | Subgroup analyses from indirect comparisons of RCTs with placebo | Similar or different in disease severity or risk | Clinically important or valid surrogate | Level 1 plus Multiple comparisons, post hoc data dredging Underpowered subgroups Misclassification into subgroups |
| 3 | Indirect comparison with placebo from RCTs | Similar or different in disease severity or risk | Unvalidated surrogate | Surrogate outcomes may not capture all good or bad effects of treatment |
| 4 | Indirect comparison of nonrandomized studies | Similar or different in disease severity or risk | Clinically important | Confounding by indication, compliance, or time Unknown or unmeasured confounders Measurement error Limited database, or coding systems not suitable for research |

estimate of how many patients or events constitute a reasonable number for analysis.

### Levels of evidence for safety

These are shown in Table 2.1.4. There are always going to be problems concerning rare, but serious, adverse events. The inverse rule of three tells us that, if we have seen no serious adverse events in 1500 exposed patients, then we can be 95% sure that they do not occur more frequently than 1 in 500 patients (1500/3, or $n/3$) [8].

**Table 2.1.4** Levels of evidence for safety for class effect

| Level | Type of study | Advantages | Criteria for validity |
|---|---|---|---|
| 1 | RCT | Only design that permits detection of adverse effects when the adverse effect has similar frequency to the event the treatment is trying to prevent | Underpowered for detecting adverse events unless specifically designed to do so |
| 2 | Cohort | Prospective data collection, defined cohort | Critically depends on follow-up, classification, and measurement accuracy |
| 3 | Case-control | Cheap and usually fast to perform | Selection and recall bias may provide problems, and temporal relationships may not be clear |
| 4 | Phase 4 studies | Can detect rare but serious adverse events if sufficient patients recruited | No control or unmatched control Critically depends on follow-up, classification, and measurement accuracy |
| 5 | Case series | Cheap and usually fast | Often small sample size; selection bias may be a problem; no control group |
| 6 | Case report(s) | Cheap and usually fast | Often small sample size; selection bias may be a problem, no control group |

Randomized trials of efficacy will usually be underpowered to detect rare, serious adverse events, and we will usually have to use other study designs. In practice the difficulty will be that, soon after new treatments are introduced, there will be a paucity of data from these other types of study. Only rarely will randomized trials powered to detect rare adverse events be conducted; an example is coxib trials looking at gastrointestinal bleeding.

Most new treatments are introduced after being tested on perhaps a few thousand patients in controlled trials. As an example, to be sure that a drug did *not* cause hepatic damage occurring at 1 in 15,000 we would need to have studied 45,000 patients without seeing a case. Particular caution is necessary for drugs to be used in chronic disease. This is especially the case if the trials were short-term and when other diseases and treatments are likely in these patients.

*Compliance*

A difficult issue this, with a fragmented literature. But we do know that, while compliance is usually high in clinical trials, it may be lower in practice, especially for preventive treatment. Treatment schedules that are likely to improve compliance (once a day, for instance) might be important.

*Cost*

Economic studies are complicated beasts, and we need to treat this evidence with caution. Assumption of a class effect is usually done to justify choosing the cheapest drug in terms of acquisition (prescribing) costs. Terrific if this means that the costs of achieving the same ends are minimized. It may not be like that, and health economics in class effects need to be carefully thought through.

## Problems

The correct design of a trial is situation-dependent. In some circumstances very complicated designs have to be used to ensure sensitivity and validity.

### No gold standard

There may be circumstances in which there is no established treatment of sufficient effectiveness to act as a gold standard against which to measure a new treatment, as is often the case in chronic pain. Clearly, the use of placebo or no-treatment controls is of great importance, especially when effects are to be examined over prolonged periods of weeks or months. But it is paradoxically these very circumstances in which ethical constraints act against using placebo or non-treatment controls because of the need to do *something*.

In acute conditions, conversely, there is often little problem with using placebos, since the failure of placebo (or any treatment) can be dealt with by prescribing additional therapies ('escape' analgesia) that should work, as is done in trials of acute pain or migraine.

### Are these patients like mine?

Clearly, people have to have a condition to demonstrate the efficacy of treatment, or to have a reasonable chance of developing a condition to have a reasonable chance of demonstrating the efficacy of a preventative intervention or strategy. Meticulous attention to trial design is necessary to be able to show differences, and it is always worth looking at a study to see how ill patients are, or how severe is their condition at the start. The relevant question is 'are these patients like mine?'.

## Commentary

What makes a trial relevant is governed by many factors. For the most part, when we consider a trial designed to show efficacy, it has to live up to rigorous standards. If not, then it could give the wrong answer. There is simply no escape from recognizing that we need to understand the basics of good trial design if we are not to be misled. That is especially the case when we look at papers that try to demonstrate equivalence between two treatments, or where folks make hurried assumptions about class effects to justify choosing interventions with lower acquisition costs, and ignore differences in efficacy, effectiveness, or safety.

## References

1. Carroll, D. *et al.* (1996). Randomization is important in studies with pain outcomes: systematic review of transcutaneous electrical nerve stimulation in acute post-operative pain. *British Journal of Anaesthesia* **77**, 798–803.
2. Ernst, E. and White, A.R. (1998). Acupuncture for back pain: a meta-analysis of randomised controlled trials. *Archives of Internal Medicine* **158**, 2235–41.
3. Moseley, J.B. *et al.* (2002). A controlled trial of arthroscopic surgery for osteo-arthritis of the knee. *New England Journal of Medicine* **347**, 81–8.
4. Walach, H. *et al.* (1997). Classical homeopathic treatment of chronic headaches. *Cephalalgia* **17**, 119–26.
5. McAlister, F.A. and Sackett, D.L. (2001). Active-control equivalence trials and antihypertensive agents. *American Journal of Medicine* **111**, 553–8.
6. Moher, D. *et al.* (1994). Statistical power, sample size, and their reporting in randomized controlled trials. *Journal of the American Medical Association* **272**, 122–4.
7. McAlister, F.A. *et al.* (1999). Users' guides to the medical literature XIX Applying clinical trial results B. Guidelines for determining whether a drug is exerting (more than) a class effect. *Journal of the American Medical Association* **282**, 1371–7.
8. Eypasch, E. *et al.* (1995). Probability of adverse events that have not yet occurred: a statistical reminder. *British Medical Journal* **311**, 619–20.

# 2.2 Outputs and utility

Understanding clinical trials and systematic reviews and meta-analyses involves understanding not only how trials are conducted and what constitutes a good or bad trial, but also how to comprehend and use results from a trial. Any time we read a clinical trial report or a systematic review we need to think not about one or two factors, but many.

For instance, we tend to think of clinical trials as having numbers attached to them, measuring outcomes (e.g. reduction in cholesterol with statin) and statistical significance (e.g. a significant reduction in cholesterol with statin). When we analyse systematic reviews we have become accustomed to meta-analysis, where we do sums on clinical trials with numbers. This would be a quantitative review.

We can also do qualitative reviews, where it may have been impossible to pool results from different trials because, for instance, different outcomes were measured. What we might then do is to say that we have trials measuring different things, but they all showed a statistically significant benefit in the different things measured. In qualitative reviews we end up vote-counting, in which each trial has one 'vote'. We count up positives, negatives, and neutrals. The problem with this is that one large, well-conducted trial can be outvoted by more small, poorly conducted trials. Vote-counting can lead us astray because it takes no account of either the size of the trial or the size of the treatment effect in a trial.

For quantitative reviews, even if trials and review are impeccably conducted, we have to get our heads around how the results are described. This can be not just in one way but many, often statistical. We have to understand the results before we can use them, and how those results are reported affects our comprehension.

There is probably no single 'best' way of reporting results so that everyone will comprehend them. We are all very different in our tastes. It is not surprising that we vary in the facility with which our minds grasp and manipulate different concepts. Some of us will be happiest with complex statistical concepts. Others, and Bandolier is one of those, are happiest with the simplest representations. In this section we will try to avoid being judgemental about different outputs, but will point out where there can be difficulties.

## The meaning of words

### Output

'Quantity produced or turned out; data after processing by a computer.' This dictionary definition differentiates between two different and important qualities of results of clinical trials. One, and perhaps that most useful to practitioners, is the quantity of benefit or harm a treatment is going to produce in patients like those in the trial or review. If the subject were a car, it would be equivalent to measuring how fast it would go, or the fuel economy. The other is a statistical result, often a comparison with some other intervention, perhaps placebo. Again, if the subject were a car, this would tell us whether this car went faster than another car, or had better or worse fuel efficiency.

But we can drive only one car at a time. It might be nice to know that my car is more fuel-efficient than yours, but it is the car I am driving, and I want to know how many litres per 100 kilometres, or miles per gallon, my car does, because otherwise I might run out of petrol. If our best evidence comes from randomized trials and systematic reviews, then one of the most important things is how that trial or review gives us the result. From a clinical point of view we want to know how much benefit (or harm) a treatment will produce, and results of data-processing might not be much help.

### Utility

'Usefulness: the power to satisfy the wants of people in general.' If systematic reviews are to be useful, and therefore used, they have to present results in ways that are immediately accessible to ordinary professionals. Rapid understanding is important for busy people. Trying to work out what a hazard ratio or an effect size means in terms of treating the patient in front of us will not make for an easy morning surgery.

## Defining outputs

Most of the outputs that we use for reporting trials and reviews have their origins in epidemiology, the domain where we look for small effects in large populations—things like aspirin after a heart attack, or reducing cholesterol. Most of the activity of medicine is, conversely, about large effects in small populations, such as hip replacements for osteoarthritic joints, or pain relief for migraine, or antibiotics for infection.

Table 2.2.1 is a hypothetical trial of ibuprofen in acute pain. Not worrying too much at this stage about any other features or even the result itself, we will use this trial to present some of the more common definitions for presentation of results where information was available in dichotomous form. Dichotomous means the patient either had the outcome or did not, and we have the numbers for each result. In this trial, for instance, 22 of 40 patients given ibuprofen had adequate pain relief compared with only 7 of 40 given placebo. The term, experimental event rate (EER), is used to describe the rate at which good events occur with ibuprofen (22/40 or 55%) and 'control event rate' (CER) describes the rate at which good events occur with placebo (7/40 or 18%).

### Odds ratios

Table 2.2.1 shows first how to compute odds. Odds refers to the ratio of the number of people *having* the good event to the number *not having* the good event, so the experimental event odds are 22/18 or 1.2. The odds ratio is the ratio of the odds with experimental treatment to that of control, or here 1.2/0.21 = 5.7. There are different ways of computing odds ratios that give slightly different answers in different circumstances. Values greater than 1 show that experimental is better than control and, if a 95% confidence interval is calculated, statistical significance is assumed if the interval does not include 1.

Some would change this around and compute the odds ratios from the point of view of the patients *not* having adequate pain relief. The experimental event odds would be 18/22 or 0.82, and the control event odds would be 33/7 or 4.7. The odds ratio then would be 0.82/4.7 = 0.17.

For ibuprofen versus placebo the odds ratio is 5.7 or 0.17. Pick the bones out of that. How would you use that, other than knowing that an odds ratio that was far from 1 meant that ibuprofen was better than placebo?

**Table 2.2.1** Hypothetical acute pain trial: EER is experimental event rate; CER is control event rate; and NNT is number needed to treat

| | | At least 50% pain relief | |
|---|---|---|---|
| Treatment | Total number of patients treated | Number achieving | Number not achieving |
| Ibuprofen 400 mg | 40 | 22 | 18 |
| Placebo | 40 | 7 | 33 |
| **Calculations made from these results** | **Values** | | |
| Experimental event rate (EER, event rate with ibuprofen) | 22/40 = 0.55 or 55% | | |
| Control event rate (CER, event rate with placebo) | 7/40 = 0.18 or 18% | | |
| Experimental event odds | 22/18 = 1.2 | | |
| Control event odds | 7/33 = 0.21 | | |
| Odds ratio | 1.2/0.21 = 5.7 | | |
| Relative risk (EER/CER) | 0.55/0.18 = 3.1 | | |
| Relative risk increase (100(EER − CER)/CER) as a percentage | 100((0.55 − 0.18)/0.18) = 206% | | |
| Absolute risk increase or reduction (EER − CER) | 0.55 − 0.18 = 0.37 (or 37%) | | |
| NNT (1/(EER − CER)) | 1/(0.55 − 0.18) = 2.7 | | |

### Relative risk or benefit

Relative risk is a bit easier on the brain. It is simply the ratio of EER to CER, here 0.55/0.18 (or 55/18 for percentages), and is 3.1. Again values greater than 1 show that experimental is better than control and, if a 95% confidence interval is calculated, statistical significance is assumed if the interval does not include 1. Odds ratios and relative risk tend to concur when event rates are low, but not when event rates are high. Table 2.2.2 shows this for a series of hypothetical examples where the experimental event rate is always three times higher than the control event rate. The relative risk is always 3, but the odds ratio varies from 2.8 to 12. There is disagreement between eminent statisticians about which of these is 'best'. We (and Bandolier) use relative risk whenever possible, but wouldn't pick a fight with someone who preferred odds ratios.

Again, knowing that the relative risk is 3.1 is not intuitively useful. Both relative risk and odds ratio are important ways of ensuring that there is statistical significance in our result. Unless there is statistical significance, we should not be using a treatment except in exceptional circumstances. So,

**Table 2.2.2** Calculated odds ratios and relative risk at different event rates

| Event rates | | | |
|---|---|---|---|
| Experimental | Control | Odds ratio | Relative risk |
| 3 | 1 | 2.8 | 3.0 |
| 6 | 2 | 2.8 | 3.0 |
| 12 | 4 | 3.0 | 3.0 |
| 24 | 8 | 3.3 | 3.0 |
| 48 | 16 | 4.3 | 3.0 |
| 60 | 20 | 5.3 | 3.0 |
| 90 | 30 | 12.0 | 3.0 |

whatever else we do in the way of data manipulation, statistical significance of one or other of these tests gives us the right to move on.

*Relative risk reduction or increase*
The relative risk reduction is the difference between the EER and CER (EER – CER) divided by the CER and is usually expressed as a percentage. In Table 2.1.1 the relative risk increase is 206%. If the number of events is smaller with treatment, then the relative risk reduction is calculated by subtracting the CER from EER in the equation.

*Absolute risk increase or reduction*
If we subtract the CER from the EER (EER – CER) then we have the absolute risk increase (ARI), the effect due solely to ibuprofen, and nothing else. The language here doesn't quite work because it was originally taken from the world of epidemiology where reducing risk (cholesterol lowering, etc.) is all. The absolute risk reduction (ARR) is CER – EER, when events occur more often with control than they do with treatment.

*Number needed to treat (NNT)*
For every 100 patients with acute pain treated with ibuprofen, 37 (= 55 – 18) will have adequate pain relief because of the ibuprofen we have given them. Clearly then, we have to treat 100/37, or 2.7 patients with ibuprofen for one to benefit because of the ibuprofen they have been given. That's what NNT is (Table 2.2.1). This has immediate clinical relevance because we immediately know what clinical and other effort is being made to produce one result with a particular intervention.

The best NNT would be 1, where everyone got better with treatment and nobody got better with control, and NNTs close to 1 can be found with antibiotic treatments for susceptible organisms, for instance. Higher NNTs represent less good treatment, and the NNT is a useful tool for comparing two similar treatments. When doing so the NNT must always specify the comparator (e.g. placebo, no treatment, or some other treatment), the therapeutic outcome, and the duration of treatment necessary to achieve that outcome. If these are different, you probably should not be comparing NNTs. It is also worth mentioning that prophylactic interventions that produce small effects in large numbers of patients will have high

NNTs, perhaps 20–100. Just because an NNT is large does not mean it will not be a useful treatment.

We can use the same methods for adverse events, when numbers needed to treat become numbers needed to harm (NNH). Here small numbers are bad (more frequent harm) and larger numbers good. When making comparisons between treatments, the same provisos apply as for NNT—the need to specify the type of harm, the comparator, and the dose and duration of therapy.

For both NNT and NNH we should recognize that we are working with an unusual scale running from 1 (everyone has the intended outcome with treatment and none with control) to −1 (no one has outcome with treatment and everyone has it with control), with infinity as the midpoint where we divide by zero when experimental event rate equals control event rate. Once NNTs or NNHs are much above 10, the upper confidence interval gets closer to infinity and the upper and lower intervals look unbalanced.

## Other outputs

There are many other outputs that people use for trials and epidemiological studies. These include effect size and p-values, which deserve a quick look. We don't find these useful, but there will always be circumstances in which they are the appropriate outputs.

### Effect size

As used in meta-analysis, this is the standardized observed effect. By standardizing the effect, the effect size becomes dimensionless (helpful when pooling data). The effect size then becomes:

- a generic term for the estimate of effect for a study;
- a dimensionless measure of effect that is typically used for continuous data when different scales are used to measure an outcome. It is usually defined as the difference in means between the intervention and control groups divided by the standard deviation of the control or both groups.

The effect size can be just the difference between the mean values of the two groups, divided by the standard deviation, as below, but there are other ways to calculate effect size in other circumstances.

Effect size = (mean of experimental group − mean of control group)/ standard deviation

Generally, then, the greater the impact of an intervention, the larger the effect size. The usual interpretation of this statement is that anything greater than 0.5 is large, 0.5–0.3 is moderate, 0.3–0.1 is small, and anything smaller than 0.1 is trivial.

### p-Values

A p-value is the probability (ranging from zero to one) that the results observed in a study (or results more extreme) could have occurred by chance. Conventionally, we accept a p-value of 0.05 or below as being statistically significant. That means a chance of 1 in 20, which is not very unlikely. This convention has no solid basis, other than being the number chosen many years ago because it seemed like a good idea at the time, and not specifically for medical interventions. When many comparisons are being made, statistical significance can occur just by chance. A more stringent rule is to use a *p*-value of 0.01 (1 in 100) or below as statistically significant, though some folk get hot under the collar when you do it.

### Outputs and circumstance

In order to see how the different outputs look, we can return again to a hypothetical trial of analgesic and placebo, though for convenience we use 1000 patients per group because we want to explore a range of possible results. In Table 2.2.3 we show six possible results in which the absolute proportion of patients benefiting with ibuprofen and placebo varies wildly, but the relative proportions stay the same.

Table 2.2.3 shows that the relative risk and relative risk increase can stay almost exactly the same in the face of huge changes in NNT, absolute risk increase, and the absolute percentages of patients benefiting. It explains why statistical outputs like relative risk may be great for measuring statistical significance, but lack utility in everyday practice.

These are clearly different trials or conditions, where the event rate with placebo varies between 1% and 36% in 1000 patients. Indeed, if these trials were part of a systematic review, this would be an obvious case where we would expect clinical heterogeneity in the condition (diagnosis), or its severity, or in patients recruited for the trials, or outcomes measured, or time over which the outcomes were measured. What is interesting is that using *statistical* tests for heterogeneity, this is a 'perfect' result, giving a *p*-value of 1.0. It underlines the fact that most statistical tests for heterogeneity are usually wrong, and even the one that is right is useless at detecting whether a group of trials is homogeneous or not [1].

### Confidence intervals

Confidence intervals provide a range about the observed effect size. This range is such that we know how likely it is to capture the true but unknown value for the population in a study. The definition of a confidence interval is a range of values for a variable of interest constructed so that this range has a specified probability of including the true value of the variable. The specified probability is called the confidence level, and the end points of the confidence interval are called the confidence limits.

**Table 2.2.3** Hypothetical trials with 1000 patients each given active or placebo. Definitions are as for Table 2.2.1

| Number with outcome | | | EER (%) | CER (%) | Relative risk | Relative risk increase (%) | Absolute risk increase (%) | NNT |
|---|---|---|---|---|---|---|---|---|
| Trial | Active | Placebo | | | | | | |
| 1 | 800 | 360 | 80 | 36 | 2.2 | 122 | 44 | 2.3 |
| 2 | 400 | 180 | 40 | 18 | 2.2 | 122 | 22 | 4.6 |
| 3 | 200 | 90 | 20 | 9 | 2.2 | 122 | 11 | 9.1 |
| 4 | 100 | 45 | 10 | 5 | 2.2 | 100 | 5 | 18.2 |
| 5 | 50 | 23 | 5 | 2 | 2.2 | 150 | 3 | 37.0 |
| 6 | 20 | 9 | 2 | 1 | 2.2 | 100 | 1 | 90.9 |

Conventionally, we create confidence intervals at the 95% level, meaning that 95% of the time properly constructed confidence intervals should contain the true value of the variable of interest for the population being studied. The confidence interval provides a range for our estimate of the true treatment effect that is plausible given the size of the difference actually observed.

A useful feature of confidence intervals is that they tell us whether or not statistical significance has been reached, just like a p-value.

- If the confidence interval *includes* the value reflecting no effect (say, 1 for relative risk or odds ratio, or infinity for NNT), this represents a difference that is statistically non-significant (for a 95% confidence interval, this is non-significance at the 5% level).
- If the confidence interval *does not include* the value reflecting no effect, this represents a difference that is statistically significant (again, for a 95% confidence interval, this is significance at the 5% level).

Thus statistical significance can be inferred from confidence intervals but, in addition, these intervals show the largest and smallest effects that are likely given the observed data. This is useful extra information.

Most people who use confidence intervals forget that they only apply to the population being studied, not the whole population. So, while a confidence interval should include the mean of the population being studied, it may not necessarily include the true mean of the whole population. It all comes down to size of sample and play of chance (of which more later).

## Some real examples

### Rizatriptan for acute migraine

A real example is an individual-patient meta-analysis of all the randomized single-dose trials of rizatriptan compared with placebo in acute migraine [2]. This is interesting because it looks at four different outcomes for migraine trials, and because it allows us to compute all the different outputs (Table 2.2.4). For clarity, the confidence intervals have been omitted, but rizatriptan was significantly better than placebo for all four outcomes.

Both odds ratios and relative benefit tell us that rizatriptan 10 mg is better than placebo, but the numerical values are not helpful. The relative risk increase looks very impressive for pain-free responses compared with headache response over 2 or 24 hours, despite fewer patients actually achieving this outcome. Absolute risk increase and NNT are more helpful, while conveying the same information in slightly different ways. Best of all for some of us is the absolute percentage of patients who will get each outcome if given 10 mg rizatriptan when they have a migraine.

### Prophylaxis for NSAID-induced gastrointestinal problems

A Cochrane review [3] examines the efficacy of misoprostol, histamine antagonists (H2A), and proton pump inhibitors (PPI) to reduce the propensity of NSAIDs to cause gastric and duodenal ulcers. Its main focus is on ulcers seen endoscopically (because that's where most of the evidence is) and on adverse events, particularly diarrhoea caused by misoprostol. This is a good review, but like many Cochrane reviews, one that concentrates on statistical outputs.

The review actually uses odds ratios for much of the reporting of results, but for completeness Table 2.2.5 shows the different outputs

**Table 2.2.4** Outputs of meta-analysis of rizatriptan 10 mg versus placebo for acute migraine

| Outcome | Number of patients with the outcome | | Output | | | | | |
| | Treatment (N = 2056) | Placebo (N = 1249) | Odds ratio | Relative benefit | Relative risk increase (%) | Absolute risk increase (%) | NNT | % patients with outcome |
| --- | --- | --- | --- | --- | --- | --- | --- | --- |
| Headache response at 2 hours | 1460 | 475 | 3.9 | 1.9 | 87 | 33 | 3.0 | 71 |
| Pain free at 2 hours | 843 | 125 | 4.5 | 4.1 | 310 | 31 | 3.2 | 41 |
| Headache response over 24 hours | 761 | 225 | 2.5 | 2.1 | 106 | 19 | 5.3 | 37 |
| Pain free over 24 hours | 514 | 87 | 3.4 | 3.6 | 257 | 18 | 5.5 | 25 |
| **Bigger or smaller numbers better** | | | **Bigger** | **Bigger** | **Bigger** | **Bigger** | **Smaller** | **Bigger** |

**Table 2.2.5** Outputs (presentation methods) of meta-analysis of prophylaxis for NSAID-induced gastroduodenal ulcer

| Treatment | Number of patients with the outcome/total | | Output | | | | | % with treatment | % with placebo |
|---|---|---|---|---|---|---|---|---|---|
| | Treatment | Placebo | Odds ratio | Relative risk | Relative risk reduction (%) | Absolute risk reduction (%) | NNT | | |
| H2A | | | | | | | | | |
| Standard dose | 48/494 | 75/487 | 0.6 | 0.6 | 33 | 5 | 17 | 10 | 15 |
| Double dose | 22/151 | 53/147 | 0.3 | 0.4 | 58 | 21 | 4.7 | 15 | 36 |
| Misoprostol | | | | | | | | | |
| 400 μg | 21/357 | 49/366 | 0.4 | 0.4 | 54 | 7 | 13 | 6 | 13 |
| 800 μg | 8/380 | 45/376 | 0.2 | 0.2 | 83 | 10 | 10 | 2 | 12 |
| PPI | 49/443 | 98/331 | 0.2 | 0.3 | 63 | 19 | 5.4 | 11 | 30 |

(presentation methods) for results for prevention of endoscopically detected NSAID-induced gastroduodenal ulcers for each treatment. All are significantly better than placebo, and confidence intervals have been omitted for clarity.

Odds ratios and relative risks were lower (better), at 0.2–0.3 for PPI, double doses of histamine antagonists, and 800 μg misoprostol. Relative risk reduction was higher (better) for these same three treatments. Misoprostol and standard dose histamine antagonists were less good with odds ratios and relative risks about 0.4–0.6. But looking at the NNT shows that, despite these statistical results, only PPI and double-dose histamine antagonists had the lower (better) NNT values of about 5.

Looking at the percentage figures, we find that only 2–6% of patients given misoprostol had endoscopic ulcers, with about 10% for PPI and standard dose histamine antagonist, while the worst result was for double-dose histamine antagonist with 15% of patients with ulcers.

Are you confused? Join the club. To help ourselves out the first thing to notice is what happens when we do nothing, in this case give placebo gastroprotection to patients who are taking NSAIDs. With no active prophylactic treatment there is a large variation in what happened in the review—12% of patients developed gastroduodenal ulcers in trials with 800 μg misoprostol, while 36% developed them with double-dose histamine antagonists. Part of this is to do with size (of which more later) and its effects on variability. Figure 2.2.1 shows what happens with placebo gastroprotection given with NSAIDs in individual trials.

Circles were the individual trials with double-dose histamine antagonist, and the vertical line the average result (18%) from all trials. Clearly, the high-dose histamine antagonist trials included two small trials with very high rates of ulcer development without prophylactic treatment, and with no obvious reason for it. The high rate at which things happen with placebo with small numbers of patients is why the odds ratios, relative risk, and relative risk reduction were so impressive, being relative to what happened with placebo. Even absolute risk reduction and NNT are dependent on what happened with placebo, because high rates with placebo give more scope for an effect of treatment. Actually, there was not much difference between double-dose and standard dose H2A, or 400 μg and 800 μg misoprostol, or PPI on the basis of these figures.

Of course, the outcome here is gastroduodenal ulcers seen on endoscopy, which is not the same as clinically relevant ulcers, which we will look at in a later section for other reasons. Perhaps we shouldn't get too excited about these results, except that they are our main guidance as to what to prescribe. Let's look at the reviewers' own conclusions [3].

Misoprostol, PPIs, and double dose H2As are effective at preventing chronic NSAID related endoscopic gastric and duodenal ulcers. Lower doses of misoprostol are less effective and are still associated with diarrhoea. Only misoprostol 800 μg/day has been directly shown to reduce the risk of ulcer complications.

So standard-dose H2A has been dismissed, despite providing lower rates of gastroduodenal ulcers than double-dose H2A, and equivalent to that obtained with PPI. Lower dose misoprostol is dismissed despite providing lower absolute rates of gastroduodenal ulcers than double-dose H2A and PPI.

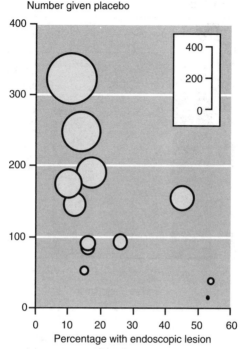

Number given placebo

Percentage with endoscopic lesion

**Figure 2.2.1**   Endoscopic gastroduodenal lesions with placebo gastroprotection in individual trials where patients are taking NSAIDs.

*Diarrhoea with misoprostol*

Now let's look at what the same review [3] said about diarrhoea with misoprostol.

Both misoprostol doses were associated with a statistically significant risk of diarrhoea. However, the risk of diarrhoea with 800 μg/day (RR = 3.05; 95% CI: 2.42–3.83) was significantly higher than that seen with 400 μg/day (RR = 1.92; 95% CI: 1.64–2.26; $p = 0.0012$).

This is impressive stuff, with high statistical significance. The actual results are shown in Figure 2.2.2, where 21% of patients on misoprostol 800 μg had diarrhoea, compared with 19% on misoprostol 400 μg. The NNHs were 7 (95% confidence interval 6–9) for 800 μg and 12 (9–16) for 400 μg. We can be reasonably sure of these results, because in each case they were obtained from over 3000 patients. The result is true: there was a *statistically* significant increase in diarrhoea with the higher dose, and the NNHs were different. But was the increase in incidence from 19% to 21% *clinically* significant?

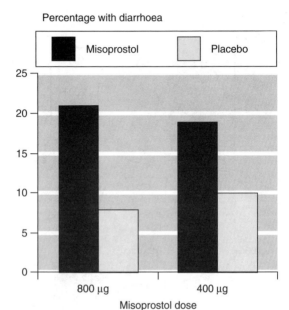

**Figure 2.2.2** Incidence of diarrhoea with misoprostol.

These examples serve to demonstrate several important points. First, it isn't easy. But it becomes much easier if we look at all the possible outputs before making any decisions. Relative statistics can mislead by overemphasizing statistical over clinical relevance. Absolute outputs tell us what happens absolutely, and the NNT tells us about the therapeutic effort needed to produce one clinically relevant result.

### Different outputs do matter

There has been research on the interpretation of numerical information and how that depends on the presentation of the information. Technically this is known as 'framing', and the effects of framing have been examined in a systematic review [4] of 12 studies published up to about 1998. Relative risk reduction or increase were outputs viewed most positively by doctors, but formal meta-analysis was not possible. Some selected studies are examined below, but the review concluded that the effects of framing on clinical practice are unknown.

### Purchasers and presentation

The importance of the way in which information is presented is emphasized by Fahey et al. [5], who gave 182 health authority members results from a randomized trial on breast cancer screening and results from a systematic

**Table 2.2.6**   Presentation of results on mammography and cardiac rehabilitation

| Information presentation | Mammography | Cardiac rehabilitation |
|---|---|---|
| Relative risk reduction | 34% | 20% |
| Absolute risk reduction | 0.06% | 3% |
| Percentage of event-free patients | 99.82% vs 99.80% | 84% vs 87% |
| Number needed to treat | 1592 | 31 |

review on cardiac rehabilitation. The results were presented to them (Table 2.2.6) in four different ways:

• relative risk reduction;
• absolute risk reduction;
• proportion of event-free patients;
• numbers of patients treated to prevent one death.

From the 140 questionnaires returned the willingness to fund either programme was influenced significantly by the way in which results were presented. Relative risk reduction produced significantly higher inclination to purchase, followed by NNT. Intriguingly, only three respondents, 'all non-executive members claiming no training in epidemiology', said that they realized that all four sets of data summarized the same results.

## Doctors and presentation

It is not only members of health authorities who are susceptible to altered perceptions of effectiveness according to the way in which the results of studies are presented to them. Two studies have looked at the effects of presentation on decisions by doctors in teaching hospitals in Canada [6] and by GPs in Italy [7]. Both used data from the Helsinki heart study.

### Hospital doctors

In the first of these studies, David Naylor and colleagues [6] compared clinicians' ratings of therapeutic effectiveness by looking at different end points presented as percentage reductions in relative risk, absolute risk, and numbers-needed-to-treat. The study was conducted using random allocation of questionnaires using relative data or absolute data, each with NNT, among doctors of various grades at Toronto teaching hospitals. They used an 11-point scale anchored at 'no effect' and running from −5 'harmful' to +5 'very effective'.

Relative risk presentation consistently showed a tendency to higher scores—that is, the intervention was interpreted as being more effective (Figure 2.2.3). Where data from a single end point, for any myocardial infarction, was examined, both relative and absolute comparison were scored consistently higher than NNT presentation of the same data. NNT reporting of the same information produced a reduction of about two points in the effectiveness scale, reducing the judgement from quite effective to one of only slight effect.

### General practitioners

This second study [7] presented information to 148 GPs using information from the trial as if it referred to five different drugs. The presentations were:

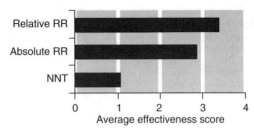

**Figure 2.2.3** Scoring effectiveness for outcome of 'any myocardial infarction' according to method of presentation of the same results.

- relative risk reduction;
- absolute risk reduction;
- difference in event-free patients;
- NNT to prevent one event;
- events reduction and mortality.

For each statement about effects, the GPs were asked to mark a 10 cm line labelled 'I would definitely not prescribe this drug' on the left and 'I would definitely prescribe this drug' on the right. The statements were presented in random sequences. The results are shown in Figure 2.2.4. Presentation as relative risk reduction produced a very large tendency towards prescribing with a mean score of 7.7 out of 10. All other presentations produced scores of between about 2.5 and 3.5.

### US and European physicians and pharmacists

A more recent study looked at US and European physicians and US pharmacists and examined how data presentation related to their willingness to prescribe a drug [8]. The same information was presented in three different ways, and overwhelmingly respondents chose data presented as relative risk reduction as that most likely to make them prescribe (Figure 2.2.5).

But three 'distracter' statements about life expectancy, cost, and hospital admission rate also attracted significant attention as first-choice determinants, and about 40% of respondents preferred those to the clinical trial results.

Interestingly, determinants were slightly different for European physicians compared with US physicians. European physicians were much

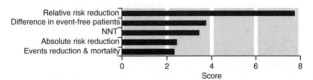

**Figure 2.2.4** GPs' willingness to prescribe scores, according to method of presenting data.

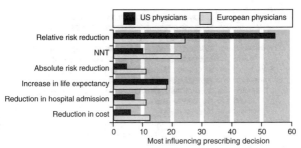

**Figure 2.2.5** Choice of information for determining prescribing decision.

more influenced by NNT and absolute risk reduction (and cost and hospital admission), and they were much less influenced by relative risk reduction. Despite this, relative risk reduction remains a potent influence on decisions, as a UK study confirmed [9].

### What GPs understand
Most consumer-oriented companies spend a lot of time finding out what their customers want, and giving it to them. There's little attention paid to the needs and wants of ordinary health-care professionals trying to provide an excellent service despite many difficulties. In one of the few such studies regarding outputs from research, GPs in Wessex were asked about their knowledge of evidence-based terms in 1996 [10].

The questionnaire asked some penetrating questions about GPs' knowledge of technical terms used in evidence-based medicine (things like odds ratios, heterogeneity, and the like). They used a very high hurdle—whether respondents understood the term and could explain it to others.

Of all the terms, the one that came out top of this stiff test was the number needed to treat (NNT), with 35% of GPs being able to understand it and explain it to others (Figure 2.2.6). Relative risk was also reasonably well understood, but odds ratios were not.

It is instructive to look at this from the other perspective, that is, how many people do *not* understand these terms. Ninety per cent of GPs have no idea how to describe or use an odds ratio. But 65–70% don't know how to describe or use an NNT or relative risk, at least according to the high standard set by this study. And that's the best result from a savvy group of GPs.

A similar study in Australia came to very similar conclusions, while also exploring the difficulties faced by GPs in putting evidence into practice [11]. What is also interesting is that GPs were able to spot that heterogeneity tests weren't worth thinking about, that odds ratios lack intuitive utility, and that publication bias is something best left to academic pointy heads to argue about because it can never be proved or disproved. All we can say is that tests to detect publication bias don't work [12].

### How randomized trials report results
Five top English-language journals were examined in 1989, 1992, 1995, and 1998 for how randomized trials reported their results [13]. Of 359 articles

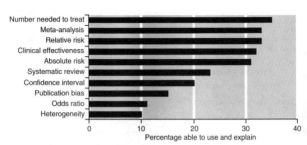

**Figure 2.2.6** GPs' ability to explain and use evidence-based medicine terms.

in total, eight (2.2%) reported NNTs and 18 (5.0%) reported absolute risk reduction.

## Commentary

There's no single answer as to which output works best for everyone, or anyone, or for particular circumstances. Graphical representations may be better than numbers in aiding comprehension of clinical trial results [14]. The main thing is to be sure that you know and understand whatever output you choose, and especially not to be swayed by things like relative risk, or odds ratios, or relative risk reduction, or whatever, when some of these can be highly statistically significant but clinically irrelevant.

Few clinical trials and few systematic reviews will give you results in the way that you want them, so there's no escaping doing some work yourself.

We have found it most useful to follow the following procedures when looking at outputs from systematic reviews and meta-analyses.

1. First check on the statistical result (relative risk or benefit, or odds ratio).
2. *If* statistically significant, proceed to calculate an NNT. Use NNT to estimate the **treatment-specific therapeutic effort** needed for one outcome, which puts some clinical relevance on the result.
3. *If* this seems sensible, look at what percentage of patients benefit from (or are harmed by) treatment, and use this figure for everyday work because this is immediately clinically relevant every time.

This procedure seems to work, if only because we can remember and use percentages quite easily, and because that is what is relevant in everyday practice. Bandolier's NNT calculation sheet follows. It can be used for clinical trials or systematic reviews. In getting to the NNT it makes us look at the real information in a trial or review, and that is probably the most useful part of trying to understand what's going on, and whether there are real benefits for patients.

The bottom line, though, is what people can use effectively in their day-to-day practice. Once statistics are done with, perhaps the best thing to remember, if there is only room for one number, is the percentage of people benefiting (or being harmed) by the treatment. Figure 2.2.7 emphasizes the differences between odds ratios, relative risks, NNTs, and percentages for two hypothetical trials.

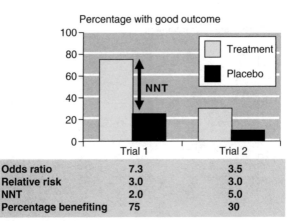

**Figure 2.2.7** Two hypothetical trials compared.

#### Bandolier's NNT worksheet

A number needed to treat (NNT) is defined by a number of characteristics. This worksheet is designed as an aide memoir for working out NNTs from papers and systematic reviews. First fill in the answers to the questions, where appropriate, plot the data on the L'Abbé plot, Figure 2.2.8 and finally do the NNT calculation.

| Question/action | Answer |
|---|---|
| **A**  What is the intervention ( dose & frequency)? | |
| **B**  What is the intervention for? | |
| **C**  What is the successful outcome (when, over what time did it occur)? | |
| **D**  How many had the intervention? | |
| **E**  How many had successful outcome with the intervention? | |
| **F**  Express as a percentage (100 × E/D) | |
| **G**  What is the control or comparator? | |
| **H**  How many people had the control? | |
| **I**  How many had successful outcome with the control? | |
| **J**  Express as a percentage (100 × I/H) | |

Now plot the percentages for the trial on the graph from the **percentages** from F and J. This can be done for different outcomes of a trial, or for individual trials in a systematic review or meta-analysis.

Now calculate the NNT using the **proportions** from F and J.

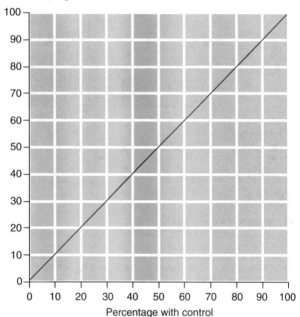

Figure 2.2.8 L'Abbé plot data.

$$NNT = \frac{1}{\boxed{F} - \boxed{J}} = \frac{1}{\boxed{\phantom{xx}} - \boxed{\phantom{xx}}}.$$

$$NNT = \frac{1}{\boxed{\phantom{xxxx}}} = \boxed{\phantom{xxxxxx}}$$

### References

1. Gavaghan, D.J. *et al.* (2000). An evaluation of homogeneity tests in meta-analyses in pain using simulations of individual patient data. *Pain* **85**, 415–24.
2. Ferrari, M.D. *et al.* (2001). Meta-analysis of rizatriptan efficacy in randomised controlled clinical trials. *Cephalalgia* **21**, 129–36.
3. Rostom, A. *et al.* (2002). Prevention of NSAID-induced gastroduodenal ulcers (Cochrane review). In: *The Cochrane Library* Issue 3, 2002. Oxford: Update Software.

4. McGettigan, P. *et al.* (1999). The effects of information framing on the practices of physicians. *Journal of General Internal Medicine* **14**, 633–42.
5. Fahey, T. *et al.* (1995). Evidence-based purchasing: understanding results of clinical trials and systematic reviews. *British Medical Journal* **311**, 1056–60.
6. Naylor, C.D. *et al.* (1992). Measured enthusiasm: does the method of reporting trial results alter perceptions of therapeutic effectiveness? *Annals of Internal Medicine* **117**, 916–21.
7. Bobbio, M. *et al.* (1994). Completeness of reporting trial results: effect on physicians' willingness to prescribe. *Lancet* **343**, 1209–11.
8. Lacy, C.R. (2001). Impact of presentation of research results on likelihood of prescribing medications to patients with left ventricular dysfunction. *American Journal of Cardiology* **87**, 203–7.
9. Cranney, M. and Walley, T. (1996). Same information, different decisions: the influence of evidence on the management of hypertension in the elderly. *British Journal of General Practice* **46**, 661–3.
10. McColl, A. *et al.* (1998). General practitioners' perceptions of the route to evidence based medicine: a questionnaire survey. *British Medical Journal* **316**, 361–5.
11. Young, J.M. and Ward, J.E. (2001). Evidence-based medicine in general practice: beliefs and barriers among Australian GPs. *Journal of Evaluation in Clinical Practice* **7**, 201–10.
12. Sterne, J.A. *et al.* (2000). Publication and related bias in meta-analysis: power of statistical tests and prevalence in the literature. *Journal of Clinical Epidemiology* **53**, 1119–29.
13. Nuovo, J. *et al.* (2002). Reporting number needed to treat and absolute risk reduction in randomized controlled trials. *Journal of the American Medical Association* **287**, 2813–14.
14. Elting, L.S. *et al.* (1999). Influence of data display formats on physician investigators' decisions to stop clinical trials: prospective trial with repeated measures. *British Medical Journal* **318**, 1527–31.

## 2.3 Placebo

Placebo means lots of different things to different people, leading to endless confusion because we all use the same word, but mean different things. The phrase 'placebo effect' is a greater nightmare, because some people use it to mean what happens when you do nothing, while others consider that using a placebo creates an effect over and above doing nothing. The key to thinking about placebo, about how we use it in trials, why we use it in trials, and what to do with results when we have them, is to take a deep breath, clear the mind, and start afresh.

We begin by talking about the technical use of placebos in clinical trials, and the extent of the placebo response, then about the mechanism, i.e. 'How does the placebo work?', and lastly about the ethics of placebo in the contexts of research and in everyday practice. Placebo is used here to mean an inert treatment, given as if it were a real treatment. The word first entered the English language through St Jerome's Latin version (the Vulgate) of the Septuagint: 'Placebo Domino in regione vivorum'. Jerome's verse was used in the Vespers of the Office for the Dead. The verse began with the word 'placebo', so in the thirteenth century *Placebo* became the name of that service. Some people attended the service and sang the *Placebo*, hoping to be rewarded by a dead person's relatives, or the relatives paid priests to sing the *Placebo* on their behalf. Placebo came then to mean a sycophant. How it acquired its current meaning is not known [1].

To set the scene ask yourself how you would design a trial to answer the question of whether or not arthroscopy is useful in knee osteoarthritis. Moseley *et al.* randomized patients to arthroscopy or to placebo surgery, which involved three incisions and anaesthesia [2]. The justification for placebo surgery was that there was no other way to control for the act of surgery itself, rather than what it may achieve, to produce pain relief [3]. This trial shows some of the problems around placebo to be addressed below, such as why placebo may be the best or indeed the only way to design trials that can answer questions credibly, how much risk is acceptable for placebo patients, albeit in a non-life-threatening context, and about the confusion between the ethics of clinical research and the ethics of clinical care. Interestingly, the knee arthroscopy trial, like its famous predecessor that used placebo surgery to investigate the efficacy of internal mammary artery ligation for angina [4], showed no benefit from the procedure.

### Clinical trials

In the early days of margarine there was an advertising slogan asking if you could tell Stork (a margarine brand) from butter. The manufacturers assumed that your ability to distinguish tastes was working well, but that they had made the tastes so similar that even with fully functioning taste discrimination you would not be able to tell the two apart. If your taste discrimination was poor or absent then you would say, incorrectly, the two spreads were indistinguishable. Saying that two things are the same when they are not, because a test is technically insensitive, is precisely the reason that placebo is so important for clinical trials.

Imagine a very simple clinical trial, a comparison of treatment A with treatment B for relief of pain after dental extraction. You need an outcome measure like pain relief. Let us say that at the end of the trial both treatments appear to work, but with exactly the same amount of pain relief (Figure 2.3.1). Does this result mean that the two treatments were genuinely equally good analgesics, or that your pain relief outcome measure was too insensitive to pick up a real difference between the two, or indeed that neither was any good? We have no way of knowing unless we change the trial design to incorporate an index of sensitivity of the measures.

Such an index of sensitivity can be a third group of patients, randomized to receive placebo rather than treatments A or B (Figure 2.3.2). If both treatment A and treatment B do well, and placebo does badly, then we can be more confident that A and B are both effective treatments, because placebo was ineffective, and that there is minimal difference between A's and B's performances in the trial.

This use of placebo as a 'negative control' as the index of sensitivity is, and rightly so, pervasive in explanatory clinical trials designed to establish the efficacy of new treatments. An alternative to the negative control is the positive control, in which a known effective treatment, treatment X, is given, ideally with one group of patients given a high dose of X and another group given a low dose (Figure 2.3.3). The index of sensitivity criterion will be met if low dose X does badly compared with high dose X. While this positive control method reduces the ethical concerns about use of placebo, to be discussed later, it is also a fudge, in that low dose X needs to be a minimally effective dose for the sensitivity index to work,

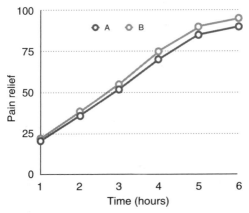

**Figure 2.3.1** Treatment A versus treatment B with no index of internal sensitivity.

A versus B: versus placcebo (negative control)

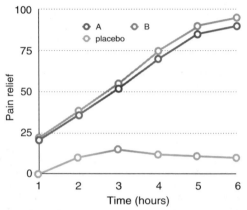

**Figure 2.3.2** Treatment A versus treatment B with placebo as the index of internal sensitivity.

A versus B: versus standard treatment (positive control)

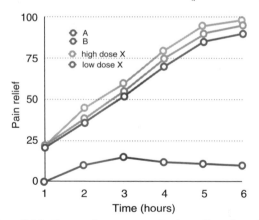

**Figure 2.3.3** Treatment A versus treatment B with two different doses of known active drug X as the index of internal sensitivity.

which then means that that patient group is receiving a less effective treatment.

An example in the pain field would be using paracetamol 500 mg as low dose X and 1000 mg as high dose X. Few trials have shown good separation at these doses. Those that do not manage to separate 500 mg from 1000 mg then have no proven index of internal sensitivity.

### Placebo response or placebo effect

This is perhaps one of the most difficult of all topics, especially with subjective outcomes such as pain or depression. If we were discussing a topic like myocardial infarction and our outcome measure was death, then we might be reasonably sure that a placebo would have no effect on the outcome. But with subjective outcomes like pain, we might guess that patients would feel better after placebo, and consequently have less pain, if the doctor or nurse were nice to them, or appeared authoritative, or if the placebo were given as a big red capsule instead of a tiny white pill, or as an injection and not a tablet. Whatever we think, proving that any or all of these influences had an effect would be difficult because very large trials would be necessary to show any effect independent of random chance. Table 2.3.1 summarizes effects that we might expect to find in various control groups [5].

It is all very complicated, and made more so by the difficulty in proving that 'negativity', or 'interaction', or 'expectation' contribute anything at all to the actual perception of pain as it is measured. We don't help ourselves by using lax, if understandable, shorthand. When we want to discuss the effect that we observe when patients are given a placebo, we call it the 'placebo effect' or placebo response. Immediately that can be retranslated as 'the effect caused by placebo'. Indirectly, of course, administration of placebo can and does result in an effect, for instance, resulting in analgesia in a pain study. The pitfall is that we jump to a simplistic causal connection, and then in turn jump to conclusions about the mechanism by which this happens. Ideas about how placebo has its effect will be discussed later. At this point just note that it is a creek where we don't have a paddle.

**Table 2.3.1**  Effects in control groups

| Control | Effects |
|---|---|
| Waiting list | Natural course of disease **minus** the negativity from nothing being done |
| Visits without treatment | Natural course of disease **plus** doctor/nurse/patient interaction |
| Placebo | Natural course of disease **plus** interaction **plus** expectation that there will be an effect |
| Active control | Natural course of disease **plus** interaction **plus** expectation **plus** actual effect |

## Common misconceptions about the response to placebo

There are a number of misconceptions about placebo, and they are worth examining because they are highly instructive.

*Misconception 1*

For every intervention, a fixed fraction of the population, usually a third, responds to placebo, whatever the outcome.

This just is not so. Table 2.3.2 lists rates of response with placebo in a number of clinical conditions in acute and chronic pain. They all measure pain, a common condition, and they all measure pain relief in some way, but at different times or at different levels.

There is a wide range of response, from 7% for the response of freedom from pain 2 hours after migraine pain of moderate or severe intensity, to 49% of patients with painful diabetic neuropathy saying their pain is at least much better after 8 weeks of treatment with a topical placebo. For some of the chronic painful conditions we have pitifully little information and the estimates may just be wrong, but even where we have large amounts of data there is wide variation. Why are we surprised? Would we not expect a large response if we do nothing to strains and sprains over a week, when a

**Table 2.3.2** Response rates with placebo in acute and chronic pain conditions

| Pain condition | Treatment | Outcome | Duration | Number given placebo | % with pain relief with placebo |
|---|---|---|---|---|---|
| Acute postoperative pain | Oral analgesics | At least 50% pain relief | 4–6 hours | 12,000 | 18 |
| Strains and sprains | Topical NSAID | At least 50% pain relief | 7 days | 3,239 | 39 |
| Migraine | Oral triptan | No pain or mild pain | 2 hours | 3,148 | 28 |
| Migraine | Oral triptan | Pain free | 2 hours | 2,661 | 7 |
| Dysmenorrhoea | Oral analgesics | At least 50% pain relief | About 1 day | 1,607 | 22 |
| Trigeminal neuralgia | Antiepileptics | At least 50% pain relief | 3–7 months | 224 | 18 |
| Diabetic neuropathy | Tricyclic antidepressant | At least 50% pain relief | 3–7 months | 200 | 36 |
| Diabetic neuropathy | Topical capsaicin | Pain at least much better | 4–8 weeks | 165 | 49 |
| Atypical facial pain | Tricyclic antidepressant | At least 50% pain relief | 3–7 months | 85 | 35 |
| Postherpetic neuralgia | Tricyclic antidepressant | At least 50% pain relief | 3–7 months | 68 | 12 |

fair proportion are going to get better anyway? People with a migraine will rarely have it next week, at least not the same attack.

The real issue here is how hard the outcome is to achieve. If we use migraine as the exemplar, there are four outcomes for pain relief from migraine that we can consider:

- no pain or mild pain at 2 hours;
- no pain at 2 hours;
- no pain or mild pain at 2 hours and pain not returned and no analgesics over 24 hours;
- no pain at 2 hours and pain not returned and no analgesics over 24 hours.

We might guess that no pain is harder to achieve than mild pain, and that 'no return of pain plus no additional analgesics over 24 hours' is more difficult to achieve than outcomes that look only at the first 2 hours. Not surprisingly, we find that 35–40% of people can obtain no pain or mild pain with placebo at 2 hours, but that only about 10% have no pain. Fewer people have a favourable outcome with placebo over 24 hours than over 2 hours (Figure 2.3.4). No surprise here then.

*Misconception 2*

The placebo response is a fixed fraction (about a third) of the maximum effect of treatment—the bigger the treatment effect, the bigger the placebo response.

This idea came from an analysis of five randomized trials in acute pain [6]. The relationship that Evans found, treatment effect and placebo response moving in the same direction, was an artefact because he used mean values of skewed TOTPAR (total pain relief) data. The relationship could not be demonstrated when median values were used [7].

Of course, it may be the case that, when the outcome is easier to achieve, both the response to placebo and the response to treatment are likely to be higher. Figure 2.3.5 is Figure 2.3.4 with the addition of the

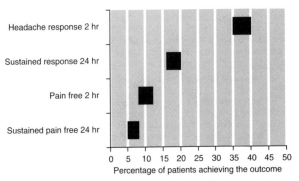

**Figure 2.3.4**  Responses to placebo in migraine using different outcome measures. Bars represent the 95% confidence interval of the response.

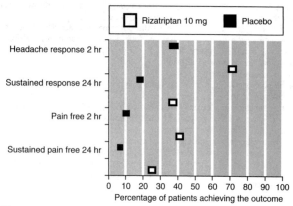

**Figure 2.3.5** Responses to placebo and rizatriptan 10 mg in migraine using different outcome measures. Bars represent the 95% confidence interval of the response.

response from rizatriptan 10 mg. There is a general relationship based on degree of difficulty of the outcome, but it is not a fixed fraction.

*Misconception 3*

The more invasive the method of delivering a treatment, the higher will be the response to placebo—injection will give bigger response than tablets.

Again this is not so. Table 2.3.3 shows that, while we have relatively small numbers of patients given intramuscular placebo, the proportion of patients having at least 50% pain relief is no bigger than with oral administration of placebo tablets. The same complete lack of any difference can be seen in an analysis of responses to placebo with different routes of administration in migraine (Table 2.3.4). Though injected placebo has been claimed to give higher response rates than oral placebo in migraine [8], this was based on an analysis of a limited data set.

*Misconception 4*

Randomization of different numbers of patients to active and placebo can affect the response to placebo.

This final misconception again comes from the migraine field. The claim was that randomization to different proportions of active treatment and placebo could affect the response to placebo. This was on the basis of one trial in which 16 patients were randomized to active treatment for every one randomized to placebo. Fifty-six patients were randomized to placebo, and the response rate at 2 hours for no pain or mild pain, or just no pain, was high (Figure 2.3.6). The answer, though, was that with 56 patients the 95% confidence interval of the response rate included that of the overall response rate from all randomization schedules.

**Table 2.3.3** Response to oral and intramuscular placebo in acute postoperative pain

| Active intervention | Route | Number given placebo | Per cent with at least 50% pain relief |
|---|---|---|---|
| **All placebo** | Oral/IM | > 12,000 | 18 |
| Aspirin 600/650 mg | Oral | 2562 | 16 |
| Ibuprofen 400 mg | Oral | 2183 | 14 |
| Paracetamol 1000 mg | Oral | 1132 | 20 |
| Paracetamol 600/650 mg plus codeine 60 mg | Oral | 432 | 20 |
| Tramadol 100 mg | Oral | 414 | 8 |
| Morphine 10 mg | IM | 460 | 16 |
| Parecoxib 20/40 mg | IM | 176 | 16 |
| Ketorolac 30 mg | IM | 183 | 23 |

**Table 2.3.4** Response to oral, intranasal, and injected placebo in acute migraine

| Route of administration | Number of trials | 2-hour headache response with placebo (number/total) | Per cent responders (95% CI) |
|---|---|---|---|
| Oral | 30 | 875/3148 | 28 (26–29) |
| Subcutaneous | 14 | 382/1257 | 30 (28–33) |
| Intranasal | 6 | 205/650 | 32 (28–35) |

Data are from patients given placebo in randomized, double-blind trials of migraine diagnosed using International Headache Society criteria and with initial pain of moderate or severe intensity.

### Where does this leave us?

The most important point to appreciate is that the response to placebo can vary hugely. While these examples all came from pain studies, we could have used data from early postoperative nausea and vomiting after general surgery (range 0–50% patients vomiting) [9], or after squint correction, where with essentially the same operation and anaesthetic technique the range was 18–88% [10], or in trials of surfactant in respiratory distress syndrome, where the range of the placebo response was 24%–69% [11], or in depression trials (13–52%) [12]. This range of response has led people to look for explanations within the trials, such as kind nurses versus unkind, or even flawed double-blinding.

The reality is that random chance alone can produce this range of response [13], and the first line of defence against such variability lies in the size of the dataset. An unimaginably large dataset will include the range, but would allow us to estimate the 'true' underlying placebo response in that setting. In Table 2.3.2 with 12,000 patients, the proportion of patients achieving at least 50% pain relief with placebo in postoperative pain is 18%.

Percentage of placebo patients with headache response at two hours

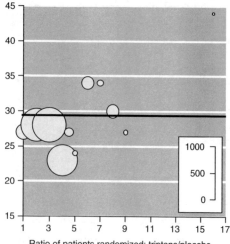

Ratio of patients randomized: triptans/placebo

**Figure 2.3.6** Different randomization rates in migraine trials. Two-hour headache response, with black horizontal line showing overall response with placebo.

If we do small trials, with just 100 patients, then random chance means that the proportion showing at least 50% pain relief with placebo could be anywhere from 0 to 50%, which obviously could have a significant impact on how we view the performance of the active drug or drugs in that trial.

Once you understand that the response can vary, and that random chance is the most important factor underlying the variability that makes small studies particularly vulnerable, then that minimizes the need to look for other explanations such as kind versus unkind nurses. The fact that much time and effort has been spent on exploring such spurious influences demonstrates just how easy it is when thinking about placebo to be navigating the creek without a paddle. The other trap has been the 'soundbites' about fixed fractions of responders and about the extent of the response. Statements suggesting that one-third of people respond to placebo or that people respond to placebo at one-third of the maximum response are common. The information above shows that both are wrong. It takes a long time to debunk widely held beliefs.

### How does placebo work?

We once ran a trial of oral morphine versus placebo in an experimental pain model, where you had to keep your arm in a bucket of icy water for as long as you could stand it. As subjects in the trial we knew that the treatment was either morphine or placebo. One of us had the treatment on one occasion, and then was constipated for a week, a very unusual event, and hence was absolutely convinced that the treatment had been morphine. It turned out that that was the placebo day. Ah, the shame of being a placebo responder!

The mysteries here are whether the placebo caused constipation and, if it did, what was the mechanism? In the absence of a better explanation it has to be the *belief* that one had received morphine that resulted in the unusual constipation. Even if you accept that belief results in the effect of the placebo, there is a long chain of biological events between belief and an effect we do not understand, and that still could be chance.

Most experiments designed to tease out the mechanism of the placebo effect are small, complicated, and with results that do not stand the test of time. Taking the analgesic effect of placebo 20 years ago researchers had the clever idea of antagonizing the analgesic action of placebo with the opioid antagonist naloxone. The hypothesis was that, if the analgesic action of placebo was mediated through the opioid system, then it would be reversed by giving naloxone. The researchers duly reported that they found such a reversal, but subsequent studies have not replicated their findings. More recently, the brain geographers with their magnificent imaging devices have shown that when placebo produces an analgesic effect the same parts of the brain light up as light up when a known analgesic is given [14, 15]. There is a common theme to these results, which is that in order to have its effect placebo uses the same biological system as an active drug, whether the effect is analgesia or constipation. We are still left with the overarching question of how an 'inert' intervention activates the system.

The curious among us take this further, and look for differences between individual humans and between humans and animals in their susceptibility to placebo. Once again experiments tackling these questions tend to be small and hence subject to our old friend the random play of chance, so that all results need to be taken with a large pinch of salt. An early observational study tried to identify the people who did respond to placebo. It found that responders tended to be older, women more often than men, church-attending but not necessarily God-believing, and with great faith in doctors and nurses. What you would expect really, if belief is the overarching switch to turn on a response to placebo.

Implicit in the idea that we can identify the believers is the principle that the belief does not waver. One way to check whether or not it is fixed is to re-challenge the same person with placebo. What you might expect in such a wolf, wolf paradigm is that, if not much really happened the first time, even though you believed it would, then your belief will wane with successive use of placebo—your response will wane. This was tested in women with dysmenorrhoea. Some brave souls received placebo on successive menstrual cycles, and the analgesic effect of the placebo decreased with successive use of the placebo [16] (Figure 2.3.7).

The idea that we differ in our faith in doctors or in other markers of trust and belief is not revolutionary. We know, for example, that there are differences in our susceptibility to hypnosis or acupuncture, and folklore has it that one-third of horses or dogs are hard to help with acupuncture, so this is not just a human issue. The fact that our belief can be context-

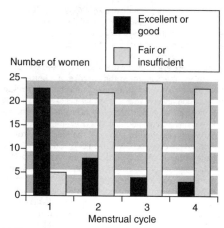

**Figure 2.3.7** Placebo response over successive menstrual cycles.

dependent, and that our response to placebo can therefore vary with context is not surprising, but it still does not explain how belief throws the switch to cause a response to placebo.

Professor Pat Wall did provide a testable explanation of the placebo mechanism [17]. He started with the link between the placebo response and the patient's expectation, and the fact that part of the response of a patient to any therapy relates to the expectation of a beneficial effect. He argued that sensory events are analysed in terms of the appropriate motor responses. For pain this would be first to remove the stimulus, second to change posture to limit further injury and optimize recovery, and third to seek safety, relief, and cure. 'If the patient's experience has taught them that a particular action is followed by relief, then they respond if they think the action has occurred.' In this scheme of thinking, the placebo is not a stimulus but an 'appropriate action', acting to terminate or cancel the pain sensation.

## Ethics of placebo

### In clinical trials

Most of us react negatively to the idea of using placebo, because 'it appears to violate the fundamental ethical principles of beneficence and non-maleficence' [3]. But if we are going to advance in medicine we need trials of our interventions. For some interventions a placebo treatment may be necessary if the trial is to answer the question posed. The arthroscopy trial mentioned at the beginning, for instance, could not have answered the question without a placebo surgery group of patients. The collision, if it is a collision, is between the ethics of our clinical care in general with the ethics of clinical research.

In clinical research trials are unethical if their design means that they cannot answer the question. In Figure 2.3.1 we could not tell if treatments A or B were both effective, or both ineffective, because there was no index of internal sensitivity. Adding a placebo group provides that index so that we would be able to tell whether treatments A or B were both effective (as in Figure 2.3.2), or both ineffective. This is the justification for using placebo in trials.

A little common sense always helps. Nobody is going to advocate using placebo in a life-threatening condition. Two obvious examples would be antibiotic trials in septicaemia or chemotherapy in cancer. In such contexts trial design that shows that one drug is as good as another (Figure 2.3.1), called equivalence trials (Chapter 2.1), can be very difficult to interpret [18]. One way round this dilemma is to add the test treatment to existing treatment, as happens in trials in epilepsy and cancer, for instance. Decisions about the legitimacy of placebo in a particular setting are not always as clear-cut as this makes it sound. If you know that statins reduce long-term cardiac risk then is it or is it not legitimate to use a placebo group in a trial of the efficacy of a new statin drug on long-term cardiac mortality? If you decide that it is not legitimate, then how do you design an equivalence trial, old statin versus new statin, that does not run into the Figure 2.3.1 problem? This takes you into a controversial area [19], controversial both because of the design problems of equivalence trials and also because cholesterol lowering is taken as a proxy of the long-term cardiac mortality.

In the circumstance where it is legitimate to use placebo, it is important to understand that being randomized to placebo does not condemn the patient to long-term suffering. The patient is free to withdraw from the trial at any point, and then receive normal treatment. Patients may be given rescue (or 'escape') medication if the trial treatment is inadequate, and that is usually done for oral medication from the first hour onwards, because it takes an hour for the medicine to get into the system. Obviously, if everyone in the placebo group drops out 1 hour after treatment, or needs to take rescue medication, and none of the active treatment patients drop out or need rescue, then you have your answer.

Ethical objections to the use of placebo in clinical trials are 'based on the requirements to minimize risks, limit the level of risks that are not offset by the potential benefits to participants, and obtain informed consent' and do not, in the view of Horng and Miller, support an absolute prohibition against the use of placebo when its use is methodologically necessary to answer clinically important questions [3]. This justification of placebo as the index of internal sensitivity, as in our Figure 2.3.1 problem with drug trials, will persist unless and until we could use a 'gold standard' active treatment as our comparator, as in Figure 2.3.3.

Imagine that we were certain that whenever and wherever amitriptyline was used it would always produce $x$ units of antidepressant activity. Then we could use it as the positive control in our design. If the amitriptyline did not produce $x$ units of improvement in the trial then we would know that the trial was faulty, a 'method failure', just as we do now if gold standard does not beat placebo. The problem is that we do not have any certainty about the $x$ units of antidepressant activity. We know that $x$ varies widely in trials [18, 12]. Perhaps the way forward is to use large pooled data sets to produce a more robust estimate, analogous to the estimate of 18% of 12,000 placebo patients achieving at least 50% postoperative pain relief (Table 2.3.2).

### In everyday practice

The ethical issues around placebo in everyday practice are different from those in clinical research. First, there should be a distinction between knowingly and unknowingly treating a patient with a placebo intervention. Knowingly doing so is deceit, which is hard to condone. Unknowing might be the use of a drug or procedure for which there is no good evidence of efficacy. The fact of the procedure itself, the fact of the prescription written, may produce improvement, particularly in a self-limiting disorder. Many of us do this, given that there is minimal risk, in our everyday practice. Indeed, the cynic would argue that much of complementary medicine is based on this principle.

## Postscript

Placebo is one of those topics that is difficult to leave without loose ends. The trouble is that trying to tuck in those loose ends tidily always makes for increasing complication. So, without trying to overcomplicate things, a few additional words.

### Getting better by oneself

People used to recover from the most serious illnesses even before modern medicine. People had plague, influenza, and other awful, frequently fatal diseases, and some got better. The body is equipped with an impressive battery of defences, and often puts up a good fight. So, when someone gets better, we have to consider that there may be a variety of reasons.

Some people believe that there is enormous power in prayer, and will ascribe an important event, like waking from a coma in ITU after several weeks, or recovering miraculously from cancer, to the prayer. They forget the power of the body to heal itself, and the power of the ITU staff, organization, and interventions to help that. It is fuzzy thinking and, though we are not discussing prayer, it is always important to remember that the body has powerful innate abilities for repair, even without outside help. If we give a placebo, then what we actually observe is just that.

### Conditions that wax and wane

Many chronic conditions are phasic; better at some times, worse at others. In order to demonstrate efficacy in clinical trials in chronic disorders, patients are recruited when the condition is worse. The clinical trial may or may not show efficacy, but one thing that it certainly will show is a large effect of placebo, for the simple reason that the next phase after the worse phase is a better one.

It is likely, then, that response to placebo will vary with time. This can be seen in restless legs syndrome trials. Here new trials of longer duration up to 12 weeks show a progressive improvement with placebo, probably for exactly this reason (see Bandolier's restless legs syndrome site for updates).

There are two points. First, we should not be surprised to see reasonably large effects with placebo treatment in some chronic conditions, but that is only to be expected. Second, if we compare effects seen with placebo, or different treatments, we should probably be wary about doing so when the duration of studies is very different, at least until we have a good hard look at what happens with placebo.

### Some things don't change
There are some constants. An example is a blood constituent, for instance, like cholesterol. Doing nothing (or giving placebo) has no effect at all on serum cholesterol (total or lipid fractions) in trials that last for years. Figure 2.3.8 takes data from all randomized trials over 12 weeks' duration, and with reasonable numbers (at least 100 patients) [20]. The effect of placebo is exactly zero after a few months, or as long as 5 years.

There is an important thought here, that we should probably not expect large effects of placebo treatment on objective outcomes outside phasic conditions. We know that cholesterol levels can vary over a day, or perhaps over a year in individuals, perhaps by up to 10% or so, but averaged out over a clinical trial there is no measurable response with placebo.

### Nice is better
Discussion of placebo or placebo effect sometimes gets entangled with discussion about being nice to people, or doing nice things. It is pretty

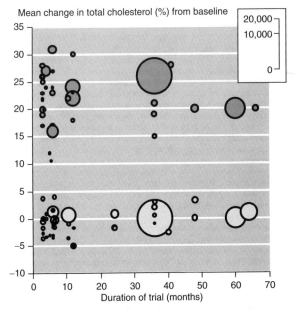

**Figure 2.3.8**  Percentage reduction in total cholesterol with time with statin (darker symbols) or placebo (lighter symbols).

obvious that doing nice things is better than being neutral, or even nasty. A few examples help.

*Room with a view*

Patients undergoing cholecystectomy in a Pennsylvania hospital had post-operative care on one of two floors, with rooms looking at either a brown brick wall, or a small stand of deciduous trees [21]. Rooms were identical apart from the view, and records were examined only for the period in the year when there were leaves on the trees.

Patient records were matched for all sorts of possible confounding factors, and then the 23 pairs of patient records were given to an experienced nurse to abstract information on number of days in hospital, analgesic and drug history, complications, and nurses' comments on patients' well-being.

Patients with the tree view spent 1 day less in hospital, used predominantly oral analgesics after the first day (with half of the number of injections), and had many fewer negative comments on their postoperative progress from nurses caring from them (one per patient compared with four per patient for the brick wall view). All these were statistically significant at the 1 in 100 level. Postoperative complications were lower in tree view patients, but not significantly so.

*The importance of being positive*

A randomized trial of a positive attitude in GP consultations was made by a single GP in consultations where no firm diagnosis could be made [22]. All such symptomatic patients could have one of four consultations:

1. a positive consultation in which the patient was given a firm diagnosis, given a prescription, and told that it would certainly make them better;
2. a positive consultation in which the patient was given a firm diagnosis and told that they required no prescription to get better;
3. a negative consultation in which they were told (honestly) 'I cannot be certain what is the matter with you', given a prescription, and told 'I am not sure that the treatment I am about to give you will have an effect';
4. a negative consultation in which they were told 'I cannot be certain what is the matter with you', followed by 'and therefore I will give you no treatment'.

Negative consultations were closed by the GP telling patients to come back after a few days if they felt no better. Wherever a prescription was given, it was 3 mg thiamine hydrochloride. Two weeks after the consultation each patient was sent a card asking:

- Did you get better?
- How many days after seeing the doctor did you get better?
- Did you need any further treatment?

Patients in whom no firm diagnosis could be made had a variety of complaints. The commonest complaint in the 200 patients was cough, sore throat, nasal congestion, or cold (in 81 patients), pain in abdomen, back, leg, head, chest, ear, muscles, arm, breast, and neck (in 69), giddiness (9), and tiredness (8).

A positive consultation produced a higher proportion of patients (64%) getting better than with a negative consultation (39%). There was no effect of giving a prescription. Overall, the number needed to treat (NNT) with a positive consultation was 4.0 (2.6 to 8.6) for one patient to get better within 2 weeks.

The only treatment used in this study was that of a positive consultation in patients who were symptomatic but in whom no firm diagnosis could be made. Sixty four per cent of such patients got better with a positive consultation. We should not be surprised that a positive attitude has an effect; a positive attitude is clearly not a placebo, and is more than doing nothing.

## Commentary

Placebo is not simple nor is it necessarily as powerful as was claimed 50 years ago [23], rather it is a by-product of how we conduct clinical trials, and a recognition that, either through faulty diagnosis or the power of the body to heal itself, people improve without anything being done to them or for them. Doing nothing isn't the cause.

Placebo need not be confusing. Keep thinking that it is what happens when we do nothing, and most times that maintains a balanced view of the world of clinical trials. Bear in mind that doing nothing often involves doing something, being nice to people or having time for them. Being nice to people or patients or providing nice surroundings are positive interventions, and not placebo. It is also worth remembering that, while placebo use in trials is justified to prove a point, we don't use placebo in the real world.

## References

1. Aronson, J. (1999). Please, please me. *British Medical Journal* **318**, 716.
2. Moseley, J.B. *et al.* (2002). A controlled trial of arthroscopic surgery for osteoarthritis of the knee. *New England Journal of Medicine* **347**, 81–8.
3. Horng, S. and Miller, F.G. (2002). Is placebo surgery unethical? *New England Journal of Medicine* **347**, 137–9.
4. Cobb, L.A. *et al.* (1959). An evaluation of internal-mammary-artery ligation by a double-blind technic. *New England Journal of Medicine* **260**, 1115–18.
5. Kalso, E. and Moore, R.A. (2000). Five easy pieces on evidence-based medicine (2). *European Journal of Pain* **4**, 321–4.
6. Evans, F.J. (1974). The placebo response in pain reduction. In *Advances in neurology* (ed. J.J. Bonica), Vol. 4, pp. 289–96. Raven Press, New York.
7. McQuay, H. *et al.* (1996). Variation in the placebo effect in randomised controlled trials of analgesics: all is as blind as it seems. *Pain* **64**, 331–5.
8. de Craen, A.J.M. *et al.* (2000). Placebo effect in the acute treatment of migraine: subcutaneous placebos are better than oral placebos. *Journal of Neurology* **247**, 183–8.
9. Tramèr, M. *et al.* (1996). Omitting nitrous oxide in general anaesthesia: meta-analysis of intraoperative awareness and postoperative emesis in randomized controlled trials. *British Journal of Anaesthesia* **76**, 186–93.
10. Tramèr, M. *et al.* (1995). Prevention of vomiting after paediatric strabismus surgery: a systematic review using the numbers-needed-to-treat method. *British Journal of Anaesthesia* **75**, 556–61.
11. Sinclair, J.C. and Bracken, M.B. (1994). Clinically useful measures of effect in binary analyses of randomized trials. *Journal of Clinical Epidemiology* **47**, 881–9.
12. Walsh, B.T. *et al.* (2002). Placebo response in studies of major depression. *Journal of the American Medical Association* **287**, 1840–7.
13. Moore, R.A. *et al.* (1998). Size is everything—large amounts of information are needed to overcome random effects in estimating direction and magnitude of treatment effects. *Pain* **78**, 209–16.

14. Petrovic, P. *et al.* (2002). Placebo and opioid analgesia—imaging a shared neuronal network. *Science* **295**, 1737–40.
15. Wager, T.D. *et al.* (2004). Placebo-induced changes in fMRI in the anticipation and experience of pain. *Science* **303**, 1162–7.
16. Fedele, L. *et al.* (1989). Dynamics and significance of placebo response in primary dysmenorrhea. *Pain* **36**, 43–7.
17. Wall, P. (1999). *Pain: the science of suffering.* Weidenfeld and Nicolson, London.
18. Engel, L.W. *et al.* (2002). *The science of the placebo.* BMJ Press, London.
19. Evans, D. (2003). *Placebo. The belief effect.* HarperCollins, London.
20. Edwards, J.E. and Moore, R.A. (2003). Statins in hypercholesterolaemia: a dose-specific meta-analysis of lipid changes in randomised, double blind trials. *BMC Family Practice* **4**, 18.
21. Ulrich, R.S. (1983). View through a window may influence recovery from surgery. *Science* **224**, 420–1.
22. Thomas, K.B. (1987). General practice consultations: is there any point in being positive? *British Medical Journal* **294**, 1200–2.
23. Beecher, H.K. (1955). The powerful placebo. *Journal of the American Medical Association* **159**, 1602–6.

# 2.4  Bias in clinical trials

This chapter contains information about several sorts of bias that occur in clinical trials. It is a useful guide when examining a systematic review, or a single clinical trial, but not observational studies or studies of diagnostic tests. Some sources of bias have been mentioned previously, such as randomization and blinding, but we add them here again for completeness. Table 2.4.1 lists the different sources of bias, and each is dealt with briefly. Later in this chapter two aspects are dealt with in a little more depth, dealing with the spectre of publication bias, and some comments on industry bias and how that works.

## Sources of bias

### Randomization

The process of randomization is important in eliminating selection bias in trials. If the selection is done by a computer, or even the toss of a coin, then any conscious or subconscious attitude of the researcher is avoided.

Some of the most influential people in evidence-based thinking showed how inadequate design exaggerated the effect measured in a trial. They compared trials in which the authors reported adequately concealed treatment allocations with those in which treatment was either inadequate or not clearly described, as well as examining the effects of exclusions and double-blinding.

The results were striking and sobering, as Table 2.4.1 shows. Odds ratios were exaggerated by 41% in trials in which there was an inadequate concealment of treatment allocation, and by 30% when the process of concealing allocation was not clearly stated.

The amount of bias arising from failure to randomize is one reason why many systematic reviews exclude non-randomized trials and why restricting systematic reviews to include only randomized studies makes sense for reviews of effectiveness. There are many, many examples where non-randomized studies have led reviews to come to the wrong conclusion.

The randomization effect is particularly strong where a review counts votes (a study is positive or negative) rather than combines data in a meta-analysis. It applies especially to studies in alternative therapies. In the example of transcutaneous nerve stimulation (TENS) for postoperative pain relief (Table 2.1.1), randomized studies overwhelmingly showed no benefit over placebo, while non-randomized studies did show benefit. Put another way, almost all the positive trials were not randomized, while almost all the negative ones were randomized.

### Blinding

The importance of blinding is that it avoids observer bias. If neither patient nor observer knows which treatment a patient has received, then no systematic overestimation of the effect of any particular treatment is possible. Non-blinded studies overestimate treatment effects by an average of 17% (Table 2.4.1).

### Reporting quality

Because of the large bias expected from studies that are not randomized or not blind, a scoring system [1] that is highly dependent on randomization

**Table 2.4.1** Sources of bias

| Source of bias | Effect on estimate of treatment efficacy | Size of the effect | References |
|---|---|---|---|
| Randomization | Increase | Non-randomized studies overestimate treatment effect by 41% with inadequate method, 30% with unclear method | Schultz, K.F. et al. (1995). Empirical evidence of bias: dimensions of methodological quality associated with estimates of treatment effects in controlled trials. *JAMA* **273**, 408–12. |
| Randomization | Increase | Completely different result between randomized and non-randomized studies | Carroll, D. et al. (1996). Randomization is important in studies with pain outcomes: systematic review of transcutaneous electrical nerve stimulation in acute postoperative pain. *British Journal of Anaesthesia* **77**, 798–803. |
| Blinding | Increase | 17% | Schultz, K.F. et al. (1995). Empirical evidence of bias: Dimensions of methodological quality associated with estimates of treatment effects in controlled trials. *JAMA* **273**, 408–12. |
| Blinding | Increase | Completely different result between blind and non-blind studies | Ernst, E. and White, A.R. (1998). Acupuncture for back pain: a meta-analysis of randomised controlled trials. *Archives of Internal Medicine* **158**, 2235–41. |
| Reporting quality | Increase | About 25% | Khan, K.S. et al. (1996). The importance of quality of primary studies in producing unbiased systematic reviews. *Archives of Internal Medicine* **156**, 661–6. Moher, D. et al. (1998). Does quality of reports of randomised trials affect estimates of intervention efficacy reported in meta-analyses? *Lancet* **352**, 609–13. |
| Duplication | Increase | About 20% | Tramèr, M. et al. (1997). Effect of covert duplicate publication on meta-analysis; a case study. *BMJ* **315**, 635–40. |

**Table 2.4.1**  (contd.)

| Source of bias | Effect on estimate of treatment efficacy | Size of the effect | References |
|---|---|---|---|
| Geography | Increase | May be large for some alternative therapies | Vickers, A. *et al.* (1998). Do certain countries produce only positive results? A systematic review of controlled trials. *Controlled Clinical Trials* **19**, 159–66. |
| Size | Increase | Small trials may overestimate treatment effects by about 30% | Moore, R.A. *et al.* (1998). Quantitative systematic review of topically-applied non-steroidal anti-inflammatory drugs. *BMJ* **316**, 333–8. |
| | | | Moore, R.A. *et al.* (1998). Size is everything—large amounts of information are needed to overcome random effects in estimating direction and magnitude of treatment effects. *Pain* **78**, 217–20. |
| Statistical | Increase | Not known to any extent, probably modest, but important especially where vote-counting occurs | Smith, L.A. *et al.* (2000). Teasing apart quality and validity in systematic reviews: an example from acupuncture trials in chronic neck and back pain. *Pain* **86**, 119–32. |
| Validity | Increase | Not known to any extent, probably modest, but important especially where vote-counting occurs | Smith, L.A. *et al.* (2000). Teasing apart quality and validity in systematic reviews: an example from acupuncture trials in chronic neck and back pain. *Pain* **86**, 119–32. |
| Language | Increase | Not known to any extent, but may be modest | Egger, M. *et al.* (1997). Language bias in randomized controlled trials published in English and German. *Lancet* **350**, 326–9. |
| Publication | Increase | Not known to any extent, probably modest, but important especially where there is little evidence | Egger, M. and Davey Smith, G. (2000). Under the meta-scope: potentials and limitations of meta-analysis. In *Evidence based resource in anaesthesia and analgesia* (ed. M Tramèr). BMJ Publications, London. |

and blinding will also correlate with bias. Trials of poor reporting quality consistently overestimate the effect of treatment [2, 3]. We describe a scoring system in a later chapter with a range of 0 to 5 based on randomization, blinding, and withdrawals and drop-outs. Studies scoring 2 or less consistently show greater effects of treatment than those scoring 3 or more.

### Duplication

Results from some trials are reported more than once. This may be entirely justified for a whole range of reasons. Examples might be a later follow-up of the trial, or a re-analysis. Sometimes though, information about patients in trials is reported more than once without that being obvious, or overt, or referenced. Only the more impressive information seems to be duplicated, sometimes in papers with completely different authors. A consequence of covert duplication is to overestimate the effect of treatment [4, 5].

### Intention to treat

Suppose 100 patients are randomized and enter a trial, but results are only reported on 50 of them because the other 50 dropped out or withdrew from treatment (a per-protocol analysis). What happened to the other 50 patients? Did they withdraw because of lack of efficacy, or because of adverse effects? Were there different reasons for withdrawal for treatment and control? If results are not reported and analysed according to all patients who entered the study, called intention to treat analysis, then bias may occur because we only see results in patients in whom the treatment worked or was tolerated.

### Geography

Vickers and colleagues [6] showed that trials of acupuncture conducted in East Asia were universally positive, while those conducted in Australia/ New Zealand, North America, or Western Europe were positive only about half the time. Randomized trials of therapies other than acupuncture conducted in China, Taiwan, Japan, or Russia/USSR were also overwhelmingly positive, and much more so than in other parts of the world (Table 2.4.2).

This may be a result of a historical cultural difference, but it does mean that care should be exercised where there is a preponderance of studies from these cultures. Again, this is particularly important for alternative therapies, and it is probably one of the best arguments for the existence of publication bias. Do we really believe that every single acupuncture trial in China comes up with a positive result, or is it unacceptable for negative results that are contrary to accepted belief to be published?

### Size

The importance of size was discussed in an earlier section. Yet clinical trials can often be ridiculously small. The record is a randomized study on three patients in a parallel group design. But when are trials so tiny that they can be ignored? Many folk take a pragmatic view that trials with fewer than 10 patients per treatment arm should be ignored.

Size can be associated with bias. There are examples where sensitivity analysis in meta-analysis has shown small trials to have a larger effect of

**Table 2.4.2**   Proportion of randomized trials of any intervention, and acupuncture trials, from different parts of the world

| Country | Randomized or controlled trials | | Acupuncture trials | |
|---|---|---|---|---|
| | Number | Positive (%) | Number | Positive (%) |
| England | 107 | 75 | 20 | 60 |
| China | 109 | 99 | 36 | 100 |
| Japan | 120 | 89 | 5 | 100 |
| Russia/USSR | 29 | 97 | 11 | 91 |
| Taiwan | 40 | 95 | 6 | 100 |

treatment than bigger trials (Table 2.4.1). The degree of variability between trials of adequate power is still substantial, because trials are powered to detect that there is a *difference* between treatments, rather than *how big* that difference is. The random play of chance can remain a significant factor despite adequate power to detect a difference.

### Statistics and data manipulation

Despite the best efforts of editors and peer reviewers, some papers are published that are just plain wrong. Wrong covers a multitude of sins, but two are particularly important.

Statistical incorrectness can take a variety of guises. It may be as simple as the data presented in a paper as statistically significant not being significant. It can often take the form of inappropriate statistical tests [7]. It can be data trawling, where a single statistical significance is obtained and a paper written round it. Reams could be written about this, but the simple warning is that readers or reviewers of papers have to be cautious of results of trials, especially where vote counting is being done.

But also beware the power of words. Even when statistical testing shows no difference, it is common to see the results hailed as a success. While that may sound silly when written down, even the most cynical of readers can be fooled into drawing the wrong conclusion. Abstracts are notorious for misleading in this way.

Data manipulation is a bit more complicated to detect. An example would be an intervention where we are not told what the start condition of patients is, nor the end, but that at some time in between the rate of change was statistically significant by some test with which we are unfamiliar. This is done only to make positive that which is not positive, and the direction of the bias is obvious (Table 2.4.1). Again, this is crucially important where vote counting is being done to determine whether the intervention works or not.

### Validity

Do individual trials have a design (apart from issues like randomization and blinding) that allows them to adequately measure an effect? What constitutes validity depends on the circumstances of a trial, but studies often lack validity. A validity scoring system applied to acupuncture for head and neck pain demonstrated that trials with lower validity were more likely to say that the treatment worked than those that were invalid [7]. A validity scoring system derived for pain trials is described later, because it is particularly relevant to trials and reviews of complementary therapy where pooling data is less likely, and vote counting of positive and negative trials more likely.

### Language

Too often the search strategy for a systematic review or meta-analysis restricts itself to the English language only. Authors whose language is not English may be more likely to publish positive findings in an English language journal, because these would have a greater international impact. Negative findings would be more likely to be published in non-English language journals [8].

### Publication

Finally, there is the old chestnut of publication bias. This is usually thought to be the propensity for positive trials to be published and for negative trials not to be published. It must exist, and there is a huge literature about publication bias [9].

That not all studies are published is well known [10]. All researchers wil have started projects that have not been completed, because once begun they were obviously flawed or because completion was impossible (lack of recruitment to a clinical trial, for instance). Some perfectly good studies will have been completed, but not written up or, if written, refused publication, though failure to publish is often investigator based [11].

While this is clearly the case across the broad sweep of scientific and clinical research, in any particular case we can have no idea whether there are trials completed but unpublished. Authors of systematic reviews will often go to great lengths to discover unpublished trials by writing to authors, experts in the field, and to manufacturers, or will extensively search abstracts for studies that may have been started but remain unpublished. The problem is that what is unknown remains unknowable.

It is worth having some reservations about the fuss that is made, though. Partly this stems from the failure to include assessments of trial validity and quality. Most peer reviewers would reject non-randomized studies or those where there are major failings in methodology. These trials will be hard to publish. Much the same can be said for dissertations or theses. One attempt to include theses [12] found 17 dissertations for one treatment. Thirteen were excluded because of methodological problems, mainly lack of randomization, three had been published and were already included in the relevant review, and one could be added. It made no difference.

Funnel plots, which plot some outcome of individual trials against size of the trial, are not likely to be helpful. One often quoted, of magnesium in acute myocardial infarction [13], can more easily be explained by the fact that many of the trials in the meta-analysis were trivially too small to detect any effect and should never have been included in a meta-analysis in the first place (Figure 2.4.1).

But these are quibbles. If there is sufficient evidence available, from large numbers of large, well conducted trials, then publication bias is not likely to

Number given placebo

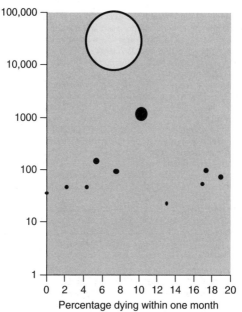

**Figure 2.4.1**  Size and baseline risk in trials included in a meta-analysis of magnesium in acute myocardial infarction (dark symbols) and a large randomized trial (light symbol).

be a problem. Where there is little information, from small numbers of low-quality trials, then it becomes more problematical.

### Dealing with the spectre of publication bias

A number of methods have been proposed to detect publication bias, and these have been extensively reviewed [10, 14, 15]. The power of statistical or graphical tests to detect publication bias has been shown to be limited [16, 17]. The only sensible and conservative approach is to assume that, in any particular case, there will be unpublished studies, however heroic our efforts to discover them.

Thornton and Lee [14] examined 12 methods for detecting and correcting for publication bias, and found limitations with all of them. Other authors [10, 16, 18] have come to similar conclusions about methods that attempt to correct for possible publication bias.

In summary then, we know that some studies are not published, that unpublished studies may alter the results of a meta-analysis, and that we have no robust method for detecting or correcting for possible publication bias. We need to deal with this uncertainty.

*Rosenthal file drawer*

The failure of statistical methods to reliably detect and correct for unpublished studies leaves us with the problem of dealing with the possible consequences of the unknowable. One of the most useful approaches is to use the amount of known information and the size of the effect in that known information to calculate how much negative unpublished information is needed to overturn what is known.

Rosenthal proposed calculating the number of null studies (no difference between experimental and control) that would be required to overcome a statistically significant result [19]. This is attractive because it demonstrates whether the amount of unpublished material needed to overturn a result would be implausibly large or plausibly small. Rosenthal suggested that results of a meta-analysis became resistant to publication bias when the number of new, filed, or unretrieved trials (unpublished) with a null result required to change a result to bare statistical significance was five times the extant number of trials plus 10 (fail-safe number). This was considered a conservative level of tolerance, suggesting that 'file drawers' had more than that number of unpublished studies, and the addition of 10 meant that the minimum number of unpublished studies that could be filed away was 15 (five times a single study, plus 10).

The problems with the Rosenthal solution are twofold. First, a number of statisticians will argue about the validity of the method. More importantly, it is almost impossible to calculate, because it depends on statistical outcomes of trials, such as effect size or relative risk. For most of us, therefore, this is of limited use.

*A back-of-envelope solution*

However, there is one remarkably easy way of thinking about publication, based on having an NNT available. Look again at Table 2.2.1 with our hypothetical trial in acute pain, with a calculated NNT for ibuprofen of 2.7, based on a total size of 80 patients, 40 given ibuprofen 400 mg and 40 given placebo. Now suppose that there is one identical trial, but it is one in which the effect of ibuprofen is identical to that with placebo, and then a second such negative (zero effect) trial, and then a third, and so on (Table 2.4.3). The effect of every trial with zero effect is to double the size of the NNT, because the absolute risk difference halves every time you do it.

The beauty is that you can do this for any data set, whether it be clinical trial or meta-analysis. You can declare what you think of as a useful NNT, and do a swift calculation to see how many negative data sets would be needed for the NNT to rise above that level. In the case above, for instance, two small, unpublished negative trials would produce an NNT of 8, not very good for pain relief. But if this were a meta-analysis of ibuprofen, as in Table 2.4.4, with many thousands of patients, then I would need vast numbers (well over 100 average acute pain trials) of zero effect trials, with over 10,000 patients in them, to overturn it and what is the likelihood of that?

The likelihood of non-publication of negative trials is a product of how effective a treatment is, and how much information there is. When there is lots of information on an effective therapy, the existence of huge numbers of negative trials can be discounted. Where there is only a small amount of information, and there is limited efficacy, one or two moderate-sized

**Table 2.4.3** Effect of increasing numbers of negative (zero effect) trials on NNT

| | Number with pain relief/total number (%) | | | |
|---|---|---|---|---|
| | **Original trial** | **Additional trial 1** | **Additional trial 2** | **Additional trial 3** |
| Placebo | 7/40 (18%) | 7/40 (18%) | 7/40 (18%) | 7/40 (18%) |
| Ibuprofen 400 mg | 22/40 | 7/40 (18%) | 7/40 (18%) | 7/40 (18%) |
| **Cumulative totals** | | | | |
| Placebo | 7/40 (18%) | 14/80 (18%) | 21/120 (18%) | 28/160 (18%) |
| Ibuprofen 400 mg | 22/40 (55%) | 29/80 (36%) | 36/120 (30%) | 44/160 (28%) |
| **NNT** | **2.7** | **5.4** | **8.1** | **10.8** |

negative or less good studies could overturn it. Try it out on some of the interventions in Table 2.4.4.

### Special case of outcome reporting bias

It is now being recognized that not all outcomes measured in clinical trials are reported. In surveys of studies funded by government agencies in

**Table 2.4.4** Results of meta-analyses providing NNTs

| Intervention | Condition | Outcome | Number of patients | NNT |
|---|---|---|---|---|
| Statin | Secondary and primary prevention | Prevent fatal or non-fatal heart attack or stroke | 44,748 | 19 |
| Statin | Older people | Prevent major coronary event | 25,499 | 23 |
| Aspirin | Previous myocardial infarction | Prevent vascular event | 20,006 | 28 |
| Aspirin | Secondary prevention | Prevent any vascular event | 6300 | 18 |
| Ibuprofen 400 mg | Acute pain | At least half pain relief | 4700 | 2.4 |
| Finasteride for haematuria | Older men with BPH and haematuria | Prevent recurrence of haematuria | 165 | 2.0 |
| Finasteride for haematuria | Older men with BPH and haematuria | Prevent prostatic surgery | 165 | 6.1 |
| Anti-TNF antibodies | Spondylarthropathy | 50% improvement in disease activity | 150 | 2.0 |

Canada [20], and in a selection of clinical trials in journals [21], there was failure to report all outcomes of efficacy and harm. Those that were reported in published accounts of the trials tended to be more likely to be statistically significant than those that were not published. So even in published trials there can be outcome reporting bias. A survey of authors [21] suggested that a major reason was space constraints in journals, though other reasons included outcomes not being clinically important, or not being statistically significant.

Registration of clinical trial protocols may be one way of dealing with publication bias. Details of all new clinical trials will also be publicly registered in advance, so that patients and clinicians will have information about how to enrol. Both requirements are likely to be adopted by the worldwide pharmaceutical industry during 2005. Moreover, from July 2005 member journals of the International Committee of Medical Journal Editors will require, as a condition of publication of a trial, that it was registered in a public trials registry before patient enrolment [22]. Such a policy, if extended, should remove much of the disquiet about possible unpublished trials, and should increase transparency in performance and reporting of clinical trials.

Limitations of space on publication are likely to continue to be a problem. Most journals restrict authors to 3000 to 4000 words, though increasingly tables and additional material can be published electronically. Many clinical trials performed by industry are available (at least internally and to regulatory authorities) as clinical trial reports. One analysis of 40,000 patients in 31 clinical trials had over 180,000 pages of data in clinical trial reports of 23 of those trials, and extensive clinical trial summaries for the other eight [23].

At the time of writing we do not know whether incomplete trial reporting makes any difference to a trial result, though it does make life difficult for those performing systematic review and meta-analysis. This is a topic to bear in mind as our knowledge develops.

### Industry bias

For-profit sponsorship of clinical trials is thought to lead to results that cast the sponsor's product in a more favourable light. This industry or sponsorship 'bias' is a rather loose term, because there are several possible ways in which that bias can be exerted. Recent years have seen many publications on the topic, some of which are reprised briefly in Table 2.4.5. Most of these papers have examined studies funded by the pharmaceutical companies, and compared them with trials not funded by the pharmaceutical industry. While many papers have reported on various different aspects of suspected for-profit sponsorship bias, none had a prior specification of minimum criteria of trial quality, validity, or size when comparing for-profit with non-profit sponsorship, and none declared prior intent to compare like with like, in terms of drug, dose, condition, duration, or outcomes used (Table 2.4.5).

If we do not compare like with like, what can that possibly tell us? Not a lot. What we want to know is whether trials funded by industry produce a different result from those funded from another source, like a medical research council, or charity. There are examples where the criteria of quality, validity, and size were met, where the same interventions were compared, and where for-profit sponsorship did not influence the result.

and size or a prior intent to compare like with like).

| Reference | Design/methods | Subject | Relevant findings |
|---|---|---|---|
| Als-Nielsen, B. et al. (2003). Association of funding and conclusions in randomised drug trials: a reflection of treatment effects or adverse effects. JAMA **290**, 921–8 | Observational study of 370 RCTs included in meta-analyses from selected Cochrane reviews | Range of diseases | Before and after adjusting for study quality and sample size, sponsored trials significantly more likely to recommend sponsored drug compared with trials funded by non-profit organizations |
| Baker, C.B. et al. (2003). Quantitative analysis of sponsorship bias in economic studies of antidepressants. Br. J. Psychiatry **183**, 498–506 | Observational study of cost or cost-effectiveness studies of antidepressants found by systematic searching | Depression | Clear relationship between outcome of study and pharmaceutical sponsorship |
| Barnes, D.E. and Bero, L.A. (1998). Why review articles on the health effects of passive smoking reach different conclusions. JAMA **279**, 1566–70 | Systematic review and secondary analysis | Health effects of passive smoking | Industry-sponsored studies were significantly more likely to reach favourable conclusions compared with non-industry sponsored studies |
| Bekelman, J.E. et al. (2003). Scope and impact of financial conflicts of interest in biomedical research: a systematic review. JAMA **289**, 454–65 | Systematic review of quantitative studies on the financial relations between industry, scientists, and academia | Financial relations | A large proportion of scientists and institutions receive industry funding |
| Bhandari, M. et al. (2004). Association between industry funding and statistically | Observational study of a consecutive series of 332 RCTs published in 8 leading | Surgical, drug, and other interventions | Before and after adjusting for treatment effect and double-blinding, sponsored |

(contd.)

**Table 2.4.5** (contd.)

| Reference | Design/methods | Subject | Relevant findings |
|---|---|---|---|
| significant pro-industry findings in medical and surgical randomized trials. *Can. Med. Assoc. J.* **170**, 477–80 | surgical and 5 medical journals | | trials significantly more likely to recommend sponsored drug compared with trials funded by non-profit organisations |
| Chard, J.A. et al. (2000). Epidemiology of research into interventions for the treatment of osteoarthritis of the knee joint. *Ann. Rheum. Dis.* **59**, 414–18. | Systematic review of all research and all treatments | Osteoarthritis of the knee | Industry-sponsored studies were significantly more likely to produce positive findings compared with non-industry sponsored studies |
| Cho, M.K. and Bero, L.A. (1996). The quality of drug studies published in symposium proceedings. *Ann. Intern. Med.* **124**, 485–9 | Systematic review of a random selection of original clinical drug articles from 625 symposium proceedings | Not mentioned | Significantly more articles with industry funding (98%) reported favourable results for the drug of interest compared with non-industry funded articles (79%) |
| Clifford, T.J. et al. (2002). Funding source, trial outcome and reporting quality: are they related? Results of a pilot study. *BMC Health Services Research* **2**, 18 | Observational study of a convenience sample of 100 RCTs from 5 leading medical journals between 1999 and 2000 | Not mentioned | Trial outcome was not found to be associated with funding source. 30/44 sponsored studies, 30/44 mixed and non-industry, 15/28 studies with not-for-profit funding favoured new product |
| Dieppe, P. et al. (1999). Funding clinical research. | Analysis of meta-analyses published in 8 high | Osteoarthritis of the knee | Meta-analyses sponsored by industry more likely to beneficial effect |

| Reference | Study type | Subject | Findings |
|---|---|---|---|
| *Lancet* **353**, 1626 | impact medical journals between 1993 and 1998 | | compared with meta-analyses conducted with other sources of funding or where sources were not disclosed |
| Djulbegovic, B. et al. (2000). The uncertainty principle and industry-sponsored research. *Lancet* **356**, 635–8 | Systematic review of RCTs | Multiple myeloma | Sponsored trials failed to maintain equipoise, 74% of studies favoured new therapies over existing ones. Industry trials more likely to use inactive controls |
| Finucane, T.E. and Boult, C.E. (2004). Association of funding and findings of pharmaceutical research at a meeting of a medical professional society. *Am. J. Med.* **117**, 842–5 | Review of abstracts presented at an annual meeting of a medical society | Any | Research funding from pharmaceutical companies associated with study findings supporting use of drugs marketed by sponsors |
| Friedman, L.S. et al. (2004). Relationship between conflicts of interest and research results. *J. Gen. Intern. Med.* **19**, 51–6. | Manuscripts published in 1 year published in two medical journals | Any | Studies whose authors have conflicts of interest are more likely to present positive findings |
| Hartmann, M. et al. (2003). Industry-sponsored economic studies in oncology vs studies sponsored by nonprofit organisations. *Br. J. Cancer* **89**, 1405–8 | Systematic review of health economic publications | Oncology | Sponsored trials were more likely to involve cost minimization analyses, less likely to explore diagnostic screening methods, and more likely to reach positive qualitative conclusions on cost |
| Kemmeren, J.M. et al. (2001). Third generation oral contraceptives and risk of venous thrombosis: meta-analysis. *BMJ* **323**, 131–4 | Review of case-control and cohort studies conducted before 1995 | Third generation contraceptives and venous thrombosis | Pooled OR of venous thrombosis from studies funded by industry 1.3 (1.0 to 1.7), compared with 2.3 (1.7 to 3.2) for non-industry sponsored studies |

(contd.)

**Table 2.4.5** (contd.)

| Reference | Design/methods | Subject | Relevant findings |
|---|---|---|---|
| Koepp, R. et al. (1999). Meta-analysis of tacrine for Alzheimer disease: the influence of industry sponsors. *JAMA* **281**, 2287 | Response to published study | Alzheimer's disease | Misfounded criticism of effects of industry funding in a systematic review of tacrine |
| Kjaergard, L.L. and Als-Nielsen, B. (2002). Association between competing interests and authors' conclusions: epidemiological study of randomised clinical trials published in the BMJ. *BMJ* **325**, 249 | Systematic review of RCTs published in the BMJ | 12 medical specialties | Authors' conclusions significantly favoured experimental drug where financial competing interests were declared. Other competing interests not associated |
| Lexchin, J. et al. (2003). Pharmaceutical industry sponsorship and research outcome and quality: systematic review. *BMJ* **326**, 1167–70 | Systematic review of studies, meta-analyses, reviews of reviews, and clinical trials | Range of diseases | 16 studies on funding source and outcome. 14 favoured product of sponsor (8 significantly so). Two studies showed no difference |
| Montgomery, J.H. et al. (2004). An analysis of the effect of funding source in randomized clinical trials of second generation antipsychotics for the treatment of schizophrenia. *Control. Clin. Trials* **25**, 598–612 | Systematic review of RCTs of second generation antipsychotics | Schizophrenia | Industry bias may occur in RCTs in schizophrenia |
| Procyshyn, R.M. et al. (2004). Prevalence and outcomes of pharmaceutical industry-sponsored clinical trials involving clozapine, risperidone or olanzapine. *Can. J. Psychiatry* **49**, 601–6 | Systematic review of three drugs used in any clinical circumstance | Not mentioned | Reported outcomes of sponsored trials favour manufacturer's product |

| Rochon, P.A. et al. (1994). A study of manufacturer-supported trials of nonsteroidal anti-inflammatory drugs in the treatment of arthritis. Arch. Intern. Med. **154**, 157–63 | Systematic review of RCTs of NSAIDs published between 1987 and 1990 | NSAIDs for arthritis | 56 trials. 71% reported sponsored drug as comparable with comparator, and 29% as superior (authors felt claims supported by findings), 87% reported sponsored drug as safer (authors felt claims supported in only 55%) |
| Stelfox, H.T. et al. (1998). Conflict of interest in the debate over calcium-channel antagonists. N. Engl. J. Med. **338**, 101–6 | Systematic review of articles and secondary survey of authors | Calcium channel blockers | Authors with financial relationships with pharmaceutical companies were significantly more likely to reach positive conclusions |
| Thomas, P.S. et al. (2002). Sponsorship, authorship, and accountability. Lancet **359**, 351 | Systematic review of trials of inhaled steroids | Asthma | Funded trials tended to favour sponsor's drug |
| Turner, C. and Spillich, G.J. (1997). Research into smoking or nicotine and human cognitive performance: does the source of funding make a difference? Addiction **92**, 1423–6 | Articles about nicotine and cognitive performance taken from a review | Effects of nicotine on cognitive performance | Funded authors tended to conclude an improvement in cognitive function. Non-funded authors were split on conclusions about effects |
| Wahlbeck, K. and Adams, C. (1999). Sponsored drug trials show more favourable outcomes. BMJ **318**, 465 | Sensitivity analysis conducted within a Cochrane review | Clozapine versus atypical antipsychotics for schizophrenia | Chance of relapse significantly in favour of clozapine in sponsored trials, equivocal results from non-sponsored trials |
| Yaphe, J. et al. (2001). The association between funding by commercial interests and study outcome in randomised controlled drug trials. Fam. Pract. **18**, 565–8 | Observational study of RCTs published in 5 leading medical journals between 1992 and 1994 | Not mentioned | Positive outcomes were found in 181/209 sponsored trials compared with 62/96 trials funded by non-profit organizations |

Industry-sponsored outcome trials of statins all showed similar risk reduction [24, 25], as did the large, independent Heart Protection Study [26]. Neither was there any significant difference in the effects of finasteride 5 mg daily for benign prostatic hyperplasia between a systematic review where the majority of trials were industry-funded [27] and the MTOPS trial primarily funded by the National Institutes of Health [28].

Most clinical trials of drugs are performed by industry, usually for regulatory purposes, so a comparison between industry and non-profit sponsorship is unlikely. A different approach is to examine results when a drug is involved in trials as the investigational drug, when any bias would be expected to inflate its effects, and when it is involved in similar trials as an active comparator, when any bias should work to deflate its effects. This method of investigating opposing potential biases has been applied to acute pain and migraine studies. The results (Table 2.4.6) showed no major difference.

The problem is that we have large amounts of opinion, but relatively little hard evidence. We do know that, for acute pain and migraine and some other clinical areas, there is no signal for major bias in studies performed by industry.

### Spotting commercial bias (marketing)

Even if clinical trials are not biased, that doesn't mean that pharmaceutical companies or other commercial organizations (or charities, or government) don't have their own agendas. Those agendas involve selling their products, and that means marketing. Marketing in turn means putting their products in the best light, given that most pharmaceutical marketing is highly regulated. What companies can and do do is to find the best trial in a bunch and concentrate on that one.

Two examples, again from acute pain. These are chosen so as not to upset anyone, because they involve rofecoxib (now withdrawn) and valdecoxib (never actively marketed for acute pain). In the rofecoxib example (Figure 2.4.2), the study with the filled symbol was the one chosen to highlight for comparison with valdecoxib. In the diclofenac example, the study with the filled symbol was the one chosen for comparison with rofecoxib. Each was chosen because it put another analgesic in a bad light, yet each of the chosen trials was uncharacteristic of other trials of the same drug at the same dose, in the same type of patients.

### Commentary

There are many sources of bias. What is so terrific is that we know about so many, and are getting to grips with more, like outcome reporting bias. This should not be seen as nihilistic, but as part of a process for making things better. Those of us who read many papers, especially older ones, recognize the mistakes that used to be prevalent, but now are uncommon in good studies in good journals. The problem is that poor studies still slip through. By knowing about sources of bias we can be vigilant, and know both when to be impressed, and when to be unimpressed.

### References

1. Jadad, A.R. *et al.* (1996). Assessing the quality of reports of randomized clinical trials: is blinding necessary? *Controlled Clinical Trials* **17**, 1–12.
2. Khan, K.S. *et al.* (1996). The importance of quality of primary studies in producing unbiased systematic reviews. *Archives of Internal Medicine* **156**, 661–6.
3. Moher, D. *et al.* (1998). Does quality of reports of randomised trials affect estimates of intervention efficacy reported in meta-analyses? *Lancet* **352**, 609–13.

**Table 2.4.6**   Method of opposing potential biases applied to acute pain and migraine trials

| Drug & dose | Drug status | Outcome | Number of | | NNT | p-value |
|---|---|---|---|---|---|---|
| | | | Trials | Patients | | |
| Aspirin 600/650 mg | Investigational | At least 50% pain relief over 6 hours | 8 | 567 | 5.1 (3.6–8.3) | 0.54 |
| | Comparator | | 42 | 3287 | 4.5 (4.0–5.1) | |
| Ibuprofen 400 mg | Investigational | At least 50% pain relief over 6 hours | 15 | 1584 | 2.5 (2.2–2.8) | 0.7 |
| | Comparator | | 26 | 2585 | 2.5 (2.3–2.8) | |
| Acetaminophen 1000 mg | Investigational | At least 50% pain relief over 6 hours | 7 | 651 | 3.6 (2.9–4.6) | 0.34 |
| | Comparator | | 10 | 1316 | 4.1 (3.4–5.1) | |
| Rofecoxib 50 mg | Investigational | At least 50% pain relief over 6 hours | 13 | 1900 | 1.9 (1.8–2.1) | 0.68 |
| | Comparator | | 4 | 548 | 2.0 (1.7–2.2) | |
| Sumatriptan 100 mg | Investigational | Headache response | 2 | 563 | 7.5 (4.7–18) | 0.75 |
| | Comparator | 1 h | 5 | 1743 | 7.6 (5.8–11) | |
| | Investigational | Headache response | 6 | 1453 | 3.0 (2.6–3.5) | 0.05 |
| | Comparator | 2 h | 6 | 1986 | 3.6 (3.1–4.3) | |
| | Investigational | Pain free | 1 | 131 | 6.7 (3.7–33) | 0.35 |
| | Comparator | 2 h | 6 | 1991 | 4.8 (4.2–5.6) | |
| Sumatriptan 50 mg | Investigational | Headache response | 2 | 861 | 10.3 (6.3–29) | 0.75 |
| | Comparator | 1 h | 2 | 471 | 12.3 (6.3–186) | |
| | Investigational | Headache response | 4 | 1081 | 3.6 (3.0–4.5) | 0.03 |
| | Comparator | 2 h | 2 | 471 | 6.3 (4.0–15) | |
| | Investigational | Pain free | 2 | 612 | 9.1 (5.9–19) | 0.44 |
| | Comparator | 2 h | 2 | 471 | 7.1 (5.3–11) | |

Analyses are based on whether the drug was a test drug ('investigational', when the drug was the primary focus of the trial), or active comparator ('comparator', when the same drug was used as an active comparator in a trial with a different test drug).

4. Tramèr, M.R. *et al.* (1997). Impact of covert duplicate publication on meta-analysis: a case study. *British Medical Journal* 1997 **315**, 635–9.
5. Von Elm, E. *et al.* (2004). Different patterns of duplicate publication. An analysis of articles used in systematic reviews. *Journal of the American Medical Association* **291**, 974–80.
6. Vickers, A. *et al.* (1998). Do certain countries produce only positive results? A systematic review of controlled trials. *Controlled Clinical Trials* **19**, 159–66.
7. Smith, L.A. *et al.* (2000). Teasing apart quality and validity in systematic reviews: an example from acupuncture trials in chronic neck and back pain. *Pain* **86**, 119–32.

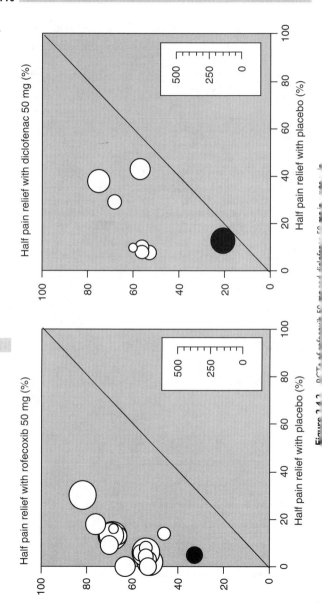

**Figure 14.1** RCTs of rofecoxib 50 mg and diclofenac 50 mg in acute pain.

8. Egger, M. *et al.* (1997). Language bias in randomised controlled trials published in English and German. *Lancet* **350**, 326–9.

9. Egger, M. and Davey Smith, G. (2000). Under the meta-scope: potentials and limitations of meta-analysis. In *Evidence based resource in anaesthesia and analgesia* (ed. M. Tramèr). BMJ Publications, London 45–56.

10. Song, F. *et al.* (2000). Publication and related biases. *Health Technology Assessment* **4**, no 10.

11. Dickersin, K. and Min, Y.I. (1993). Publication bias: the problem that won't go away. *Annals of the New York Academy of Science* **703**, 135–46.

12. Vickers, A.J. and Smith, C. (2000). Incorporating data from dissertations in systematic reviews. *International Journal of Technology Assessment in Health Care* **16**, 711–13.

13. Egger, M. and Smith, G.D. (1995). Misleading meta-analysis. Lessons from 'an effective, safe, simple' intervention that wasn't. *British Medical Journal* **310**, 752–4.

14. Thornton, A. and Lee, P. (2000). Publication bias in meta-analysis: its causes and consequences. *Journal of Clinical Epidemiology* **53**, 207–16.

15. Pham, B. *et al.* (2001). Is there a 'best' way to detect and minimize publication bias? *Evaluation and the Health Professionals* **4**, 109–25.

16. Sterne, J.A. *et al.* (2000). Publication and related bias in meta-analysis: power of statistical tests and prevalence in the literature. *Journal of Clinical Epidemiology* **53**, 1119–29.

17. Macaskill, P. *et al.* (2001). A comparison of methods to detect publication bias in meta-analysis. *Statistics in Medicine* **20**, 641–54.

18. Terrin, N. *et al.* (2003). Adjusting for publication bias in the presence of heterogeneity. *Statistics in Medicine* **22**, 2113–26.

19. Rosenthal, R. (1979). The 'file drawer problem' and tolerance for null results. *Psychological Bulletin* **86**, 638–41.

20. Chan, A-W. *et al.* (2004). Outcome reporting bias in randomized trials funded by the Canadian Institutes of Health Research. *Canadian Medical Association Journal* **171**, 735–40.

21. Chan, A-W. and Altman, D.G. (2005). Identifying outcome reporting bias in randomised trials on PubMed: review of publications and survey of authors. *British Medical Journal* **330**, 753–6.

22. DeAngelis, C.D. *et al.* (2004). Clinical trial registration: a statement from the International Committee of Medical Journal Editors. *Journal of the American Medical Association* **292**, 1363–4.

23. Moore, R.A. *et al.* (2005). Tolerability and adverse events in clinical trials of celecoxib in osteoarthritis and rheumatoid arthritis: systematic review and meta-analysis of information from company clinical trial reports. *Arthritis Research and Therapy* **7**, R644–R665 (http://arthritis-research.com/contents/7/3/R644).

24. LaRosa, J.C. *et al.* (1999). Effect of statins on risk of coronary disease. A meta-analysis of randomized controlled trials. *Journal of the American Medical Association* **282**, 2340–6.

25. Sever, P.S. *et al.* (2003). Prevention of coronary and stroke events with atorvastatin in hypertensive patients who have average or lower-than-average cholesterol concentrations, in the Anglo-Scandinavian Cardiac Outcomes Trial—Lipid lowering arm (ASCOT-LLA): a multicentre randomised controlled trial. *Lancet* **361**, 1149–58.

26. Heart Protection Study Collaborative Group (2002). MRC/BHF Heart Protection Study of the cholesterol lowering with simvastatin with 20 536 high-risk individuals: a randomised placebo-controlled trial. *Lancet* **360**, 7–22.

27. Edwards, J.E. and Moore, R.A. (2002). Finasteride in the treatment of clinical benign prostatic hyperplasia: a systematic review of randomised trials. *BMC Urology* **2**, 14.

28. McConnell, J.D. *et al.* (2003). The long-term effect of doxazosin, finasteride, and combination therapy on the clinical progression of benign prostatic hyperplasia. *New England Journal of Medicine* **349**, 2387–98.

## 2.5 Clinical trial validity

What constitutes trial validity is a difficult concept. The dictionary definition of valid is that which is sound or defensible, or having a premise from which the conclusion follows logically. We know it when we see it, or more particularly when our eyes are opened to its absence. Validity is always situation-dependent, but criteria might include severity of illness at the start of a trial, the dose or intensity of the intervention, the duration of the intervention, or the duration of observation.

### Duration of treatment or observation

Some validity criteria are fairly obvious. For example, the importance of the duration of an intervention is seen in a trial of TENS for chronic pain, where a single 10-minute low-intensity treatment period was tried, in the face of evidence that it takes weeks rather than minutes to work. The importance of duration of observations can be seen in, for instance, 5-alpha-reductase inhibitors in benign prostatic hyperplasia, where effects on prostate volume or urine flow continue to improve over several years [1] rather than weeks or months (Figure 2.5.1). Clearly, a trial that compared a 5-alpha-reductase inhibitor with a treatment that worked very quickly, like alpha-blockers, would be bound to show that alpha-blockers were better over the short term than 5-alpha-reductase inhibitors. When long-term trials over 4 years are conducted, they show equal efficacy [2]. The decision then is whether other long-term benefits of 5-alpha-reductase inhibitors, such as reduced prostate volume, are more valuable, and for which man with benign prostatic hyperplasia.

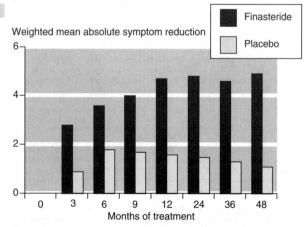

**Figure 2.5.1** Long-term symptom improvement with 5-alpha-reductase inhibitors.

There is an even better example of how duration of a study can lead to different results. A systematic review of 164 short-term (2–6 weeks) randomized trials of statins for cholesterol-lowering demonstrated a convincing dose response for six statins investigated [3]. It was a large meta-analysis, well done, using good studies, with 24,000 participants on statins and 14,000 on placebo, and showed a strong dose-response for LDL-cholesterol reduction.

A different analysis of statin efficacy [4] used a different strategy. It selected longer duration studies, of at least 12 weeks, arguing that statins were for long-term use, so long-term effects were the best measure of efficacy. The analysis, with 43,000 people on statins and 24,000 on placebo, showed no convincing dose-response for any lipid subfraction. The results for total cholesterol with different doses of simvastatin, both fixed and adjusted, is shown in Figure 2.5.2, with information on 17,000 patients. There was no dose-response for simvastatin in longer-term trials.

There are other problems with the duration of studies that relate to the natural tendency of some conditions to wax and wane in intensity, a process not often well understood. Restless legs syndrome (RLS) affects a significant proportion of older people, with a spectrum of bothersomeness that at one

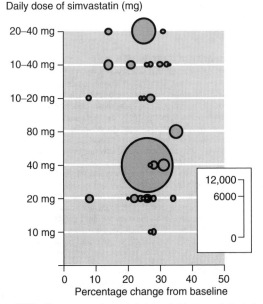

**Figure 2.5.2**  Dose-response for total cholesterol with simvastatin in studies of 12 weeks or longer.

extreme is distressing, with considerable interference with sleep and consequent day-time drowsiness. There are relatively few studies of drug therapy, and these have been summarized on the Bandolier RLS website (*www.jr2.ox.ac.uk/bandolier/booth/booths/RLS.html*). Most of these trials have been of short duration, and in short-duration RLS trials placebo is not very effective. Thus in one 4-week cross-over trial, no placebo patient achieved a suitably low symptom score that would indicate a success [5]. By contrast, in a 12-week study, 40% of people with RLS given placebo were much or very much improved [6], and there was a clear tendency for RLS to improve spontaneously with time.

The natural history of RLS has barely been studied, but the indication is that the condition waxes and wanes. For inclusion in trials patients had to fulfil various criteria, including a minimum amount of bothersomeness and frequency of RLS attacks. Some patients were probably recruited when their symptoms were at a peak, and while doing nothing they got better. Doing nothing for long enough would result in high success rates. Measuring efficacy in the short term would probably show interventions at their best, compared with placebo. Longer duration trials would tend to show the same intervention as being less effective, for no other reason than that placebo was doing better.

What duration constitutes validity in RLS trials? In the present state of knowledge it is probably shorter-, rather than longer-term studies, of 6 weeks or less rather than 12 weeks or longer. It also suggests that therapy might best be used when symptoms are bad, and used in short bursts rather than continually. For the moment we have to wait and see what further research tells us.

### Dose or intensity of intervention

It is commonly understood that efficacy and harm from interventions vary with the intensity or dose. The dose-response for efficacy may be different from the dose-response for harm, and often there is a therapeutic window in which efficacy is maximized, and harm minimized. This will usually be the therapeutic dose used. Clearly, trials, or meta-analysis of trials, should concentrate on the therapeutic dose. An example of how dose changes the value of a therapy can be seen for sildenafil for erectile dysfunction [7]. Efficacy increases with dose; common adverse events increase also, but differently (Figure 2.5.3).

Sildenafil is frequently used where dose is optimized by using a starting dose of 50 mg, continuing if there is effect but no adverse effects, reducing the dose to 25 mg if there is effect but also adverse effects, or increasing to 100 mg if effects are suboptimal and there are no adverse effects. The result is that dose optimization for each patient provides good effect with low adverse effects. The way in which dose is used is important, therefore, and the validity of trials of sildenafil is governed by the dose, and dose regimen, used.

### Patient condition

Acute pain trials demonstrate the importance of the condition of patients at the start of a trial. It is quite difficult to measure an analgesic effect in the absence of pain. In acute pain trials, patients have to have pain of at least moderate intensity before they can be given a test intervention. Figure 2.5.4

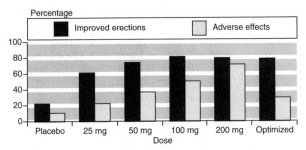

**Figure 2.5.3**  Dose-response for efficacy and adverse events with sildenafil for erectile dysfunction.

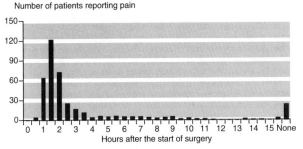

**Figure 2.5.4**  Time after operation start when 410 patients having minor orthopaedic procedures reported pain of at least moderate intensity.

shows what happened to 410 patients after minor orthopaedic surgery that lasted about 20 minutes [8]. A trained nursing sister was with them so that when pain was of at least moderate intensity they could enter a clinical trial.

Most of them needed an analgesic by about 3 hours, but some didn't need an analgesic until 12 hours or more had elapsed, and 23 (6%) didn't need any analgesia at all. But unless that process was carried out, some patients would have entered analgesic trials who did not have, or would not have had, any pain.

### The problem with averages

Many, if not most, clinical trials report average results for groups of patients. In trials of cholesterol reduction, they might give us the average percentage reduction in total or subfraction cholesterol, rather than, say, the number or percentage of patients who have achieved a target level. Some give both, but that is rare.

In clinical trials it is common to find that some patients do very well, and others have almost no response to treatment. This mirrors clinical experience, and is what we expect. For instance, in the RLS example above [5], patients at baseline had RLS symptom scores mainly between 20 and 30 points out of a maximum of 40 points. On ropinirole 9/22 of patients had almost complete resolution of their RLS symptoms, while 8/22 had almost no change (Figure 2.5.5). The paper reports a 50% average reduction in symptom score; this is the average of those doing very well, those doing very badly, and those with intermediate response. At best only 4/22 patients had an average response.

That might sound daft at first glance, but it is repeated endlessly in clinical trials. Another example comes from an individual patient analysis of 1330 patients given 50 mg of rofecoxib for moderate or severe levels of acute pain following third molar extraction [9]. Pain relief was scored over various times up to 24 hours after the dose, and the percentage of the maximum pain relief possible calculated over 6, 8, 12, and 24 hours (Figure 2.5.6). A quarter or more had virtually no pain relief (under 10%), and about a third in all had less than 20% pain relief. About half had good pain relief (over 50% of maximum pain relief, a high hurdle in acute pain studies). Again, some people do quite well, some do very badly, yet traditionally clinical trials have reported an average result. Again, the average figure for percentage of maximum pain relief for all 1330 patients was between 40% and 50%, almost where there were fewest patients.

There is a case for saying that validity in a trial is smudged when averages are used as the only way results are reported. The common experience of some patients doing very well and others doing less well should be

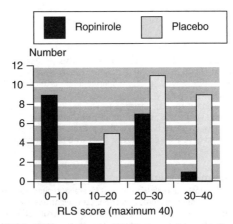

**Figure 2.5.5** RLS scores after 4 weeks of treatment with ropinirole dose-titration and placebo.

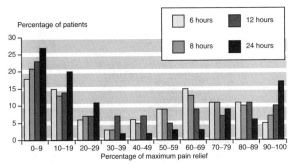

**Figure 2.5.6** Percentage of maximum pain relief with 50 mg rofecoxib in patients with moderate or severe pain over 6 to 24 hours.

respected, and should be valued highly, because individual health-care professionals deal with individual patients, and averages are inadequate in helping professionals covey the likely benefits of therapy.

### Equal on average is not equal for everyone

This fascinating title comes from a thoughtful commentary [10] on an even more thoughtful and useful trial [11] examining the effectiveness of SSRIs in a naturalistic trial in primary care. The trial was conducted in two primary care practice networks in the USA and was designed to resemble real-world practice. The decision to start an antidepressant was based strictly on physician judgement that there was clinical depression, rather than specific criteria for diagnosis. Patients and physicians knew what was being taken because blinding would have obscured typical patient management. All decisions about discontinuation, switching, or dose change were made by physician and patient, with no pre-set criteria. There was no interaction between information gathering and physicians, who were un-influenced by any results.

Apart from very obvious exclusions, adult patients with clinical depression were randomized (with adequate concealment) to initial doses of paroxetine (20 mg), fluoxetine (20 mg), or sertraline (50 mg). Drugs were free to patients. After enrolment, they were interviewed by telephone and questionnaire at several time points over 9 months. The primary outcome was SF-36 mental component summary, but a battery of other measures was used. Compliance (switching, discontinuation) was assessed.

Patients were predominantly white women with major depression, with an average age of 46 years. All three SSRIs showed substantial improvements in depression and other outcomes. There were no differences between treatments for any outcome, using any definition of intention to treat or per protocol analysis, or with any subgroup analysis. In the whole sample, the proportion meeting criteria for major depression fell from 74% at baseline to 26% at 9 months. Rapid initial benefit was followed by slow continued improvement.

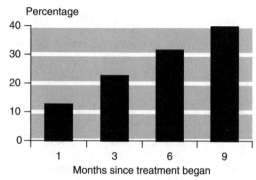

**Figure 2.5.7**  Stopping or switching antidepressants.

Patients initially randomized to one particular treatment frequently changed treatment to one or more of the others. By the time 9 months had elapsed, only 44% were still taking the original treatment to which they had been randomized. Some (about 15%) were lost to follow-up after baseline measurement or when on randomized treatment. Others either switched to another antidepressant or stopped treatment because of adverse effects or lack of efficacy, again without any difference between the three SSRIs (Figure 2.5.7).

The trial sought to mimic clinical practice, and found no practical difference between the three SSRIs. It also found that clinical practice, in which dose or drug changes were done on the basis of patient–physician interaction as they would be in real life, resulted in many patients stopping or switching drugs. It showed that, while the drugs were similar on average, individual patients benefited from particular drugs, and that the fact that they were equal on average meant that they were not equal for every patient.

### Scoring trials for validity

The foregoing shows that trying to develop any sort of scoring system for validity of trials will be difficult, though it may not be impossible in particular circumstances. The Oxford Pain Validity Scale (OPVS) was designed specifically to examine issues regarding validity in pain trials [12] and is described in detail in Table 2.5.1. It uses eight criteria (16 points total) to be applied to randomized trials. The criteria include blinding, size, statistics, drop-outs, credibility of statistical significance and authors' conclusions, baseline measures, and outcomes in order to examine whether a trial might be considered valid or not.

The scale was applied in a systematic review of back and neck pain. The conclusions of the original authors were found to be incorrect in two of 13 trials (and, as an aside, this is not an uncommon problem in clinical trial reporting, or even systematic reviews, where frank errors change the results). Using reviewers' conclusions, more valid trials were significantly more likely to have a negative conclusion (Figure 2.5.8).

**Table 2.5.1** Oxford Pain Validity Scale (OPVS). The OPVS should be only be used on trials that: (1) are randomized; (2) have a start group size ≥ 10 for all groups relevant to the review question

| Item | | Score (circle one number per item) | Comments |
|---|---|---|---|
| 1. Blinding | Was the trial convincingly double-blind? | 6 | i.e. states double-blind and how this was achieved, e.g. double-dummy, identical appearance, etc. |
| | Was the trial convincingly single-blind or unconvincingly double-blind? | 3 | i.e. states single-blind and how this was achieved, e.g. observer-blind, patient-blind, etc. |
| | Was the trial either not blind or the blinding is unclear? | 0 | |
| 2. Size of trial groups | Was the start group start size ≥ 40? | 3 | Not all groups in the trial will necessarily be relevant to the review question. Rate this item using the smallest group that is relevant to the review question |
| | Was the start group start size 30 to 39? | 2 | |
| | Was the start group start size 20 to 29? | 1 | |
| | Was the start group start size 10 to 19? | 0 | |
| 3. Outcomes | Look at pre hoc list of most desirable outcomes relevant to the review question: Did the paper include results for at least one pre hoc desirable outcome, and use the outcome appropriately? | 2 | NB. If the trial has not reported the results of any measures relevant to the review question (even if it described them in methods) it should be excluded from the review |
| | There were no results for any of the pre hoc desirable outcomes, or, a pre hoc desirable outcome was used inappropriately | 0 | |

(cont)

**Table 2.5.1** (cont.)

| Item | | Score (circle one number per item) | Comments |
|---|---|---|---|
| **4. Demonstration of internal sensitivity** | Look at the baseline levels for the outcomes relevant to the review question: For all treatment groups, baseline levels were sufficient for the trialist to be able to measure a change following the intervention (e.g. enough baseline pain to detect a difference between baseline and post-treatment levels). Alternatively, did the trial demonstrate internal sensitivity? | 1 | One way to demonstrate internal sensitivity is by having an additional active control group in the trial that demonstrates a significant difference from placebo (i.e. the trial design is able to detect a difference). For example, by having an extra group treated with an analgesic known to be statistically different from placebo, and by demonstrating this difference. Alternatively, internal sensitivity can be demonstrated with a dose response |
| | For all treatment groups, baseline levels were insufficient to be able to measure a change following the intervention, or, baseline levels could not be assessed, or internal sensitivity was not demonstrated | 0 | |
| **5. Data analysis** | (1) Definition of outcomes. Did the paper define the relevant outcomes clearly, including where relevant, exactly what 'improved', 'successful treatment', etc. represented? | 1 | There must be at least one outcome measure defined clearly to score 1. This item refers to any outcome measure relevant to the review question, not just pre hoc desirables |
| | The paper failed to define the outcomes clearly. | 0 | |
| | (2) Data presentation: location and dispersion. Did the paper present either mean data with standard deviations, or dichotomous outcomes, or median with range, or sufficient data to enable extraction of any of these? | 1 | |

| | | |
|---|---|---|
| The paper presented none of the above | 0 | |
| (3) Statistical testing. | | |
| Did the trialist choose an appropriate statistical test, with correction for multiple tests where relevant? | 1 | Corrections for multiple testing must be put in place when a series of tests or measures have been carried out on the same patient group |
| Inappropriate statistical tests were chosen and/or multiple testing was carried out, but with no correction, or, no statistics were carried out | 0 | |
| (4) Handling of drop-outs. | | |
| The drop-out rate was either ≤ 10%, or was >10% and includes an intention-to-treat analysis in which drop-outs were included appropriately | 1 | |
| The drop-out rate was >10% and drop-outs were not included in the analysis, or, it is not possible to calculate a drop-out rate from data presented in the paper | 0 | |

**Total score**

**Author conclusion:** Trial positive/trial negative
**Reviewer conclusion:** Trial positive/trial negative

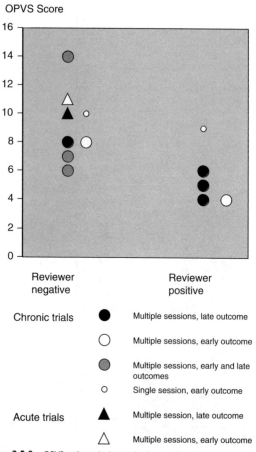

**Figure 2.5.8** OPVS scale applied to trials of acupuncture for chronic neck and back pain.

## Commentary

The validity of any clinical trial is crucial to whether or not the evidence that it contains is of value to a reader. There are many different aspects to validity, and there is no universally applicable checklist that can be used to determine whether a trial is valid. A simple rule is to ask whether the patients in the trial are like those you treat, whether the treatment being tested is like one you use, and whether the outcomes presented are ones you can understand, value, and use.

## References

1. Edwards, J.E. and Moore, R.A. (2002). Finasteride in the treatment of clinical benign prostatic hyperplasia: a systematic review of randomised trials. *BMC Urology* **2**, 14. (*http://www.biomedcentral.com/1471–2490/2/14*).

2. McConnell, J.D. *et al.* (2003). The long-term effect of doxazosin, finasteride, and combination therapy on the clinical progression of benign prostatic hyperplasia. *New England Journal of Medicine* **349**, 2387–98.

3. Law, M.R. *et al.* (2003). Quantifying effect of statins on low density lipoprotein cholesterol, ischaemic heart disease, and stroke: systematic review and meta-analysis *British Medical Journal* **326**, 1423.

4. Edwards, J.E. and Moore, R.A. (2003). Statins in hypercholesterolaemia: a dose-specific meta-analysis of lipid changes in randomised, double blind trials. *BMC Family Practice* **4**, 18. (*http://www.biomedcentral.com/1471–2296/4/18*).

5. Adler, C.H. *et al.* (2004). Ropinirole for restless legs syndrome. A placebo-controlled crossover trial. *Neurology* **62**, 1405–7.

6. Trenkwalder, C. *et al.* (2004). Ropinirole in the treatment of restless legs syndrome: results from the TREAT RLS 1 study, a 12 week randomised placebo controlled study in 10 European countries. *Journal of Neurology, Neurosurgery, and Psychiatry* **75**, 92–7.

7. Moore, R.A. *et al.* (2002). Sildenafil (Viagra) for male erectile dysfunction: a meta-analysis of clinical trial reports. *BMC Urology* **2**, 6. (*http://www.biomedcentral.com/1471–2490/2/6/*).

8. McQuay, H.J. *et al.* (1982). Some patients don't need analgesics after surgery. *Journal of the Royal Society of Medicine* **75**, 705–8.

9. Moore. R.A. *et al.* (2005). Acute pain: individual patient meta-analysis shows the impact of different ways of analysing and presenting results. *Pain* **116**, 322–31.

10. Simon, G. (2001). Choosing a first line antidepressant. Equal on average does not mean equal for everyone. *Journal of the American Medical Association* **286**, 3003–4.

11. Kroenke, K. *et al.* (2001). Similar effectiveness of paroxetine, fluoxetine and sertraline in primary care. *Journal of the American Medical Association* **286**, 2947–95.

12. Smith, L.A. *et al.* (2000). Teasing apart quality and validity in systematic reviews: an example from acupuncture trials in chronic neck and back pain. *Pain* **86**, 119–32.

# 2.6 Quality scoring and appraisal

By now it should be evident that, if clinical trials, and by extrapolation systematic reviews and meta-analyses of clinical trials, are not done properly, any results they produce will be worthless. This section looks at several checklists that can help examine quality issues in clinical trials and systematic reviews of clinical trials that we read and want to critically appraise. It will begin with looking at clinical trials, and then move on to systematic reviews and meta-analysis.

As an aside, all sorts of checklists of critical appraisal tools have been produced for different study architectures. Few have been validated. Many are more complex than the studies they assess. The approach here is to use the best simple checklists, and to also mention an important initiative aimed at improving the quality of papers in the journals we read, by making sure that all useful information is contained in them. Not everyone would necessarily agree with the use of checklists at all or what is contained in them. But mostly that is pointy-headed academic waffle, and the checklists help those of us wanting to understand and use evidence to avoid the rubbish and concentrate on the good, or at least know when there is an absence of good evidence.

## Clinical trial quality

### Oxford quality score

The major sources of bias in clinical trials of efficacy are lack of proper randomization, lack of proper blinding, and failure to account for all the patients entered into a trial. The Oxford five-point scoring system [1] uses these three criteria, full details of which are given in Table 2.6.1. Briefly, it asks three questions.

1. Is the trial randomized (1 point)? Additional point if method is given and appropriate.
2. Is the trial double-blind (1 point)? Additional point if method given and appropriate.
3. Were withdrawals and drop-outs described and assigned to different treatments (1 point)?

Trials that scored 3 or more were relatively free of bias and could be trusted. Lower scores were shown to be associated with increased treatment effects—they were biased [2, 3]. This means that, if you are reading a clinical trial that scores 3 or more points out of five, then you can be reasonably sure that you are not being misled because of bias. If the trial scores 2 points or less, then you have to ask yourself why you are bothering.

The really neat thing about the Oxford scale is that is quick and simple to use. It is also portable. Once you get the hang of it you carry the three items in your head, and you don't need protocols or complex charts that take forever.

### CONSORT statement

The CONSORT statement is an important research tool that takes an evidence-based approach to improve the quality of reports of randomized trials. The statement is available in several languages and has been endorsed by prominent medical journals such as *The Lancet, Annals of Internal Medicine*, and the *Journal of the American Medical Association*. Although

Table 2.6.1 Oxford scoring system for clinical trial quality

## Oxford scale for quality scoring controlled trials

This is not the same as being asked to review a paper. It should not take more than 10 minutes to score a report and there are no right or wrong answers.
Please read the article and try to answer the following questions (see attached instructions):

1. Was the study described as randomized (this includes the use of words such as randomly, random, and randomization)?
2. Was the study described as double-blind?
3. Was there a description of withdrawals and drop-outs?

**Scoring the items:**
Give a score of 1 point for each 'yes' and 0 points for each 'no'. There are no in-between marks

Give 1 additional point if:
- On question 1, the method of randomization was described and it was appropriate (table of random numbers, computer generated, coin tossing, etc.) and/or
- On question 2 the method of double-blinding was described and it was appropriate (identical placebo, active placebo, dummy, etc.)

Deduct 1 point if:
- On question 1, the method of randomization was described and it was inappropriate (patients were allocated alternately, or according to date of birth, hospital number, etc.) and/or
- On question 2 the study was described as double-blind but the method of blinding was inappropriate (e.g. comparison of tablet vs. injection with no double dummy)

**Advice on using the scale**

1. Randomization
   If the word randomized or any other related words such as random, randomly, or randomization are used in the report, but the method of randomization is not described, give a positive score to this item. A randomization method will be regarded as appropriate if it allowed each patient to have the same chance of receiving each treatment and the investigators could not predict which treatment was next. Therefore methods of allocation using date of birth, date of admission, hospital numbers, or alternation should not be regarded as appropriate
2. Double-blinding
   A study must be regarded as double-blind if the word double-blind is used (even without description of the method) or if it is implied that neither the care-giver nor the patient could identify the treatment being assessed
3. Withdrawals and drop-outs
   Patients who were included in the study but did not complete the observation period or who were not included in the analysis must be described. The number and the reasons for withdrawal must be stated. If there are no withdrawals, it should be stated in the article. If there is no statement on withdrawals, this item must be given a negative score (0 points)

papers about CONSORT have been published in a number of journals, probably the best place to find information is on the CONSORT internet site (*www.consort-statement.org*). Reporting randomized trials according to CONSORT criteria provides something of a guarantee of integrity in the reported results of research, and that is of value not only to researchers, but also to peer reviewers, journal editors, health-care providers, health policy makers, not to mention those of us who want to try and understand research without being misled.

CONSORT comprises a checklist and flow diagram to help improve the quality of reports of randomized controlled trials. It offers a standard way for researchers to report trials. The checklist (Table 2.6.2) includes items, based on evidence, that need to be addressed in the report; the flow diagram provides readers with a clear picture of the progress of all participants in the trial, from the time they are randomized until the end of their involvement. The intent of CONSORT is to make the experimental process more clear, flawed or not, so that users of the data can more appropriately assess its validity for their purposes.

## Scoring system for reviews

The purpose is to evaluate the scientific quality (i.e. adherence to scientific principles) of research overviews (review articles) published in the medical literature. It is not intended to measure literary quality, importance, relevance, originality, or other attributes of overviews.

The index [4] (Table 2.6.3) is for assessing overviews of primary ('original') research on pragmatic questions regarding causation, diagnosis, prognosis, therapy, or prevention. A research overview is a survey of research. The same principles that apply to epidemiological surveys apply to overviews: a question must be clearly specified; a target population identified and accessed; appropriate information obtained from that population in an unbiased fashion; and conclusions derived, sometimes with the help of formal statistical analysis, as is done in 'meta-analyses'. The fundamental difference between overviews and epidemiological surveys is the unit of analysis, not the scientific issues that this index addresses.

Since most published overviews do not include a methods section it is difficult to answer some of the questions in the index. Base your answers, as much as possible, on information provided in the overview. If the methods that were used are reported incompletely relative to a specific item, score that item as 'partially'. Similarly, if there is no information provided regarding what was done relative to a particular question, score it as 'can't tell', unless there is information in the overview to suggest either that the criterion was or was not met.

For question 8, if no attempt has been made to combine findings, and no statement is made regarding the inappropriateness of combining findings, check 'no'. If a summary (general) estimate is given anywhere in the abstract, the discussion, or the summary section of the paper, and it is not reported how that estimate was derived, mark 'no' even if there is a statement regarding the limitations of combining the findings of the studies reviewed. If in doubt mark 'can't tell'.

For an overview to be scored as 'yes' on question 9, data (not just citations) must be reported that support the main conclusions regarding the primary question(s) that the overview addresses.

**Table 2.6.2**  CONSORT: checklist of items to include when reporting a randomized trial

| Paper section & topic | Item | Description | Reported on page number |
|---|---|---|---|
| **Title & abstract** | 1 | How participants were allocated to interventions (e.g. 'random allocation', 'randomized', or 'randomly assigned') | |
| **Introduction** | | | |
| Background | 2 | Scientific background and explanation of rationale | |
| **Methods** | | | |
| Participants | 3 | Eligibility criteria for participants and the settings and locations where the data were collected | |
| Interventions | 4 | Precise details of the interventions intended for each group and how and when they were actually administered | |
| Objectives | 5 | Specific objectives and hypotheses | |
| Outcomes | 6 | Clearly defined primary and secondary outcome measures and, when applicable, any methods used to enhance the quality of measurements (e.g. multiple observations, training of assessors) | |

(contd.)

**Table 2.6.2** (contd.)

| Paper section & topic | Item | Description | Reported on page number |
|---|---|---|---|
| Sample size | 7 | How sample size was determined and, when applicable, explanation of any interim analyses and stopping rules | |
| Randomization: sequence generation | 8 | Method used to generate the random allocation sequence, including details of any restrictions (e.g. blocking, stratification) | |
| Randomization: allocation concealment | 9 | Method used to implement the random allocation sequence (e.g. numbered containers or central telephone), clarifying whether the sequence was concealed until interventions were assigned | |
| Randomization: implementation | 10 | Who generated the allocation sequence, who enrolled participants, and who assigned participants to their groups | |
| Blinding (masking) | 11 | Whether or not participants, those administering the interventions, and those assessing the outcomes were blinded to group assignment. When relevant, how the success of blinding was evaluated | |
| Statistical methods | 12 | Statistical methods used to compare groups for primary outcome(s); methods for additional analyses, such as subgroup analyses and adjusted analyses | |

| **Results** | | |
|---|---|---|
| Participant flow | 13 | Flow of participants through each stage (a diagram is strongly recommended). Specifically, for each group report the numbers of participants randomly assigned, receiving intended treatment, completing the study protocol, and analysed for the primary outcome. Describe protocol deviations from study as planned, together with reasons |
| Recruitment | 14 | Dates defining the periods of recruitment and follow-up |
| Baseline data | 15 | Baseline demographic and clinical characteristics of each group |
| Numbers analysed | 16 | Number of participants (denominator) in each group included in each analysis and whether the analysis was by 'intention-to-treat'. State the results in absolute numbers when feasible (e.g. 10/20, not 50%) |

(contd.)

**Table 2.6.2** (contd.)

| Paper section & topic | Item | Description | Reported on page number |
|---|---|---|---|
| Outcomes & estimation | 17 | For each primary and secondary outcome, a summary of results for each group, and the estimated effect size and its precision (e.g. 95% confidence interval) | |
| Ancillary analyses | 18 | Address multiplicity by reporting any other analyses performed, including subgroup analyses and adjusted analyses, indicating those pre-specified and those exploratory | |
| Adverse events | 19 | All important adverse events or side-effects in each intervention group | |
| **Discussion** | | | |
| Interpretation | 20 | Interpretation of the results, taking into account study hypotheses, sources of potential bias or imprecision, and the dangers associated with multiplicity of analyses and outcomes | |
| Generalizability | 21 | Generalizability (external validity) of the trial findings | |
| Overall evidence | 22 | General interpretation of the results in the context of current evidence | |

**Table 2.6.3** The Oxman and Guyatt index for systematic reviews

| The Oxman & Guyatt index of scientific quality | | | |
|---|---|---|---|
| 1 | Were the search methods used to find evidence on the primary question(s) stated? | No | Partially | Yes |
| 2 | Was the search for evidence reasonably comprehensive? | No | Can't tell | Yes |
| 3 | Were the criteria used for deciding which studies to include in the overview reported? | No | Partially | Yes |
| 4 | Was bias in the selection of studies avoided? | No | Can't tell | Yes |
| 5 | Were the criteria used for assessing the validity of the included studies reported? | No | Partially | Yes |
| 6 | Was the validity of all the studies referred to in the text assessed using appropriate criteria? | No | Can't tell | Yes |
| 7 | Were the methods used to combine the findings of the relevant studies (to reach a conclusion) reported? | No | Partially | Yes |
| 8 | Were the findings of the relevant studies combined appropriately relative to the primary question of the overview? | No | Can't tell | Yes |
| 9 | Were the conclusions made by the author(s) supported by the data and/or analysis reported in the overview? | No | Partially | Yes |
| 10 | How would you rate the scientific quality of this overview? | | | |

| Flaws | | | | | | |
|---|---|---|---|---|---|---|
| **Extensive** | | **Major** | | **Minor** | | **Minimal** |
| 1 | 2 | 3 | 4 | 5 | 6 | 7 |

The score for question 10, the overall scientific quality, should be based on your answers to the first nine questions. The following guidelines can be used to assist with deriving a summary score: if the 'can't tell' option is used one or more times on the preceding questions, a review is likely to have minor flaws at best and it is difficult to rule out major flaws (i.e. a score of 4 or lower). If the 'no' option is used on questions 2, 4, 6 or 8, the review is likely to have major flaws (i.e. a score of 3 or less, depending on the number and degree of the flaws).

The guide has been applied to systematic reviews of pain topics [5] and the results are worth noting because they teach us much about the need for scepticism when reading systematic reviews. Seventy reports were included in the quality assessment. The earliest report was from 1980. Over two-thirds appeared after 1990. Reviews considered between two and 196 primary studies (median 28). Sixty reviews reached positive conclusions, seven negative, twelve uncertain, and one did not manage any conclusion. All were based on published data only (no individual patient data analysis).

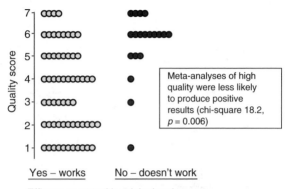

**Figure 2.6.1** Applying Oxman and Guyatt to systematic reviews of pain therapies.

The median agreed overall Oxman and Guyatt score for the systematic reviews was 4 (range 1 to 7). Systematic reviews of high quality were significantly less likely to produce positive results (Figure 2.6.1). Sixteen of 19 systematic reviews with negative or uncertain results had overall quality scores above the median, compared with only 20 of the 60 with positive results. Systematic reviews restricted to RCTs were significantly less likely to produce positive conclusions (19 of 31) than those that included other study architectures (41 of 49). All conclusions from systematic reviews of psychological interventions were positive. In only one of those reviews was quality scored above the median. All abstracts scored below the median, and 6 of 8 abstracts received the minimum possible score.

### QUOROM statement for meta-analysis of clinical trials

Although guidelines for reporting systematic reviews have been suggested, a consensus across disciplines about how they should be reported has only recently been developed. Following a recent initiative to improve the quality of reporting of randomized controlled trials (CONSORT statement) a conference referred to as the 'quality of reporting of meta-analyses' [QUOROM] was held to address issues relating to systematic reviews of randomized trials. The QUOROM conference participants were clinical epidemiologists, clinicians, statisticians, and researchers who conduct meta-analysis as well as editors from the UK and North America who are interested in systematic reviews.

This conference resulted in the creation of the QUOROM statement (Table 2.6.4), which consists of a checklist and flow diagram. The checklist consists of 18 items, including eight evidence-based ones. The checklist encourages

**Table 2.6.4** The QUOROM statement: improving the quality of reports of meta-analyses of randomized controlled trials: the QUOROM statement checklist

| Heading | Subheading | Descriptor | Reported? (Y/N) | Page number |
|---|---|---|---|---|
| Title | | Identify the report as a meta-analysis (or systematic review) of RCTs | | |
| Abstract | | **Describe:** | | |
| | Objectives | The clinical question explicitly | | |
| | Data sources | The databases (i.e. list) and other information sources | | |
| | Review methods | The selection criteria (i.e. population, intervention, outcome, and study design); methods for validity assessment, data abstraction, and study characteristics, and quantitative data synthesis in sufficient detail to permit replication | | |
| | Results | Characteristics of the RCTs included and excluded; qualitative and quantitative findings (i.e. point estimates and confidence intervals); and subgroup analyses | | |
| | Conclusion | The main results | | |
| Introduction | | **Describe:** | | |
| | | The explicit clinical problem, biological rationale for the intervention, and rationale for review | | |
| Methods | Searching | The information sources, in detail (e.g. databases, registers, personal files, expert informants, agencies, hand-searching), and any restrictions (years considered, publication status, language of publication) | | |
| | Selection | The inclusion and exclusion criteria (defining population, intervention, principal outcomes, and study design) | | |
| | Validity assessment | The criteria and process used (e.g. masked conditions, quality assessment, and their findings) | | |
| | Data abstraction | The process or processes used (e.g. completed independently, in duplicate) | | |

(contd.)

**Table 2.6.4** (contd.)

| Heading | Subheading | Descriptor | Reported? (Y/N) | Page number |
|---------|------------|------------|-----------------|-------------|
| | Study characteristics | The type of study design, participants' characteristics, details of intervention, outcome definitions, and how clinical heterogeneity was assessed | | |
| | Quantitative data synthesis | The principal measures of effect (e.g. relative risk), method of combining results (statistical testing and confidence intervals), handling of missing data; how statistical heterogeneity was assessed; a rationale for any *a priori* sensitivity and subgroup analyses; and any assessment of publication bias | | |
| Results | Trial flow | Provide a meta-analysis profile summarizing trial flow | | |
| | Study characteristics | Present descriptive data for each trial (e.g. age, sample size, intervention, dose, duration, follow-up period) | | |
| | Quantitative data synthesis | Report agreement on the selection and validity assessment; present simple summary results (for each treatment group in each trial, for each primary outcome); present data needed to calculate effect sizes and confidence intervals in intention-to-treat analyses (e.g. $2 \times 2$ tables of counts, means and SDs, proportions) | | |
| Discussion | | Summarize key findings; discuss clinical inferences based on internal and external validity; interpret the results in light of the totality of available evidence; describe potential biases in the review process (e.g. publication bias); and suggest a future research agenda | | |

authors to provide readers with information regarding searches, selection, validity assessment, data abstraction, study characteristics, quantitative data synthesis, and trial flow. A flow diagram is also suggested to provide information about the progress of randomized trials throughout the review process from the number of potentially relevant trials identified, to those retrieved and ultimately included.

## Commentary

It is worth remembering that no scale or checklist on its own can guarantee that a result is not fraudulent, or mistaken, or achieved just by random chance. Some very large studies looking at rare events may have thousands of patients, but will accumulate only a few tens of events. However clever we think we are, we can be mistaken, but the chances of being mistaken are very much reduced by using a few simple scales or checklists.

## References

1. Jadad, A.R. *et al.* (1996). Assessing the quality of reports of randomized clinical trials: is blinding necessary? *Controlled Clinical Trials* **17**, 1–12.
2. Khan, K.S. *et al.* (1996). The importance of quality of primary studies in producing unbiased systematic reviews. *Archives of Internal Medicine* **156**, 661–6.
3. Moher, D. *et al.* (1998). Does quality of reports of randomised trials affect estimates of intervention efficacy reported in meta-analyses? *Lancet* **352**, 609–13.
4. Oxman, A.D. and Guyatt, G.H. (1991). Validation of an index of the quality of review articles. *Journal of Clinical Epidemiology* **44**, 1271–8.
5. Jadad, A.R. and McQuay, H.J. (1996). Meta-analyses to evaluate analgesic interventions: a systematic qualitative review of their methodology. *Journal of Clinical Epidemiology* **49**, 235–43.

# 2.7   Systematic reviews and meta-analysis of clinical trials

Systematic reviews should identify and review all the relevant studies, and are more likely to give a reliable answer. They use explicit methods and quality standards to reduce bias. Their results are the closest we are likely to get to the truth in the current state of knowledge, though much depends on how many clinical trials exist and how good and how large they are. Systematic reviews (and meta-analysis, the statistical combining of information from many trials) are our best defence against making incorrect decisions based on inadequate data.

The questions a systematic review should answer for us are:

- How well does an intervention work (compared with placebo, no treatment, or other interventions in current use)—or can I forget about it?
- Is it safe?
- Will it work and be safe for the patients in my practice?

Clinicians live in the real world and are busy people, and need to synthesize their knowledge of a particular patient in their practice, their experience and expertise, and the best external evidence from systematic review. They can then be pretty sure that they are doing their best. But the product of systematic review and particularly meta-analysis—often some sort of statistical output—is not usually readily interpretable or usable in day-to-day clinical practice.

This section is all about quality control, about how systematic reviews deal with the potential problem of bias in clinical trials, and how they provide their results for us to understand and use. The job of a systematic review is to pull all the nuggets from piles of dross, not to give us one big pile of dross that may or may not have some nuggets in it. What we seek, but unfortunately do not always get, is a good review of good trials. Too often we get bad reviews, even bad reviews of good trials (Figure 2.7.1).

The ideal is a good review of good trials. If we have a good review of bad trials, it can analyse why those trials are bad, and perhaps suggest what would constitute a good trial, and so we move forward. If we have a bad review of good trials, it should have at least identified the trials that already exist, so we or others could repeat it and do a better job. The worst of all possible worlds is a bad review of bad trials, when the chances are we will be misled. Later in this section we will look at a few examples as a guide.

### Searching for relevant trials

To produce valid reviews of evidence, the reviews need to be systematic. To be systematic they need to include all relevant randomized controlled trials, or whatever other reports are available and identified as targets for the review. Identifying all the relevant trials is a 'fundamental challenge' [1]. The advent of the Cochrane Library with its CDROM or Internet database of about 450,000 controlled trials has made this much easier in recent years. We now have many more and easier electronic ways of searching,

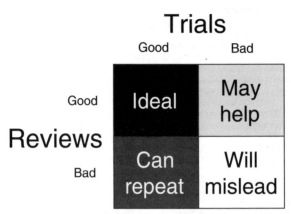

**Figure 2.7.1**   Trials and reviews—hopes and expectations.

including PubMed (*www4.ncbi.nlm.nih.gov/entrez*), with searching freely and easily available over the Internet.

The first obstacle faced by any reviewer is finding out how many eligible RCTs exist. Commonly, the total is unknown, unless it is a new drug intervention, when all the trials will usually have been done with industrial sponsorship. Thus, only for newer interventions are reviewers likely to be sure that they have found all the RCTs available. Otherwise, the only way to find how many RCTs there are would be to scan every record in every language, in every available bibliographic database; to search by hand all non-indexed journals, theses, proceedings, and textbooks; to search the reference lists of all the reports found; and to ask investigators of previous RCTs for other published or unpublished information [2]. In practice, constrained by time and cost, reviewers have to compromise, and then hope that what they have found is a representative sample of the unknown total population of trials. The more comprehensive the searching the more trials will be found, and any conclusions will then be stronger. Comprehensive searches can be very time-consuming and costly, so again this emphasizes the necessary compromise, where the target is the highest possible yield for given resources.

Retrieval bias is the failure to identify reports that could have affected the results of a systematic review or meta-analysis [3]. This failure may be because trials are still ongoing, or completed but unpublished (publication bias) or because, although published, the search did not find them. Trying to identify unpublished trials by asking researchers had a very low yield [4], and was not cheap. Registers of ongoing and completed trials are another way to find unpublished data, but such registers are rare though increasingly becoming available.

## Quality control

Systematic reviews of inadequate quality may be worse than none, because faulty decisions may be made with unjustified confidence. Quality control in the systematic review process, from literature searching onwards, is vital, and the QUOROM statement on publication of systematic reviews should enable journals to publish better systematic reviews, of higher methodological quality. How to judge the quality of a systematic review is encapsulated in the questions [5]:

1. Were the question(s) and methods stated clearly?
2. Were the search methods used to locate relevant studies comprehensive?
3. Were explicit methods used to determine which articles to include in the review?
4. Was the methodological quality of the primary studies assessed?
5. Were the selection and assessment of the primary studies reproducible and free from bias?
6. Were differences in individual study results explained adequately?
7. Were the results of the primary studies combined appropriately?
8. Were the reviewers' conclusions supported by the data cited?

This is all very methodological, and important, stuff. But the key to systematic review is to avoid allowing bias to creep in and colour the results.

## Garbage in, garbage out

For the avoidance of doubt, the bottom line is that wherever bias is found it almost always results in a large overestimation of the effects of treatments. Poor trial design makes treatments look better than they really are. It can even make them look as if they work when actually they do not. This is why good guides to systematic review suggest strategies for bias minimization by avoiding including trials with known sources of bias. They further suggest performing sensitivity analysis to see whether different trial designs are affecting results in a systematic review.

But this advice is ignored more often than not. It is ignored in reviews, and it is ignored in decision-making. The result is that decisions are being made on incorrect information, and they will be wrong. There is no alternative to having some rudimentary knowledge of potential sources of bias and how badly it can hurt.

## Sensitivity analysis

Systematic reviewers should take potential sources of bias into account when performing their reviews, as well as any other feature of clinical trials or the patients in whom they are conducted that might affect results. One simple way of checking for unknown (or unknowable) bias is to perform a sensitivity analysis. Here are some examples of sensitivity analyses that are worth looking for in systematic reviews and meta-analyses.

- Trial quality: perhaps examining whether results in trials of higher or lower methodological quality give different results (say Oxford quality score 3/5 or more versus those of 2 or less). While systematic reviews should be looking only at trials of better quality to avoid bias, there may be cogent reasons for using trials of lower reporting quality. If so, then sensitivity analysis should be mandatory. If the lower quality trials are to be combined with higher quality trials, you need to know that they are not giving different, often better, results that distort the overall conclusion.

- Trial validity: perhaps examining whether results are different in trials of higher or lower validity score.

- Size of trial: often there are larger and smaller trials, with most patients in a smaller number of larger trials. It is a simple task to ask whether the larger number of smaller trials have different results from the smaller number of larger trials.

- Dose or intensity of therapy: it might be obvious that dose is an important variable but, if dissimilar doses were combined in a meta-analysis, this might distort the overall conclusions for the dose that you usually use. Comparing different doses, or higher versus lower doses should make sense.

- Patient characteristics: clearly if patients differ in the type or severity of disorder, they may react differently to therapy, though they may not. Checking by using a sensitivity analysis according to some measure of severity is sensible. One way of looking at this in trials of prevention is to examine the rate at which events occur in the control population.

- Type of intervention: most systematic reviews and meta-analyses that look at different types of intervention analyse results for each separately, but some do not. Analysis by different types of intervention is a form of sensitivity analysis.

- Duration: comparing results of longer trials with those of shorter trials may be important in some circumstances.

- Outcomes: meta-analyses sometimes combine different outcomes. That may be permissible, but if done should be preceded by a sensitivity analysis to examine whether different outcomes are producing different levels of measured efficacy.

- Different comparators: while this is not often an issue, it can be that different comparators are combined in meta-analysis.

- When studies were done: especially when a systematic review finds clinical trials spanning many decades, it may be that changes over time means that trials may not be comparable. Performing a sensitivity analysis according to age of trial probably makes sense.

- If the results of sensitivity analyses are the same, then that is fine and we can safely pool data. If they are not, we have something to explain and might wish to be cautious about results from pooled data. Reviewers who use sensitivity analysis are usually doing a good job. Reviews that don't mention sensitivity analysis are to be looked at closely to see whether it should have been done.

The one thing to be borne in mind is that sensitivity analysis can only be performed where there is sufficient information. If we have too few studies, then we end up salami-slicing small numbers of trials, and run the distinct risk of coming up with incorrect conclusions based on too little data.

### Homogeneity and heterogeneity

When we have been discussing sensitivity analyses, we have been discussing the propensity of clinical trials to be similar or different. If clinical trials are looking at the same intervention, in similar populations, at the same intensity, using the same outcomes, over the same period of time, then we would probably conclude that they were much the same. This is a definition of clinical homogeneity. Clinical heterogeneity would occur when one or more of the characteristics were different, for instance looking at completely different doses, or the same dose in completely different patients.

But in meta-analysis, the terms homogeneity and heterogeneity have other, statistical, meanings.

### Homogeneity

Clinical homogeneity means that, in trials included in a review, the participants, interventions, and outcome measures are similar or comparable. Studies are considered statistically homogeneous if their results vary no more than might be expected by the play of chance. Statistical tests used to detect statistical homogeneity would say that 10% of a perfectly homogeneous data set could be heterogeneous, because that is the usual set point for the tests.

### Heterogeneity

Heterogeneity refers to variability or differences between studies in the estimates of effects. A distinction should be made between 'statistical heterogeneity' (differences in the reported effects), 'methodological heterogeneity' (differences in study design), and 'clinical heterogeneity' (differences between studies in key characteristics of the participants, interventions, or outcome measures). Where there are large differences of a clinical or methodological nature between studies, the simplest question to ask is whether there is any good reason for pooling data from these studies in a meta-analysis, where heterogeneity is known to exist.

More difficult is the occurrence of statistical heterogeneity where there is methodological and clinical homogeneity. Statistical tests of heterogeneity are used to assess whether the observed variability in study results (effect sizes) is greater than that expected to occur by chance. These tests have low statistical power, and the boundary for statistical significance is usually set at 10%, or 0.1. Some people think that, if these tests are used, then a value of 1%, or 0.01 makes more sense. An analysis of the performance of commonly used tests shows that the Breslow–Day test performs most consistently [6], though the Cochrane Collaboration now uses the $I^2$ test [7].

It is difficult to know what to make of statistical heterogeneity in the face of apparent solid clinical homogeneity. We tend to find it when we have small, and perhaps not so good, clinical trials, where some form of clinical heterogeneity exists of which we are unaware. It may, of course, be chance.

## Graphical methods used in meta-analysis

When data from different trials are to be pooled in a meta-analysis, it is useful to have some graphical representation giving an overall impression of the results available. There are various formats, all with their benefits, and some are easier to understand than others.

### L'Abbé plots

A paper by Kristen L'Abbé and colleagues [8] is one of the most sensible and understandable ever written on systematic reviews. The authors suggest a simple graphical representation of the information from trials. Each point on a L'Abbé scatter plot is one trial in the review. The proportion of patients achieving the outcome with the experimental intervention is plotted against the event rate in controls. Figure 2.7.2 gives a representation of a L'Abbé plot, but we will see some real examples later in this section.

For treatments, trials in which the experimental intervention was better than the control will be in the upper left of the plot, between the y-axis and the line of equality. If experimental was no better than control then the trial will fall on the line of equality, and if control was better than experimental then the trial will be in the lower right of the plot, between the x-axis and the line of equality. Symbol size should be proportional to trial size, with a scale for trial size included.

These plots give a quick indication of the level of agreement among trials. If the points are in a consistent group we have some confidence that what we are seeing is a homogeneous effect. But if points are spread all over the graph, and especially if they cross the line of equality, then that should make us concerned about the intervention, or the patients being treated and their condition. This can also be called heterogeneity.

### Forest plot

A Forest plot involves a vertical representation of the overall point estimate for a measure of effect size in individual trials (odds ratio, relative risk, mean difference between treatment and control), usually and preferably with larger symbols for larger trials. Lewis and Clarke give a terrific history

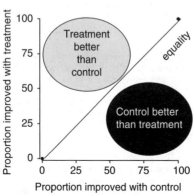

**Figure 2.7.2** Representation of a L'Abbé plot.

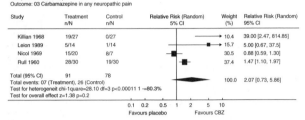

Review: Carbamazepine for acute and chronic pain
Comparison: 01 Neuropathic Pain
Outcome: 03 Carbamazepine in any neuropathic pain

| Study | Treatment n/N | Control n/N | Relative Risk (Random) 5% CI | Weight (%) | Relative Risk (Random) 95% CI |
|-------|---------------|-------------|------------------------------|------------|-------------------------------|
| Killian 1968 | 19/27 | 0/27 | | 10.4 | 39.00 [2.47, 814.85] |
| Leion 1989 | 5/14 | 1/14 | | 15.7 | 5.00 [0.67, 37.5] |
| Nicol 1969 | 15/20 | 8/7 | | 30.5 | 0.88 [0.59, 1.30] |
| Rull 1960 | 28/30 | 19/30 | | 37.4 | 1.47 [1.10, 1.97] |
| Total (95% CI) | 91 | 78 | | 100.0 | 2.07 [0.73, 5.86] |

Total events: 07 (Treatment), 26 (Control)
Test for heterogeneit chi-1quare=28.10 df=3 p<0.00011 1 -=80.3%
Test for overall effect z=1.38 p=0.2

0.1  0.2   0.5    1    2    5   10
Favours placebo         Favours CBZ

**Figure 2.7.3**  Typical forest plot.

of this representation of data [9]. The plot was not called a 'forest plot' in print for some time, and the origins of this title are obscured by history and myth. At the September 1990 meeting of the breast cancer overview, Richard Peto jokingly mentioned that the plot was named after the breast cancer researcher Pat Forest, and, at times, the name has been spelt 'Forest plot.' However, the phrase actually originates from the idea that the typical plot appears as a forest of lines.

In a forest plot the horizontal line represents the 95% confidence interval around the estimate. A different symbol (usually a diamond) represents the pooled effect size, with the horizontal arms of the diamond showing the confidence interval. In addition, a vertical line is likely to represent the point of no difference (relative risk or odds ratio of 1, for instance), and if the diamond and vertical line do not intersect, that demonstrates statistical significance.

Forest plots produced by RevMan (the statistical package used by the Cochrane Collaboration) and other packages usually have other useful information, and an example is shown in Figure 2.7.3, for carbamazepine in neuropathic pain [10]. Other examples will be shown later in this section.

### Sheldon plot

This representation of data is named after the man we first saw use it. The effect size of a number of different interventions is plotted horizontally. Each group in a trial is represented, with its symbol proportional to the number of patients in the group. A typical example is seen in Figure 2.7.4, looking at prevalence rates of depression found for five different methods of diagnosis in just under 6700 patients in whom the overall rate of depression was about 30% [11]. Many studies were very small, and this also contributed to the wide variation, which was from under 10% to over 60%.

Sheldon plots are useful ways of looking at data when there is no common comparator (like placebo). They are not quantitative tools. But they do generate a useful overall impression of the weight and strength of evidence (or lack of it), often in difficult situations that other methods cannot reach.

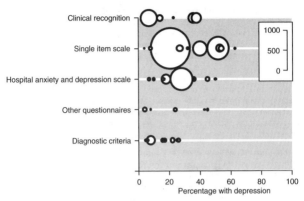

**Figure 2.7.4** Typical Sheldon plot. Prevalence rates (%) in depression for five diagnostic methods.

## Examples of systematic reviews and meta-analysis

The only way to hone one's skills in understanding evidence in systematic reviews and meta-analysis is to look at some to understand weaknesses rather than strengths. So it is useful to pick some out because they exemplify where all of us, readers and writers of systematic reviews and meta-analysis, can be misled. Where possible we have reviews available in longer form on the Internet version of Bandolier.

### Finasteride and haematuria

You will find a systematic review in *Bandolier* **111**, published in May 2003. It includes RCTs and observational data, but RCT data is limited to three open studies of low quality (scores of 2 out of a maximum of 5), so possibly biased, and with durations of 12 and 48 months. There were only 165 men in these trials. NNTs were 2 for preventing recurrence of haematuria, and 6 for preventing surgery.

By now you should be less than happy with the amount and quality of the data available, but much may have happened in 3 years. You need to know if there is more data, because a single additional large and double-blind study could overturn the results (Table 2.4.4). A quick check of PubMed using finasteride and (haematuria or hematuria) revealed no new trials, but an editorial in 2004 that may be helpful in putting what is already known in perspective.

### Acupuncture for tennis elbow

A review [12] sought randomized studies of patients with pain resulting from tennis elbow, essentially with pain originating from the common origin of the extensor tendon, and with needle acupuncture as the primary intervention. Excluded were other elbow problems and patients concurrently receiving other treatments. Of 53 articles screened, the authors chose to include six, combined in a qualitative 'best evidence synthesis'.

- Of these six included trials, one was not properly randomized.
- Of the remaining five trials, two were not double-blind.
- Of the remaining three, one had results only immediately after treatment (not much use in a chronic condition, and duration of the condition was about 10 months in some of the trials).

That left two randomized, double-blind trials, both of which reported results 2 or 3 months after treatment. Both compared real acupuncture with sham acupuncture (using different needle points, for instance). Both reported outcomes roughly equivalent to half pain relief, and the rates were similar in both treatment arms. So, by applying simple rules about known sources of bias, we refute what this meta-analysis claimed, that there was 'strong evidence' to support acupuncture for tennis elbow.

### Same patients, same intervention, same outcomes

A meta-analysis [13] of placebo-controlled studies in homeopathy published in 1997 sought to provide proof that it worked. It concluded that 'the results of our meta-analysis are not compatible with the hypothesis that clinical effects of homeopathy are completely due to placebo [but]...we found insufficient evidence from these studies that homeopathy is clearly efficacious for any single clinical condition'.

The analysis sought all the trials on homeopathy, in any condition, and with any homeopathic remedy at any dilution, that fulfilled the following inclusion criteria:

1. controlled studies;
2. parallel group design;
3. randomized, or with descriptions of double-blinding that meant they had to have been randomized;
4. written reports (including abstracts, theses, etc.);
5. had data on outcomes that could be extracted for data analysis.

It found 89 trials, breaking down like this:

- The median number of patients studied in each trial was 60.
- There were 24 clinical categories.
- There were four types of homeopathy.
- There were 50 classes of homeopathic remedy.

This was not a particularly homogeneous bunch of trials. The number of trials in each clinical class, and the number where homeopathy beat placebo are shown in Table 2.7.1. Overall, homeopathy beat placebo in only 42% of the trials. So one conclusion is that, in 6 out of 10 trials, homeopathy did not show any benefit over placebo.

The overall odds ratios favoured homeopathy. The odds ratio was 2.5 (2.1 to 2.9) for all 89 trials, though lower at 1.7 (1.3 to 2.1) for high-quality trials. The problem is that the studies were such a mixed bag in terms of intervention, patients, outcomes, and especially trial quality. A subsequent meta-analysis of meta-analyses [14] included six re-analyses of the original meta-analysis. These showed that more rigorous study design was associated with less effect, making the overall effect insignificant.

A further 11 systematic reviews published between 1997 and 2001 were located. They were carried out in different conditions with different homeopathic remedies. Conditions included postoperative ileus, delayed-onset muscle soreness, migraine, influenza, asthma, rheumatic conditions, and osteoarthritis. The number of patients for each condition was as small

**Table 2.7.1** Trials in homeopathy

| Clinical class | Number of trials | |
| --- | --- | --- |
| | Total | Homeopathy beats placebo |
| Allergy | 7 | 4 |
| Dermatology | 9 | 3 |
| Gastroenterology | 9 | 3 |
| Musculoskeletal | 6 | 2 |
| Neurology | 7 | 4 |
| Obstetrics & gynaecology | 10 | 5 |
| Chest infection, asthma, ENT | 15 | 4 |
| Rheumatology | 7 | 4 |
| Surgery & anaesthesia | 12 | 4 |
| Miscellaneous | 7 | 4 |

as 150 and as large as 3400. None of these systematic reviews provided any convincing evidence that homeopathy was effective for any condition. The lesson was often that the best-designed trials had the most negative result.

*Are these patients like ours?*

One of the best examples comes from a meta-analysis of anaesthetic techniques [15] with 141 trials including 9559 patients and looking at death after surgery. There were 247 deaths within 30 days of operation recorded in 35 trials. Overall, the analysis concluded that anaesthesia that included neuraxial blockade resulted in fewer deaths compared with general anaesthesia alone, with an odds ratio of 0.7 (95% CI, 0.5 to 0.9) and an NNT to prevent one death of 98 (60 to 270).

There were nine trials with at least 10 deaths per trial, shown in Figure 2.7.5 as a L'Abbé plot. For only three of these smaller trials was there a large effect of neuraxial blockade plus general anaesthesia, and in these three there was an extraordinarily high death rate in the general anaesthetic group of over 15%. For six other trials in which the death rate with general anaesthetic alone was below 15%, the death rates with neuraxial blockade plus general anaesthetic and general anaesthetic alone were about the same. As a series of analyses in Table 2.7.2 shows, all the statistical effect was in five studies with fewer than 100 patients each, which had death rates with general anaesthetic alone of over 10%.

The question that perhaps we should be asking is which patients are like ours—those with death rates for operations below 10% or those with death rates over 10%? Almost certainly the former. And, given that the trials with high death rates were conducted mostly over 25 years ago, and mostly in communist block countries, it might give slightly more pause for thought.

A second question is which representation (forest or L'Abbé plot) enables the clinical heterogeneity evident in these trials to be identified. It could be argued that both do the job, but it is much clearer in the L'Abbé plot.

Mortality (%) with neuraxial blockade

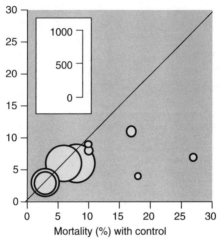

**Figure 2.7.5** L'Abbé plot of mortality in trials of anaesthetic technique.

There is an interesting twist to this. A later publication of a large RCT of much the same anaesthetic technique comparison, where death was the primary outcome, makes one think even more. In this RCT [16] most of the deaths did not occur in the operating room, nor within 48 hours of surgery, but between 1 and 4 weeks later (Figure 2.7.6). Almost certainly, the deaths were not directly associated with the anaesthetic technique and that asks further questions about the value of deaths within 30 days as a valid outcome in the original meta-analysis.

### Nicotine replacement therapy (NRT)

A Cochrane review [17] is typically thorough because the Cochrane Tobacco Addiction Group has its own ongoing register of trials that is being constantly updated. It included randomized trials in which NRT was compared to placebo or no treatment, or where different doses of NRT were compared. Excluded were trials not reporting cessation rates or with follow-up of less than 6 months. The main outcome measure was abstinence from smoking after at least 6 months of follow-up. The most rigorous definition of abstinence for each trial was used, with biochemically validated rates if available.

Numbers needed to treat for nicotine replacement versus placebo or no treatment controls depended on the size of trials included in an analysis. Table 2.7.3 shows that, for patch or gum, the NNT was higher (worse) for studies with more than 500 patients than for those with fewer than 500 patients, and statistically so for gum.

**Table 2.7.2** Sensitivity analysis of deaths in trials of different anaesthetic technique

| Criteria imposed | Number of trials | Patients (% total) | Deaths/total (%) With neural blockade | Deaths/total (%) Without neural blockade | Relative risk (95% CI) | NNT (95% CI) |
|---|---|---|---|---|---|---|
| All trials | 141 | 9559 (100) | 103/4871 (2.1) | 144/4688 (3.1) | 0.7 (0.5–0.9) | 98 (60–265) |
| Trials with fewer than 10 deaths | 132 | 7067 (74) | 32/3537 (0.9) | 44/3530 (1.2) | 0.7 (0.5–1.2) | n/c |
| Trials with more than 10 deaths | 9 | 2492 (26) | 71/1334 (5.3) | 100/1158 (8.6) | 0.6 (0.5–0.8) | 30 (19–77) |
| Trials with more than 10 deaths and with more than 100 patients (death rate in controls less than 10%) | 4 | 1889 (20) | 49/1054 (4.6) | 48/835 (5.7) | 0.9 (0.6–1.4) | n/c |
| Trials with more than 10 deaths and with fewer than 100 patients (death rate in controls more than 10%) | 5 | 603 (6) | 22/280 (7.9) | 52/323 (16.1) | 0.5 (0.3–0.8) | 12 (7.5–32) |
| All trials with a death rate with control of less than 10% | 136 | 8956 (94) | 81/4591 (1.8) | 92/4365 (2.1) | 0.8 (0.6–1.1) | n/c |

n/c = NNT not calculated because no significant difference.

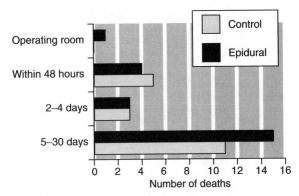

**Figure 2.7.6** Postoperative mortality and anaesthetic method [16].

Figure 2.7.7 gives us a clue to why that is. It plots the absolute risk increase obtained by subtracting placebo quit rate from nicotine quit rate for gum or patch, and plotting the absolute risk increase against the number of patients in the trial. What we see is that, for trials of fewer than 500 patients, the absolute risk increase runs from −5% to almost 30%, with many trials having absolute risk increases of 10% or more. For trials of more than 500 patients the spread is much less, from about −3% to 10%, and absolute risk increases were of the order of 0–5%.

There is another issue that Figure 2.7.7 hints at, namely why there are such huge differences in the trials. The answer, of course, is that there is considerable clinical heterogeneity, particularly in the situations where nicotine replacement was used. Many studies were in special circumstances, where perhaps the quit rates were being influenced by factors other than nicotine replacement. The authors might rightly argue that their analysis showed that nicotine replacement helped people stop smoking; after all, most of the points in Figure 2.7.7 demonstrate positive results for nicotine replacement.

**Table 2.7.3** NNTs obtained with larger or smaller trials of nicotine patch and gum

| | | Number of | | % quitting with | | |
| NRT type | Trial size | Trials | Patients | NRT | Placebo | NNT (95% CI) |
| --- | --- | --- | --- | --- | --- | --- |
| Patch | > 500 | 9 | 11, 170 | 13 | 8 | 18 (15–22) |
| Patch | < 500 | 22 | 4508 | 17 | 9 | 13 (10–17) |
| Gum | > 500 | 7 | 8509 | 13 | 9 | 25 (18–38) |
| Gum | < 500 | 41 | 8197 | 25 | 15 | 11 (9–13) |

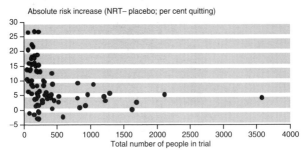

**Figure 2.7.7** Difference between nicotine patch or gum and placebo patch or gum for smoking cessation after at least 6 months.

And that is true. The trouble comes when people extrapolate from the general to the particular. In the Cochrane review, the overall NNT for one person to quit smoking compared with placebo was about 18. That would make it well worth using in primary care as a health promotion measure. But when primary care studies specifically are examined, a different result might be obtained.

Look at an example for nursing interventions for smoking cessation, and the very large differences between nursing interventions in hospital, after coronary artery bypass, for instance, and in primary care (Table 2.7.4) [18]. In hospital patients there was a significant relative benefit from nursing interventions (using both random and fixed effects models), with 7% more quitting smoking and generating an NNT of 14. That is, for every 14 patients given a nursing intervention, one more will quit smoking than would have done so without the nursing intervention. In unselected primary care patients there was no benefit from nursing interventions (using both random and fixed effects models). Nursing interventions in unselected primary care patients are probably not effective. The intervention was much the same, but the patients and setting for the intervention were not. We really have no idea whether the same holds true for nicotine replacement in primary care.

### Examples of useful meta-analyses

There are many of them. Examples would have to include some of the fantastic work done around the use of aspirin in secondary prevention, or tamoxifen in breast cancer, where large numbers of trials have been evaluated at the individual patient level to produce results that have changed practice. For the moment, though, we are going to concentrate on a series of indirect comparisons, because these can often be most helpful in making decision about policy, and making decisions about individual patients. Four examples, then, from the pages of Bandolier in Figures 2.7.8–2.7.11, which plot NNT or some measure of effect size against placebo for a series of interventions in acute pain, migraine, statins, and antiemetics in chemotherapy.

**Table 2.7.4** Smoking cessation: results for nursing interventions versus control analysed by hospital and primary care setting

| Setting | Number of studies | Number quitting/total | | % quitting (95%CI) | | Relative benefit (95%CI) | NNT (95%CI) |
|---|---|---|---|---|---|---|---|
| | | Intervention | Control | Intervention | Control | | |
| Hospital | 7 | 435/1367 | 318/1295 | 32 (30–34) | 25 (23–27) | 1.3 (1.1–1.6) | 14 (9 to 26) |
| Primary care | 3 | 111/2453 | 41/1006 | 4.5 (3.7–5.3) | 4.1 (2.9–5.3) | 0.8 (0.3–2.6) | 222 (52 to –98) |
| Combined | 10 | 546/3820 | 359/2301 | 14 (12–16) | 16 (14–18) | 1.2 (0.9–1.6) | –76 (184 to –32) |

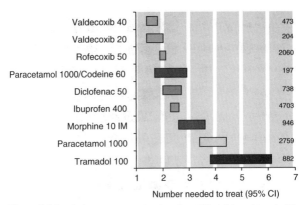

**Figure 2.7.8** Analgesics in acute pain—bars show 95% confidence interval of the NNT for at least half pain relief over 4–6 hours compared with placebo (mostly single oral dose in patients with established moderate to severe pain; dose in mg; numbers on right are number of patients in the meta-analysis).

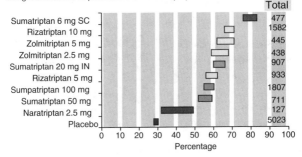

**Figure 2.7.9** Triptans for acute migraine—bars show 95% confidence interval of percentage of patients with no pain or mild pain after 2 hours (mostly single oral doses, except for single subcutaneous (SC) or intranasal (IN) dosing; dose in mg; numbers on right are number of patients in the meta-analysis).

It is great to have good data like this, but can we trust it? Well often more than one meta-analysis is done of the same data. It can be quite interesting to see whether they give the same results or not. In some of the sections above we have looked at meta-analyses and come up with different results. An example of where different analyses come up with the same result is that of rizatriptan 10 mg for acute migraine, where a series of analyses (Table 2.7.5) demonstrated considerable concordance, despite having different access to data (one looked at individual patient data; others used published trials) and using different numbers of trials and definitions of patients included in an intention-to treat analysis.

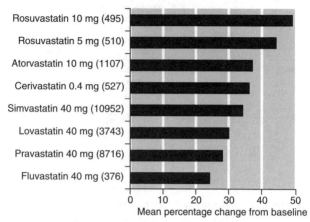

**Figure 2.7.10** Efficacy of common doses of statins in reducing LDL-cholesterol (numbers show total number of patients).

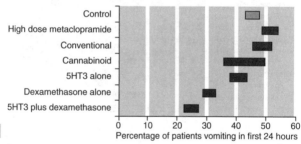

**Figure 2.7.11** Percentage of patients vomiting in the first 24 hours after chemotherapy.

### Indirect comparisons

There has been a sort of received wisdom that it is impossible to say anything about the relative efficacy of two different interventions for the same condition unless they are compared directly in head-to-head randomized controlled trials. There will be circumstances where that may well be true, but an important study [19] indicates that indirect comparisons are likely to be just as good in most cases.

If we have trials of treatment A versus placebo and treatment B versus placebo, are we able to make any comment on how good treatment A is compared to treatment B, without a trial that directly compares treatment A versus treatment B? We want to know if the relative efficacy of treatment is the same whether we compare them in a head-to-head race or if

**Table 2.7.5** Comparison of three reviews for rizatriptan 10 mg

| | Number needed to treat (95% confidence interval) for rizatriptan 10 mg | | | | |
| | At 2 hours | | Over 24 hours | |
| Meta-analysis | Headache response | Pain free | Sustained response | Sustained pain free |
|---|---|---|---|---|
| Gawel et al.[*] | 2.8 (2.6 to 3.2) | 3.2 (2.9 to 3.5) | | |
| Ferrari et al.[†] | 3.0 (2.8 to 3.4) | 3.2 (3.0 to 3.5) | 5.3 (4.6 to 6.2) | 5.5 (4.9 to 6.4) |
| Oldman et al.[‡] | 2.7 (2.4 to 2.9) | 3.1 (2.9 to 3.4) | 5.6 (4.5 to 7.4) | |

[*] Gawel, M.J. et al. (2001). A systematic review of the use of triptans in acute migraine. *Canadian Journal of Neurological Science* **28**, 30–41. This review used only tablet data from 6 trials.
[†] Ferrari, M.D. et al. (2001). Meta-analysis of rizatriptan efficacy in randomized controlled clinical trials. *Cephalalgia* **21**, 129–36. This review used data from tablets and wafers in 7 trials, but had individual data from trial records.
[‡] Oldman, A.D. et al. (2002). A systematic review of treatment for acute migraine. *Pain* **97**, 247–57. This review combined tablet and wafer from 7 trials, but probably used a different definition of intention to treat as numbers of patients differed.

each races separately against the clock (in this case, placebo). The argument against might well take the form that these were different trials, with different randomization, and perhaps in patients with different severity of disease at baseline, conducted over different periods of time, and in which different outcomes may have been measured. There may also be reservations about the amount of information available, because with smaller numbers the possibility that the random play of chance may affect the results would inevitably be greater. Any or all of these should invalidate indirect comparisons.

These are important and valid arguments. But if we have trials, in which we know that the severity of the condition is the same or very similar, conducted over the same duration, using the same outcome reported in the same way, and we have large enough amounts of information, might we not then be allowed to draw some conclusions?

In the study were 44 direct and indirect comparisons available for analysis from 28 meta-analyses. The relative risk for the direct comparison (A versus B) was compared with an imputed relative risk of A versus B from studies of A and B versus a common comparator. For some trials an odds ratio, and for others mean differences, were available.

In general, relative risks were the same for direct or indirect comparisons (Figure 2.7.12). Most of the results were similar in terms of positive, negative, or non-significant effect, with 32 of 44 indirect comparisons giving the same result as the direct comparison.

Of the 12 that were discrepant:

- eight involved sample sizes so small as to make any conclusion suspect;
- two involved minor changes to a confidence interval either side of 1, thus changing a statistical rather than any clinical conclusion;
- one was related to analysis of different doses;
- one was possibly a really different conclusion.

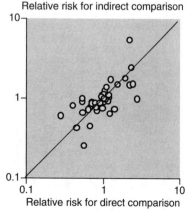

**Figure 2.7.12** Indirect versus direct comparison.

By another calculation of discrepancy, the authors indicate that three comparisons may be showing different answers, though of these one was related to analysis of different doses, and the other two could also have dose differences as complicating factors.

So there we have it, indirect comparisons are OK, and perhaps offer a more robust way forward because direct comparisons are often lacking, and certainly offer a viable alternative when direct comparisons are not available or not possible.

### Commentary

Systematic reviews and meta-analyses of clinical trials are really useful things. They allow us to see all the information on trials investigating a particular problem in one place and time. They often, if they are any good, discuss what makes a good clinical trial, to help us understand what is going on. Some of them will be misleading, either because the trials used are not good or because the review or meta-analysis is daft. But we have our antennae twitching to spot when wool is being pulled over eyes. It won't do to ignore systematic reviews and meta-analyses, and we have to learn to live with them. A dose of healthy scepticism and knowledge of some of the tools to overcome problems will be a big help in making sure that they do not flummox us.

So, one final example. Between 1996 and 2005 there have been 35 systematic reviews published on acupuncture, not counting duplicates or updates. In these 35 systematic reviews, their authors have claimed a qualified benefit of acupuncture for whatever indication in 16 reviews, and a strong positive outcome (meaning that in their view there was strong evidence that acupuncture was effective) in six (Table 2.7.6). That is, more than half of the systematic reviews claimed acupuncture to be a good thing.

Yet when one applies criteria of quality, validity, and size, one gets a different view. Throw out trials that are not randomized and blind. Throw out trials that have immediate outcomes for long-term conditions. What is left is a pitiful number of trials, and most of higher quality show no benefit. And most are small. The systematic review with the largest amount of data is on acupressure for nausea and vomiting [20], and the authors claim the systematic review supports the use of P6 acupoint stimulation. Table 2.7.7 might make one think again.

Depending on whether one is interested in fixed or random effects of the relative risk, statistical significance is lost when open studies were

**Table 2.7.6** Outcomes of systematic reviews in acupuncture

| Reviews of acupuncture | Number |
| --- | --- |
| Systematic reviews 1996–2005 | 33 |
| Any positive outcome, qualified by author | 16 |
| Any strong positive outcome | 6 |
| Any robust evidence, according to QVS criteria | 0 |

QVS, Quality, validity, size.

**Table 2.7.7** Applying quality, validity, and size to trials of acupuncture or acupressure for postoperative nausea and vomiting. Relative risk from fixed effects (upper figure) and random effects (lower figure) models

| Sensitivity analysis | Nausea | | Vomiting | | Antiemetic | |
|---|---|---|---|---|---|---|
| | Trials/patients | Relative risk (95% CI) | Trials/patients | Relative risk (95% CI) | Trials/patients | Relative risk (95% CI) |
| Randomized | 16/1826 | 0.79 (0.70 to 0.89) 0.73 (0.57 to 0.93) | 20/2187 | 0.74 (0.65 to 0.84) 0.71 (0.56 to 0.91) | 15/1492 | 0.78 (0.67 to 0.92) 0.79 (0.61 to 1.02) |
| Randomized and blind | 10/1150 | 0.84 (0.74 to 0.95) 0.78 (0.58 to 1.05) | 12/1328 | 0.83 (0.71 to 0.97) 0.84 (0.62 to 1.14) | 10/1048 | 0.81 (0.67 to 0.99) 0.83 (0.64 to 1.09) |
| Randomized, blind, over 100 pts | 5/885 | 0.90 (0.79 to 1.04) 0.82 (0.58 to 1.17) | 6/988 | 0.81 (0.67 to 0.98) 0.79 (0.55 to 1.14) | 6/848 | 0.84 (0.68 to 1.03) 0.83 (0.62 to 1.11) |
| Randomized, blind, over 100 pts, control event rate ≥20% | 5/885 | 0.90 (0.79 to 1.04) 0.82 (0.58 to 1.17) | 4/567 | 0.76 (0.62 to 0.92) 0.76 (0.54 to 1.05) | 3/444 | 0.92 (0.74 to 1.14) 0.89 (0.69 to 1.16) |

excluded, with small studies excluded, when studies with no one vomiting were excluded (because they lack sensitivity). So what starts as an exciting result finishes as one saying that P6 acupoint stimulation made no difference to nausea, or vomiting, or use of antiemetics.

Though this demonstrates, again, how sceptical one needs to be even with Cochrane reviews, it does demonstrate how useful applying quality, validity, and size criteria is to getting at the truth.

## References

1. Chalmers, I. *et al.* (1992). Getting to grips with Archie Cochrane's agenda. *British Medical Journal* **305**, 786–7.
2. Jadad, A.R. and McQuay, H.J. (1993). A high-yield strategy to identify randomized controlled trials for systematic reviews. *Online Journal of Current Clinical Trials* [Serial Online] Doc. No. 33, 3973.
3. Simes, R.J. (1987). Confronting publication bias: a cohort design for meta-analysis. *Statistics in Medicine* **6**, 11–29.
4. Hetherington, J. *et al.* (1989). Retrospective and prospective identification of unpublished controlled trials: lessons from a survey of obstetricians and pediatricians. *Pediatrics* **84**, 374–80.
5. Oxman, A.D. and Guyatt, G.H. (1988). Guidelines for reading literature reviews. *Canadian Medical Association Journal* **138**, 697–703.
6. Gavaghan, D.J. *et al.* (2000). An evaluation of homogeneity tests in meta-analysis in pain using simulations of individual patient data. *Pain* **85**, 415–24.
7. Higgins, J.P.T. *et al.* (2003). Measuring inconsistency in meta-analyses. *British Medical Journal* **327**, 557–60.
8. L'Abbé, K.A. *et al.* (1987). Meta-analysis in clinical research. *Annals of Internal Medicine* **107**, 224–33.
9. Lewis, S. and Clarke, M. (2001). Forest plots: trying to see the woods for the trees. *British Medical Journal* **322**, 1479–80.
10. Wiffen, P. *et al.* (2005). Carbamazepine for acute and chronic pain. *The Cochrane Database of Systematic Reviews* 2005, Issue 3.
11. Hotopf, M. *et al.* (2002). Depression in advanced disease: a systematic review part 1. Prevalence and case finding. *Palliative Medicine* **16**, 81–97.
12. Trinh, K.V. *et al.* (2004). Acupuncture for the alleviation of lateral epicondyle pain: a review. *Rheumatology* **43**,1085–90.
13. Linde, K. *et al.* (1997). Are the clinical effects of homeopathy placebo effects? A meta-analysis of placebo-controlled trials. *Lancet* **350**, 834–43.
14. Ernst, E. (2002). A systematic review of systematic reviews of homeopathy. *British Journal of Clinical Pharmacology* **54**, 577–82.
15. Rodgers, A *et al.* (2000). Reduction in postoperative mortality and morbidity with epidural or spinal anaesthesia: results from overview of randomised trials. *British Medical Journal* 2000 **321**, 1–12.
16. Rigg, J.R. *et al.* (2002). Epidural anaesthesia and analgesia and outcome of major surgery: a randomised trial. *Lancet* **359**, 1276–82.
17. Silagy, C. *et al.* (2001). Nicotine replacement therapy for smoking cessation (Cochrane Review). *Cochrane Database of Systematic Reviews* 2001, issue 1.
18. Moore, R.A. *et al.* (2002). Pooling data for number needed to treat: no problems for apples. *BMC Medical Research Methodology* **2**, 2. (http://www.biomedcentral.com/1471–2288/2/2).
19. Song, F. *et al.* (2003). Validity of indirect comparison for estimating efficacy of competing interventions: empirical evidence from published meta-analyses. *British Medical Journal* **326**, 472–6.
20. Lee, A. and Done, M.L. (2004). Stimulation of the wrist acupuncture point P6 for preventing postoperative nausea and vomiting. *Cochrane Database of Systematic Reviews* 2004, Issue 3.

# Section 3

# Observational studies

# 3.1 Observational studies: an introduction

Observational studies are usually cohort or case-control studies that seek associations between one feature (being overweight) and another (dying from heart disease or cancer). There are many such studies, and later in this section there are a few rules of thumb about how to treat such data. All these studies do is to provide evidence of an association (fat people are likely to die early from heart attack, say). It does not tell us that being fat causes heart attack, though we have abundant additional evidence from different sources to help substantiate the causation implicit in the association. Most of what we know about the deleterious effects of smoking on health comes from observational studies.

It is well known that medical journals try to get their contents into the public domain (meaning newspapers, TV, and radio, as well as the Internet) by issuing press releases, usually towards the week-end. These press releases are not written by hard-boiled, cautious, evidence freaks, so it is all too frequent for studies to be championed because they report apparent good or bad news (drinking cuts/increases cancer; chocolate is bad/good for you). Most, if not all of these come from two sources—animal studies (two rats and a mouse) or observational studies.

Observational studies are great for raising questions, but not for answering them or, as some clever folk once put it, 'observational studies propose, RCTs dispose' [1]. Observational studies that produce large numbers of comparisons are likely to come up with some statistically significant results if we accept a p-value of 0.05 as significant. It may be more sensible to use much more stringent levels of statistical significance, and a level of 0.001 (1 in 1000, rather than 1 in 20) has been proposed [1].

## Observational caution: causation

There are rules that we use to examine causation, and these are outlined in Table 3.1.1 (and they are important enough to be repeated in later chapters). They ask about strength of association, timing, dose-response, and other linking evidence. We need more than association to proceed to causation. It may be dark outside, and the light may be on, but putting the light on doesn't cause it to become dark outside.

## Observational caution: confounding

Confounding is where one factor that is not itself causally related to disease is associated with a range of other factors that are. Behaviours are closely related to health outcomes, but are often linked. People who eat poorly with little fruit and vegetables also tend to eat fatty foods, be overweight, take little exercise, and smoke. People who eat well with lots of fruit and vegetables also tend not to eat fatty foods, and are less likely to be overweight and smoke. Sorting the independent effect of any one factor from others is therefore going to be difficult. Increasing the significance level provides no protection against being misled by confounding associations. Confounding by indication is a special sort of bias that can arise in observational studies when patients with the worst prognosis are allocated preferentially to a particular treatment. These patients are likely to be

**Table 3.1.1** Rules of causation

| Feature | Comment |
| --- | --- |
| Consistency and unbiasedness of findings | Confirmation of the association by different investigators, in different populations, using different methods |
| Strength of association | Two aspects: the frequency with which the factor is found in the disease, and the frequency with which it occurs in the absence of the disease. The larger the relative risk, the more the hypothesis is strengthened |
| Temporal sequence | Obviously, exposure to the factor must occur before onset of the disease. In addition, if it is possible to show a temporal relationship as between exposure to the factor in the population and frequency of the disease, the case is strengthened |
| Biological gradient (dose-response relationship) | Finding a quantitative relationship between the factor and the frequency of the disease. The intensity or duration of exposure may be measured |
| Specificity | If the determinant being studied can be isolated from others and shown to produce changes in the incidence of the disease, e.g. if thyroid cancer can be shown to have a higher incidence specifically associated with fluoride, this is convincing evidence of causation |
| Coherence with biological background and previous knowledge | The evidence must fit the facts that are thought to be related, e.g. the rising incidence of dental fluorosis and the rising consumption of fluoride are coherent |
| Biological plausibility | The statistically significant association fits well with previously existing knowledge |
| Reasoning by analogy | Common sense, especially when you have other similar examples for types of intervention and outcome |
| Experimental evidence | This aspect focuses on what happens when the suspected offending agent is removed. Is there improvement? The evidence of remission—or even resolution of significant medical symptoms—following explanation obviously would strengthen the case. It is unethical to do an experiment that exposes people to the risk of illness, but it is permissible and indeed desirable to conduct an experiment, i.e. a randomized controlled trial on control measures. If fluoride is suspected of causing thyroid dysfunction, for example, the experiment of eliminating or reducing occupational exposure to the toxin and conducting detailed endocrine tests on the workers could help to confirm or refute the suspicion |

systematically different from those not treated, or treated with something else.

An example is asthmatic patients given paracetamol rather than NSAIDs for pain relief. To then argue that paracetamol causes asthma is a glorious example of confounding by indication.

The trouble with confounding associations is that we may not know they are there. Davey Smith and Ebrahim put it best [1].

We live in an associational world—people who are disadvantaged in one regard tend to be disadvantaged in other regards, since the forces that structure life chances and experience tend to ensure that some folk get the worst of all things. We showed this by producing a pairwise correlation matrix of 133 physical examination and laboratory assay variables (8778 correlations) derived from a study of over 4000 older women. This would be expected to yield 88 'significant' chance associations at the $p < 0.01$ level. In fact over 3000 such correlations were observed with a $p$ value < 0.01. In many ways it is more remarkable when things don't 'significantly' correlate with each other than when they do.

A final word on confounding. Many observational studies tell you that they have made allowances in their results for known confounding associations. They rarely say how, or give any detail that would allow a reader to replicate their calculations. Much is taken on trust.

### Observational caution: size

The one feature that is rarely commented on is size—either the number of patients or subjects in the study or, perhaps more pertinent, the number of events that have been observed. Very often cohort and other observational studies have observed very few events, so that the chance of random effects can be high, as we saw earlier with randomized trials. A Bandolier rule of thumb goes something like this.

- Fewer than 20 events: dismiss.
- 20–50 events: be very cautious.
- 50–200 events: confidence is growing.
- More than 200 events: we can probably trust these data if everything else is OK.

### Observational caution: size of the effect

The one thing they never tell us about is the size of the effect. Suppose an observational study comes up with a (statistically significant) relative risk of 1.1. So what? It is only worth knowing (even if statistically significant at the 0.001 level) if the baseline risk is large. If 10 persons in 10,000 are affected without exposure to some possibly harmful event, then with exposure the number affected goes up to 11 per 10,000, or by 1 person extra in 10,000. If the baseline risk without exposure was 10 in 100, then the additional 1 in 100 (1%) might have large clinical as well as statistical significance.

So, when looking at results of observational studies, as well as looking at the number of events, and the level of statistical significance, also look at the size of the effect. Relative risks of 2 are interesting, and at 3 and above we should probably be beginning to take them seriously. If there are 20 events, a $p$-value of only 0.05, and a relative risk of 1.2, we should probably read no further. If there were 200 events, a $p$-value of 0.001, and a relative risk of 5, then this is likely to be really, really important.

**Cohort studies**

A cohort study follows a group of people from one point in time to another and observes changes that occur during that period. The study can be retrospective, for example, reviewing all cases of breast cancer, or prospective, identifying a group of healthy people or patients and following them through time. Cohort studies may use routine data or data specially collected for the purpose of the study or both.

A cohort study is one in which subjects who presently have or don't have a certain condition, or diagnosis, or who receive a particular treatment are followed over time. They may be compared with another group who are not affected by the condition under investigation, or sometimes no comparison group may be needed, for instance, in a study of the natural history of a disease with or without treatment.

For research purposes, a cohort is any group of individuals linked in some way (by age, or sex, or occupation, or illness), who have experienced some significant life event within a given period (who have had a heart attack, or who have no disease), or who have experienced some treatment (joint replacement for arthritis, for instance). There are many kinds of cohorts, including birth (for example, all those who are born in certain years), disease, education, employment, family type. Any study in which there are measures of some characteristic of one or more cohorts at two or more points in time is cohort analysis. Cohort analysis attempts to identify cohort effects: Are changes in a dependent variable (health problems in this example) due to ageing, or are they present because the sample members belong to the same cohort (smoking)?

Cohort studies can be very powerful. Cohort studies are about the life histories of sections of populations and the individuals who comprise them. They can tell us what circumstances in early life are associated with the population's characteristics in later life, or what encourages development in particular directions and what impedes it. Much of what we know about the effects of smoking on health comes from cohort studies. Cohort studies linking health outcomes to lifestyle (diet, exercise, weight) are now common, and can be very powerful agents in helping society identify ways to improve the quality and quantity of life for individuals.

This type of research is useful for studying:

- the outcome of treatment where a randomized controlled trial is impossible, for example, the outcome of intensive care or prostatectomy. The findings of this type of study allow quality standards (for example, the readmission rate to intensive care or after prostatectomy) to be evidence-based.

- different approaches to service delivery and management where these cannot be tested by a randomized controlled trial, either because the number of units are too small to give a trial of adequate power or because the health service policy makers or managers will not allow their service to be included in such a trial. In addition, cohort studies are also a useful means of studying 'natural experiments', i.e. when changes are made in the organization or delivery for political or managerial reasons or where different patterns of care exist in similar settings as a result of history and tradition.

Often cohort studies involve exposure to a risk factor, which may be a genetic trait, an environmental exposure, a lifestyle, or specific physiological risk factors. Cohort studies are expensive because for rare diseases a large sample is needed.

### Questions to ask about a cohort study

Certain steps are required to conduct cohort studies, and the steps in the example below would be necessary for a cohort study to determine the incidence of a particular disease or death in the cohort. For other outcomes, similar criteria would be applied, specific for that purpose.

1. Define a hypothesis to be tested.
2. Define the population to be studied.
3. Take a sample of this population.
4. Evaluate the exposure status by applying a test to the sample to determine the presence or absence of a risk factor in each individual.
5. Exclude from the study individuals who already have the disease.
6. Continue to observe the sample in a follow-up, being careful to follow the cases closely to maintain a high response rate.
7. Monitor the individuals for their outcome; detect cases of disease or death.

Useful questions to ask about a cohort study to assess its quality include those below, but no formal quality test has been devised.

- Is clear information given about the way in which the cohort was recruited? (Recruitment setting, diagnostic criteria, disease severity, co-morbidity, and demographic details should be documented.)
- Were any factors that could have included or excluded more severe cases considered?
- If mortality is an outcome, what steps have been taken to ensure that all deaths have been identified?
- Were objective outcome criteria developed and used?
- Was outcome assessment blind?
- If other measures are used, have the instruments used for measurement been validated?

- Was the severity of disease taken into account in the analysis?
- Was the presence of other diseases (co-morbidity) taken into account in the analysis?
- Were more than 80% of the patients entered accounted for in results and their clinical status known?

### Features to emphasize

When appraising the recruitment of individuals into a cohort study the most important feature to note is the completeness of recruitment. All the subjects in a defined time period should be recruited. Any sampling procedure, for example, the recruitment of patients admitted only on weekdays or between 09.00 and 17.00 hours, should create suspicion that the study is biased. It can also be useful to ask, 'Where did patients go who were not admitted?', because the hospital may have referred the more difficult cases elsewhere or those referrers may have selectively referred only the mild cases to the hospital being studied.

Secondly, it is important to ensure that valid criteria are used. Inpatient mortality is an invalid criterion of the quality of the hospital care because of variations in duration of stay, and it is better to use a criterion such as the 30- or 60-day mortality. When criteria other than morbidity are used, the tools used to measure variables such as pain or quality of life should be validated measuring instruments.

Finally, in the analysis the severity of illness (the case-mix) should always be taken into account and therefore explicitly mentioned in the text. In studies of intensive care, for example, a validated system for assessing severity—the APACHE (acute physiology and chronic health evaluation) system is used. It is also essential to take into account the presence or absence of other diseases, co-morbidity, that might have influenced outcome. Robust techniques have been developed for doing this and must be used if valid results are to be obtained.

### Uses and abuses

The main abuse of a cohort study is as a means of assessing the effectiveness of a particular intervention when the more appropriate method could be a randomized controlled trial. Cohort studies are appropriate when assessing changes in service management or organization or in searching for uncommon side-effects or adverse effects of treatment.

### Cohort examples

#### Hip and knee replacement

An Australian study [2] reported on part of an ongoing prospective trial that included patients of nine orthopaedic surgeons in four Sydney hospitals. Patients with a diagnosis of osteoarthritis or rheumatoid arthritis were eligible, though here only results for osteoarthritis were reported. Preoperatively and every 3 months after the joint-replacement operation for 12 months, patients were mailed monthly WOMAC and SF-36 questionnaires to be self-administered, and reminded by telephone to complete them. WOMAC is the Western Ontario and McMaster Universities osteoarthritis index, measuring dimensions of pain, stiffness, and physical function. SF-36 is a generic quality of life questionnaire assessing 36 items in eight domains. WOMAC scoring uses 24 questions on a 1–5 scale for each question, which was transformed to a 0–100 scale, and SF-36 scores on a 0–100 scale.

There was a 67% response rate in 252 patients recruited. The 194 participants had an average age of 74 years, and 86 had osteoarthritis of the hip and 108 of the knee. The overall follow-up averaged 11 months. Disease duration averaged 10 years. Half of the patients were women.

There were significant improvements for all three areas of the WOMAC scale of physical function (Figure 3.1.1; where lower scores are better), pain, and stiffness for both hip and knee replacement. For physical functioning (Figure 3.1.1), hip replacement resulted in a beneficial reduction in the WOMAC score from 37 to 12.

There were significant improvements in the SF-36 quality of life questionnaire for most of the eight domains for both hip and knee replacement (Table 3.1.2, where higher scores are better). Bodily pain, physical functioning, and physical role functioning were most improved. Exceptions were emotional role function for both hip and knee, and general health and mental health for knee replacements, though both scores were high initially. For both of the scales the first 3 months following joint replace-

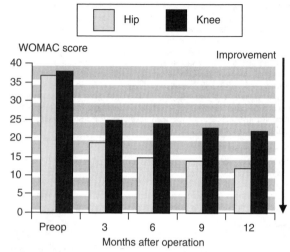

**Figure 3.1.1** Physical functioning (WOMAC). Higher scores are worse.

ment found the largest changes. Improvements tended to continue over the succeeding 9 months, but at a lower rate.

These are major beneficial changes from joint replacement surgery. A previous report [3] demonstrated that, at all ages from 55 years, hip replacement brought SF-36 scores for osteoarthritis patients back to population norms for age. Knee replacement was almost as good, except

**Table 3.1.2** Preoperative and 12 month scores in SF-36 domains (0–100) for hip and knee replacement

| SF-36 domain | Hip replacement | | Knee replacement | |
|---|---|---|---|---|
| | Preop | 12 months | Preop | 12 months |
| General health | 66 | **74** | 71 | 70 |
| Bodily pain | 33 | **73** | 33 | **57** |
| Physical function | 27 | **67** | 25 | **50** |
| Physical role function | 15 | **59** | 18 | **50** |
| Social function | 53 | **89** | 59 | **77** |
| Mental health | 71 | **82** | 70 | 77 |
| Emotional role function | 60 | 72 | 54 | 65 |
| Vitality | 47 | **68** | 47 | **59** |

Bold areas show statistical significance at 5% level. Higher scores indicate a better health state.

that, in the age group of 55–64 years, population norms were not all achieved.

For most patients having hip or knee replacement large quality of life gains will occur. With the modest cost of the operations, this will mean the cost per quality-adjusted life year will be low. The numbers in this study are low, but it is uncertain whether a randomized trial could ever be ethical, in which some patients were randomized to a group where no treatment meant they would not get better, and where they would suffer significant pain and low quality of life. Here a cohort is the only study design that makes sense. Because it examines a whole population, and finds big effects, over a reasonably long period of time, we can probably trust the results.

*Long-term outcome after head injury*

Trauma and its sequelae are major health problems, and it is one, if not the major, cause of death in children and young adults [4]. Head injury has a reported incidence of 150 to 300 per 100, 000 and is one of the most frequent injuries in trauma. A cohort study [4] conducted in Aquitaine (population 2.7 million) used data from a 1986 population-based study looking at all injuries serious enough to result in death or hospital admission. Of the 7281 patients identified, a cohort of 1005 (which included 407 head injury patients) was selected for follow-up. Head injury was defined as loss of consciousness, abnormal neurological examination, abnormalities on computerized tomography, or skull fractures. Trauma severity was rated using the abbreviated injury scale (AIS):

- AIS 1–2: short period of unconsciousness or linear skull fracture;
- AIS 3: complex skull fracture or cerebral contusion;
- AIS 4: prolonged unconsciousness or intracranial haematoma;
- AIS 5: unconsciousness > 24 hours, diffuse brain lesions, or severe mass effect.

Survivors were sent a letter 5 years after the initial trauma and were interviewed with a 200-item questionnaire at the institution or at home, or by phone, or by filling in the questionnaire at home and sending it back by post. Wherever possible, a close family member was interviewed separately to supply information on the patient's behaviour. Of the 407 head injury patients, 64 had died, 36 were lost to follow-up, and three refused to participate, so data were available on 304 patients.

Patients in the cohort were predominantly under the age of 60 years (90%), and 50–60% were under 30 years at the time of their injury. About two-thirds were male, and almost all had received their head injury in a traffic accident or fall. Almost all the patients lived at home. About 4% needed family support because of behavioural or cognitive problems, and this was permanent in about 20% of the most severe cases. Epilepsy and hemiparesis were present in 0.7% of the whole head injury cohort.

Overall good outcome depended inversely on AIS class (Figure 3.1.2). Using the Glasgow outcome score, recovery in survivors was good in 98, 97, 88, and 47% of patients in AIS 1–2, 3, 4, and 5 respectively. Five-year death rates were class-dependent, with 56% mortality in AIS class 5 (Figure 3.1.2).

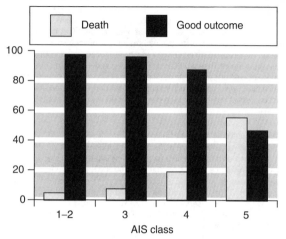

**Figure 3.1.2** Good overall outcome and 5-year death rates according to AIS score.

An impairment was defined as any loss or abnormality in body structure or function. Headaches, dizziness, memory disturbance, depressive mood, irritability, and anxiety were common. They occurred in 25% or more of patients of all AIS classes, and there was a tendency for some of these to be more severe in those in AIS 5.

A disability was defined as a change in ability to perform an activity within the range considered normal. Few patients in AIS 2–3 were affected, but disability was higher in AIS classes 4 and 5, with difficulty in walking, taking public transport, dressing, washing, and dealing with paperwork.

A handicap was defined as a disadvantage that limited the fulfilment of a role that was normal for that individual. At the time of their injury 37% of patients were working. After 5 years 15% could not work any more because of their injury.

Ninety-six patients were children at school in 1986. It was estimated that 7% of these students had problems in studying again, mostly because of behavioural changes.

These are outcomes that could only be provided by a long-term longitudinal cohort study. And they are important findings, providing good prognostic evidence for use of the Abbreviated Injury Scale.

### Case-control studies

A case-control study helps to determine whether an exposure is associated with an outcome (i.e. disease or condition of interest). First, a series of cases (a group known to have the outcome) with a set of controls (a group known to be free of the outcome) are identified. Then information is sought about which subjects in each group had the exposure, comparing the frequency of the exposure in the case group to that in the control group.

A case-control study is always retrospective because it starts with an outcome and then traces back to investigate exposures. When the subjects are enrolled in their respective groups, the investigator already knows the outcome of each subject. This, and not the fact that the investigator usually makes use of previously collected data, is what makes case-control studies retrospective.

Case-control studies are relatively quick, inexpensive, and easy. They are appropriate for studying rare diseases or outcomes. Because they start with people known to have the outcome (rather than starting with a population free of disease and waiting to see who develops it), it is possible to enrol a sufficient number of patients with a rare disease. They do require good databases, and improvement in IT systems and record-keeping in some parts of the world makes performing case-control studies much easier than formerly. In some parts of the world (with Denmark as perhaps the best example) an individual can be identified by a number used to link many different databases, and whole populations can be effectively enrolled in case-control studies. Case-control studies may also be ideal for preliminary investigation of a suspected risk factor for a common condition, or adverse event related to a drug or intervention exposure. Conclusions from a preliminary case-control study may be used to justify a more costly and time-consuming longitudinal study.

The key to the case-control study is matching controls to the cases. Controls should be chosen who are as similar as possible to the cases. Various factors (age, sex, hospital admission date, date of vaccination) can be chosen to define how controls are to be similar to the cases. Although controls must be like the cases in many ways, it is possible to over-match. Over-matching can make it difficult to find enough controls. An important technique for adding power to a study is to enrol more than one control for every case. For statistical reasons there is little gained by including more than two controls per case, but some studies enrol up to 10 controls for every case.

Case control studies can be efficient but are subject to bias.

A case control study follows well-defined steps.

1. Identify cases of the disease (or clinical events) to be studied. Ideally, all the cases in a population should be studied to lessen selection bias. New (incident) cases should be selected because previously diagnosed (prevalent) cases represent long-term survivors.

2. Recruit control subjects without disease from the same population. At least one control is needed for each case studied but two or more controls can be used to increase the statistical power. The controls should be matched for age, sex, and any other crucial factor to the cases being studied.

3. Assess cases and controls for prior exposure to the risk factor being evaluated.

4. Analyse the results. In case control studies the rate of the disease in the population is unknown.

### Case-control study examples
*Autism, febrile seizures, and epilepsy are not associated with MMR vaccination*
The lack of association of MMR vaccination with autism came from a retrospective study of all children born in Denmark between January 1991 and December 1998 [5]. In Denmark, a system of unique personal identification numbers, linked to vaccination registers, and linked information about the diagnosis of autism makes almost complete follow-up possible. A record review of 40 children with autism by a consultant in child psychiatry confirmed that 37 children met operational criteria for autism, showing that cases were properly recorded. The national Danish vaccination programme recommends first MMR vaccination at 15 months and again at 12 years.

There were 440,655 children vaccinated, and 96,648 children who were unvaccinated. The mean age of vaccination was 17 months, and 99% of children vaccinated had their first vaccination before they were 3 years of age. The proportion of vaccinated boys and girls was the same, at 82%. Table 3.1.3 shows the number and percentage of children who developed autism or autistic spectrum disorders.

Using person-years of exposure, there was no statistically significant difference between vaccinated and unvaccinated children for autism (relative risk 0.9, 95% confidence interval 0.7 to 1.2) or autistic spectrum disorders (relative risk 0.8, 0.7 to 1.1). There was no association between development of autism and age at vaccination (95% before 2 years of age) or the interval between vaccination and development of autism with no clustering at any particular time.

### Febrile seizures and epilepsy
The second study [6] used exactly the same database and patient numbers as the first [5] looking at MMR and autism. MMR vaccination status was obtained, together with information on febrile seizures or epilepsy for patients discharged from hospital, or seen in outpatients or emergency departments. There were 17,986 children with at least one febrile seizure, of which 973 occurred within 2 weeks of vaccination.

**Table 3.1.3** Number, percentage, and individual risk of autism and autistic spectrum disorders in MMR vaccinated and unvaccinated Danish children

|  | Vaccinated | Unvaccinated |
|---|---|---|
| Total | 440,655 | 96,648 |
| Number with autism | 263 | 53 |
| % with autism | 0.06 | 0.055 |
| Individual risk 1 in | 1667 | 1818 |
| Number with autistic spectrum disorder | 345 | 77 |
| % with autistic spectrum disorder | 0.078 | 0.08 |
| Individual risk 1 in | 1282 | 1250 |

The rate of first febrile seizure was higher in vaccinated than unvaccinated children, by 10% (relative risk 1.1; 95% CI 1.05 to 1.15). Febrile seizures occurred more frequently in the first and second week after MMR vaccination (relative risk 2.8; 2.6 to 3.0), but not at any time thereafter, up to 5 years. None of the following factors was associated with higher risk: siblings with febrile seizures or epilepsy; sex; birth order; gestational age at birth; birth weight; socioeconomic status; or maternal levels of education. There was additional risk in children with a previous history of febrile seizures.

Compared with children who were not vaccinated, the additional risk of febrile seizures within 14 days of MMR vaccination was one or two cases per 1000 doses of vaccine, so the risk increased from 1 per 1000 to 2–3 per 1000. For children with a history of febrile seizures the additional risk was 19 per 1000 doses, so it increased from 12 to 31 cases per 1000.

Compared with children who were not vaccinated, recurrent febrile seizures were very slightly increased in children who had one episode of febrile seizure within 14 days of vaccination (relative risk 1.2; 1.01 to 1.4), but no increased risk in those who experienced a seizure after 14 days.

Compared with children who were not vaccinated, there was no increased risk of epilepsy in children who had a febrile seizure within 14 days of MMR vaccination, or in those who had a febrile seizure after 14 days.

Both these studies are enormous and from a very important database. They used the whole population as cases and controls, over several years, and still managed only a few hundred cases of autism. Because of their size, quality, and comprehensiveness, and because they failed to find any association, we can be pretty sure that MMR is not a cause of autism from the first of these studies alone [2]. All the other evidence we have just helps.

It is also helpful to know that MMR vaccination has only a minor risk of increased febrile seizure, and none of epilepsy. MMR vaccination can produce a fever, and therefore increases the risk of a febrile seizure. The absolute risk is one or two per 1000 doses of vaccine. Children with a personal history of febrile seizures have a higher risk, of an additional 20 per 1000 doses of vaccine.

## Commentary

Observational studies can be very useful tools. The question about whether they provide the same or different answers to those from randomized trials is another question for another section. Right now, here is a brief rule of thumb for looking at observational studies and asking whether you can trust them (Table 3.1.4). There has been no testing of these rules, and others might add some points or subtract others, but they work for Bandolier.

## References

1. Davey Smith, G. and Ebrahim, S. (2002). Data dredging, bias, or confounding. They can all get you into the British Medical Journal and the Friday papers. *British Medical Journal* **325**, 1437–8.
2. Bachmeier, C.J. *et al.* (2001). A comparison of outcomes in osteoarthritis patients undergoing total hip and knee replacement surgery. *Osteoarthritis and Cartilage* **9**, 137–46.

**Table 3.1.4** Rules of thumb for looking at observational studies

| Point | Question | Reasoning |
|---|---|---|
| Recruitment | Does the study encompass a whole population? | Studies that encompass a whole population are less likely to be subjected to selection bias of any sort |
| | Were more or less severe cases selected or omitted? | Might limit the utility of any result |
| | What proportion recruited were available at follow-up? | If there is a large drop-out, then we rate the study lower and trust it less. If follow-up is good (over 80% and especially over 90%), our trust in any result increases |
| Diagnosis or case definition | Were standard criteria used, and were they objective? | For almost any condition there are standard criteria—for migraine, or arthritis, for instance. Use of standard definitions makes the study less subjective and more widely applicable |
| | Was presence of other diseases or other possible confounding factors taken into account? | Confounding is a big problem, and the more that is done to reassure us, and the more we know about absence of possible confounders, the better |
| Outcomes | How has any outcome been determined? Were standard criteria used? | More or less as above |
| | Were outcomes assessed blind? | May not be relevant, but if blinding was possible and done, it would make for a stronger case |
| Size | Were there a large number of events? | Fewer than 20 events: dismiss; 20–50 events: be very cautious; 50–200 events: confidence is growing; More than 200 events: we can probably trust these data if everything else is OK |
| Statistical significance | Was there a very high level of statistical significance reported? | $p < 0.05$ is not impressive $p < 0.01$ is better $p < 0.001$ is much, much better |
| Size of the effect | Was there a large effect (relative risk, odds ratio, hazard ratio)? | If the relative risk is (say) 1.1, then that is not impressive If it is 2.0, that is better If it is 3 and above, we really take notice |

3. March, L.M. *et al.* (1999). Outcomes after hip or knee replacement surgery for osteoarthritis. *Medical Journal of Australia* **171**, 235–8.
4. Masson, F. *et al.* (1997). Disability and handicap 5 years after a head injury: a population-based study. *Journal of Clinical Epidemiology* **50**, 595–601.

5. Madsen, K.M. *et al.* (2002). A population-based study of measles, mumps and rubella vaccination and autism. *New England Journal of Medicine* **347**, 1477–82.
6. Vestergaard, M. *et al.* (2004). MMR vaccination and febrile seizures: evaluation of susceptible subgroups and long-term prognosis. *Journal of the American Medical Association* **292**, 351–7.

## 3.2 Prevalence and incidence studies

Someone once told Bandolier that 6% of us have a rare disease. Those rare diseases are many and varied, so many and varied, in fact, that the majority of us will rarely or never have heard of more than a few of them. The figure for the percentage of us with common disease would be even more astounding, and few of us (anyone?) would have no disease or condition that wasn't (or couldn't) be medicalized, however fit, healthy, and beautiful we were.

Finding out how much disease is present is a special case for observational studies, almost certainly cohort studies. The main issues are the cases that are prevalent, or incident. Lots of people have trouble with these definitions so, for the avoidance of doubt, here they are.

- Prevalence. This is a measure of the proportion of people in a population who have a disease at a point in time, or over some period of time.
- Incidence. The proportion of new cases of the target disorder in the population at risk during a specified time interval.

For both it is usual to define the disorder, the population, the time or time period, and report the incidence as a rate.

Diagnosis is always the first key point to look for. There is the question of the diagnosis itself, whether it has been made according to some recognized scheme of diagnosis according to symptoms (the American College of Rheumatologists has definitions for arthritic disorders, or the International Headache Society for various forms of headache). There is also the question about whether every person in a cohort has been screened, or whether the diagnosis is made only on some patients complaining of certain symptoms.

It is also important to tell us how the rate is defined. For instance, if we report the number of bald Welshmen in a population (prevalence), do we give the proportion of the whole population (all people, men and women, of any age), or of adults, or of adult men, or of adult men of a specific age range? The numbers might be quite different depending on which you chose. Bandolier always remembers its old physics master who, on being given a number without units, used to ask whether it was so many elephants. So for prevalence and incidence, always remember the elephants.

A few examples of prevalence and incidence studies will help to show how useful they can be.

### Prevalence

#### Atrial fibrillation in California

This was a cross-sectional study of adults older than 20 years enrolled in a large (1.9 million) health maintenance organization (HMO) in California [1]. The enrolled population was examined to discover the number who had atrial fibrillation (AF) diagnosed in the 18 months between mid-1996 and end 1997. Patients were identified by searching for a diagnosis of atrial fibrillation in automated clinical databases, one of which included all diagnoses for inpatient and outpatient electrocardiograms. Transient atrial fibrillation after cardiac surgery was excluded, as was atrial fibrillation relating to recent-onset hyperthyroidism.

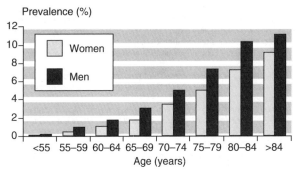

**Figure 3.2.1**   Prevalence of AF in California.

The same databases were searched for 5 years beforehand for diagnoses of valvular heart disease, stroke, atrial fibrillation, coronary heart disease, hypertension, and diabetes. Patient demographics were available, including ethnicity for almost all patients. The denominator for the prevalence calculation was the adult population of plan members, and the results were presented both for the total population and by different age ranges.

There were 17, 974 adults with atrial fibrillation, with 87% confirmed by electrocardiogram. The overall prevalence in the 1.9 million members was 0.95% (95% confidence interval, 0.94–0.96%). This increased with age from low levels in the under-55s to about 10% in the over-80s (Figure 3.2.1). Prevalence was greater in men than in women (1.1% vs 0.8%), and among patients aged over 55 was more common in white (2.2%) than black (1.5%) patients.

One interesting feature of this paper is that it exemplified how the use of electronic databases, together with coding of disease, testing of data to ensure its quality, and a bit of thought, can give interesting information on the amount of disease that we have to deal with. The paper also projected these figures on to the whole population of the USA, both now and for the next 50 years. Based on the growth in older people expected over this period, the number of people with AF in the USA was expected to grow from a current 2.3 million to 5.6 million by 2050.

### Body piercing and tattooing

If you wanted to know how common the practice of body piercing was, and searched the literature, you would find only one paper [2], examining body piercing and tattooing in undergraduates at an American university. A single-page questionnaire was refined through a pilot study, and then offered on a voluntary and anonymous basis to students over 4 months early in 2001. It asked about age and sex, and about body piercing and tattooing at various body sites, as well as about any complications associated with them. Women were specifically asked not to include pierced earlobes.

- There were 454 completed questionnaires (218 men, 236 women), about 15% of the total undergraduate population. The average age was 21 years.
- Tattoos were present in 22% of men and 26% of women undergraduates with one to three sites per individual. Common sites for men were hand or arm, backs and shoulders, and for women back. No complications were noted.
- Body piercing was present in 42% of men and 60% of women undergraduates, with 315 piercings in 229 students, with a maximum of five piercings.
- In men 31% had pierced ears, with tongue, eyebrow, nipple, genitals, and navel in 2% or fewer for each. Additionally 7% had had ear piercings removed, and tongue, nipple, and navel piercings had been removed in 2% or fewer.
- In women 29% had pierced navels, 27% had pierced ears (excluding pierced earlobes), 12% pierced tongue, and 5% pierced nipple, with genitals, nose, or lip in 2% or fewer. Additionally, 4% had had tongue piercings removed, 3% had navel piercings removed, and ear, eyebrow, nose, lip, nipple, and genital piercings had been removed in 2% or fewer.
- Complications were reported in 17% of piercings, the most common being bacterial infections, bleeding, and local trauma (Figure 3.2.2). No cases of viral infection were reported. Tongue piercing was associated with subsequent oral or dental injury in 10%.

At one level body piercing seems a simple problem, but we know of cases of very significant harm from piercing. The more people with piercings, the more likely we are to see problems, so knowing what proportion of the population is pierced and the rate of problems is helpful, even if it is, as here, from a limited and to some extent selected population.

### COPD prevalence

How many people have chronic obstructive pulmonary disease? A deceptively simple question, this, according to a systematic review of prevalence

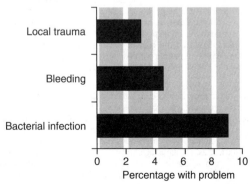

**Figure 3.2.2**  Body piercing problems.

rates [3]. It concludes that we just don't know, but it is probably more than we think. The problems are predictable, namely, the definition of the population in which we are interested, the definition of what COPD is, and how COPD is measured. What we seem to have is a number of goalposts all moving randomly in different directions.

The review used a single MEDLINE search designed to detect any studies that might have quantified the prevalence of COPD in countries or regions. Studies of interest were those that had a total population estimate or sex- or age-specific estimate of COPD and had methods sufficiently clear to establish what the sampling strategy was, what the diagnostic criteria were, and how the diagnosis was made.

The authors found 32 sources of prevalence data, most in 17 countries in the developed world. Most of the studies examined adults, but often with age restrictions and reported in both younger and older ages. Methods used to diagnose COPD included:

- Spirometry, with or without clinical examination. These studies were not uniform and usually involved some relationship of $FEV_1$ to slow or forced vital capacity, with the definition of COPD as being below some percentage of predicted. That percentage was itself variable.
- Presence of respiratory symptoms. Most of these studies used the MRC criteria of cough on most days of the week for 3 months of the year for at least 2 years.
- Patient-reported symptoms. Results here were generally derived from a patient's report of a physician's diagnosis.
- Expert opinion. This came from a WHO report on global health statistics, where disease experts made estimates based on published or unpublished studies, or informed estimates, followed by review at various stages.

Prevalence estimates varied, but the largest discrepancy was between the WHO expert opinion estimate of a world prevalence of 0.8% and all other studies where the estimate of overall prevalence was between 1% and 18%, with most between 3% and 10%. There were too many variables to determine what the differences were in different age groups, or using different diagnostic methods, but there was a tendency for prevalence to be higher in men. Estimates of prevalence where the population was large enough to be representative, in theory, of the entire population of a country are shown in Figure 3.2.3, overall, and for men and women separately. Most estimates again were between 3% and 10%.

The simple answer to our simple question is that we really don't know the prevalence of COPD with any accuracy, but it is probably more than we thought, and we probably do not pay sufficient attention to it. Definition makes a profound difference. One Italian study in a rural area in the Po valley applied various criteria used in Europe and the USA to about 2000 people aged 25 or older, and found that COPD prevalence could be as low as 11% or as high as 57%, depending on age and definition.

### Prevalence of multiple sclerosis and geography

Of course, disease prevalence is not a constant, neither in time nor place. We know that the prevalences of some infectious diseases were much higher in the past than they are now, and rates of many (such as measles in

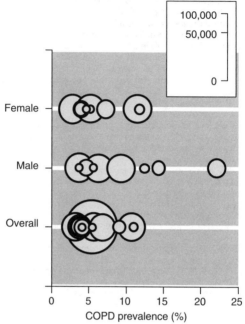

**Figure 3.2.3** Estimates of COPD prevalence in adults.

the UK) were falling long before vaccination began. We also know that many diseases, especially infectious or parasitic diseases, occur more in some parts of the world than in others. Other criteria, like diet and lifestyle, also play an enormous part in geographical variation. But sometimes geography can surprise, one example being the prevalence of multiple sclerosis.

There is considerable variation in the occurrence of MS around the world. This has been ascribed to environmental factors, like exposure to viruses or ionizing radiation, or to genetic factors. One constant, though, is that prevalence rates are higher in places closer to the poles compared with places closer to the equator. For instance, in the US the prevalence is about twice as high in North Dakota as in Florida. Here we look at two papers from the UK [4] and Australia [5].

The UK study examined the incidence and prevalence of MS in the Lothian and Borders region of Scotland in the mid-1990s, with a population of about 864,000. Incidence was examined prospectively over 3 years with cases ascertained from all neurology and neurosurgery wards in the study area. Standard diagnostic criteria were applied. There were 310 definite

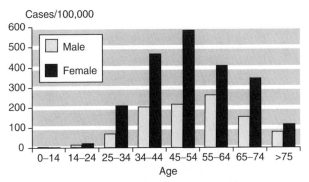

**Figure 3.2.4**   Prevalent cases in Lothian and Borders by age and sex.

cases (216 women and 94 men, sex ratio 2.3, mean age at diagnosis 34 years), giving an annual incidence of 12 (10.6 to 13.3) per 100,000. If probable cases were included also, the rate rose to 18 (16.5 to 19.8) per 100,000.

Prevalence was determined by defining a prevalent case as any person with a diagnosis of multiple sclerosis alive and normally resident in the area on 15 March 1995. Probable as well as definite cases were included. There were 1613 residents with a diagnosis of MS, giving a crude prevalence rate of 187/100,000. The sex ratio was 2.5 in favour of women and the mean age was 49 years (Figure 3.2.4).

There was a slight excess of cases in people whose surnames suggested a Scottish ancestry over that expected from the population average. Five studies of MS prevalence in Scotland have shown mean prevalence rates of about 150 to 200 cases/100,000, and have had 5–23% of names beginning with Mc or Mac. Six studies in England or Wales have prevalence rates of 90–110 cases/100,000, and have 1–2% of names suggesting Scottish ancestry. This can be suggested as forming a link between MS and genetic susceptibility in populations. However, geographical differences are also seen in the USA and in the Southern hemisphere, in largely immigrant populations with considerable mixing. That would argue against a genetic factor and more in favour of an environmental factor or factors.

The Lothian region of Scotland is about 55° of latitude N, and has a prevalence of about 180 cases of MS/100,000. England and Wales, about 50° N, have about 100 cases/100,000. Hobart is 42° S and has 74 cases/100,000, and tropical Queensland at about 18° S has 11/100,000. That describes the extent of the geographical association between latitude and MS. In Australia a study [5] has tried to unpick any relationship between ambient UV radiation and MS.

Crude MS prevalence data, age-standardized prevalence, number of MS patients, and total population information were obtained for tropical Queensland, subtropical Queensland, Western Australia, New South

Age–standardized MS prevalence per 100,000

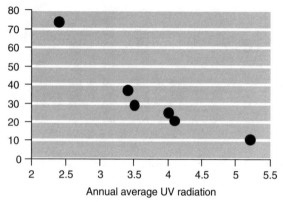

Annual average UV radiation

**Figure 3.2.5** Relationship between annual UV radiation and MS prevalence.

Wales, South Australia, and Tasmania. Cases were found from hospital records, doctors, societies, and statistical bureau. Diagnosis of MS used standard criteria.

Monthly climate data were obtained for the largest city for each region with measurements from satellite observations of atmospheric ozone and UV irradiation calculated. Annual UV irradiation was lowest in Tasmania (about 2.2 kJ/sq metre/day) and highest in tropical Queensland (5.1 kJ/sq m/day). There was a significant (1 in 100 significance) correlation between MS prevalence (and melanoma prevalence) and UV irradiation (and temperature, sunshine, and latitude; Figure 3.2.5).

This is not a comprehensive review of MS incidence and prevalence throughout the world, but rather a taste to show that it is a complicated issue—age, sex, genetics, and geography are combining here. One major feature stands out, that of the relationship with latitude. There will undoubtedly be genetic factors relating to susceptibility. There may well be a relationship to UV radiation, and the mechanism for that makes interesting reading in the Australian paper. The problem for both papers is that, while there may be statistical relationships, whether they are causal is another matter. There are more 'Macs' in Scotland, and less sunshine in Tasmania. But is this the cause of MS or even a causative factor?

## Incidence

### Perthes' disease

Perthes' disease is a developmental problem of the hip joint, usually unilateral, affecting younger children, and recognized by history, examination, and radiological changes. Literature searches provided no systematic evidence about diagnosis or treatment, but did show up some interesting population studies in the UK that can help thinking about how often it can be expected to occur, and temporal trends.

### Northern Ireland [6]

Northern Ireland has a centralized orthopaedic service where four hospitals serve children. Over a 7-year period, 313 children were diagnosed with Perthes' disease. Postcodes allowed spatial analysis by rural or urban area, and by deprivation index for each postcode district.

Analysis showed that the overall annual incidence was 11.6 per 100,000 children aged under 15 years. There were 256 boys and 57 girls (4.5 to 1), with mean age at onset of 5.7 years and 16% of cases being bilateral.

There was no relationship between incidence and settlement size or population density, but incidence was highest in children living in the most deprived areas (Figure 3.2.6). This was particularly noted for rural deprivation, where the gradient was steepest (7.1 per 100,000 to 16.1 per 100,000 for increasing deprivation), and for settlements up to 50,000 people. The relationship was not seen in larger settlements.

### Liverpool [7]

Liverpool city was the most deprived of 310 English districts in 1998, with the neighbouring districts of Knowsley ninth and Sefton 54th. There is a high incidence of Perthes' disease in the area. Children from all three districts are referred to the Alder Hey Hospital, which has maintained a Perthes' disease register since 1978. The register has been reviewed up to 1999, supplemented by computer searches of other activities in the hospital to ensure no cases were missed.

Parents of affected children were interviewed to determine the district and ward in which the children were born. Denominators for number of children under 15 in wards and districts were determined from census figures. The average ward- and district-specific rates of incidence were calculated for the periods 1976–81, 1982–89, and 1990–95.

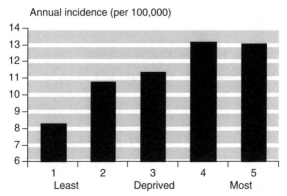

**Figure 3.2.6**   Northern Ireland—Perthes' disease incidence by deprivation index.

Incidence (per 100,000)

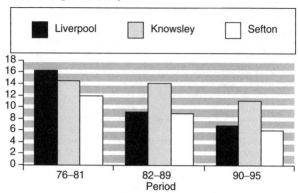

**Figure 3.2.7** Liverpool—Perthes' disease incidence by time.

There were 122 children diagnosed with Perthes' disease in Liverpool, 60 in Knowsley, and 38 in Sefton. Incidence rates declined in all three districts (Figure 3.2.7). A lower incidence of Perthes' disease was seen in Sefton, the least deprived district (Table 3.2.1). Multiple regression analysis was used to summarize various measures of social deprivation and health on ward-specific rates. Incidence increased where deprivation had increased, where the prevalence of low birth weight was highest, where free school meals were highest, and where wards had a low health index.

Both studies make general points relating to rare diseases. It is obvious that both ascertained all of the cases in their districts, and went to great lengths to do this and ensure consistency in diagnosis. They also went to great lengths to ascertain the proper denominator for their incidence calculations and determine accurately various indices of deprivation. The result is that we can look on the results with some confidence, despite the total numbers of cases being under 600.

The message for Perthes' disease is that deprivation is the key. Not just urban deprivation, but rural deprivation also, making the results important for Southern counties in the UK that are superficially affluent, but where pockets of rural deprivation occur. Liverpool and Ireland have family links,

**Table 3.2.1** Liverpool—Perthes' disease incidence by district and deprivation index

|  | Liverpool | Knowsley | Sefton |
| --- | --- | --- | --- |
| Perthes' disease per 100,000 children under 15 (1990–1995) | 8.7 | 11.3 | 4.4 |
| Deprivation index (higher values are more deprived) | 10.5 | 9.4 | 4.4 |

and there may be genetic components underlying these results. For instance, in Liverpool 6% of the population is formed by black or minority groups, but all 122 children diagnosed were white. For a population of 100,000 people where about 20% may be under 15 years, high incidence rates like those seen in Liverpool and Northern Ireland would result in two or three children with Perthes' disease every year. Less deprived areas may see only one.

### Parkinson's disease

A systematic review [8] searched to the end of 2001 for full publications of original studies providing incidence rates for idiopathic Parkinson's disease, or for Parkinsonian symptoms including Parkinson's disease in whole populations. Twenty-five incidence studies were found, looking at populations throughout the world, and with populations as low as 8000 to just under four million. The number of incident cases was between seven and about 400 in individual studies (Figure 3.2.8).

Determination of the diagnosis was mixed, with the proportion of patients seen by a specialist varying from 30% to 100%. Definition of incidence was also mixed, some studies using date of diagnosis, others date of onset, some both, and some did not give a definition. Diagnostic criteria used for defining Parkinson's disease were also mixed.

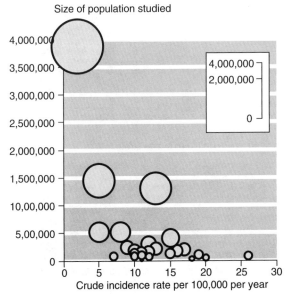

**Figure 3.2.8**    Incidence of Parkinson's disease in individual studies.

In most studies the peak incidence was between 70 and 79 years of age, though mean age of symptom onset was 60–65 years in eight studies and over 65 years in five studies. There tended to be somewhat more men than women diagnosed (rate ratio ranged from 0.9 to 2.0). The crude incidence per 100,000 per year ranged from 2 to 26 cases. Lower crude incidence rates came from populations in China, Libya, and Sardinia. Most developed countries with northern European age structures tended to have incidence rates between 12 and 20 cases per 100,000 per year.

This study not only gives some insight into the incidence of Parkinson's disease, but also an insight into the difficulty of such studies, and the need for strict criteria to ensure quality. With Parkinson's disease, which develops predominantly in older people (Figure 3.2.9), the age structure of a population would be expected to be critical to any result. A young population would have low incidence, while an older population would have a higher incidence.

The authors of the study give a list of criteria for improving the quality and consistency of incidence studies.

- Base population neither too large nor too small. Thus, for an incidence of 17 per 100,000 per year, they recommend one million person-years of surveillance, generating 60–80 cases.
- Studies should be prospective to maximize case ascertainment and accuracy.
- Multiple sources should be used to identify cases (records, secondary and primary care sources, etc., nursing homes).
- Prospective cases should be seen by an expert.
- Incident cases should be defined by specific symptoms and diagnostic criteria.
- Clear and consistent inclusion criteria applied to population. Broad screening terms should be used to avoid missing cases.
- Studies should have a period of follow-up, perhaps to determine response to therapy.
- Incidence rates should be reported by standard age strata (deciles, for instance) with confidence intervals. Crude information about the study population would be useful so that calculations are transparent.

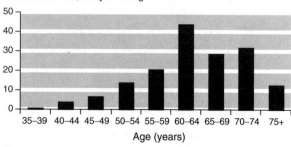

Incidence/100,000/year in age strata

**Figure 3.2.9** Parkinson's disease—incidence and age.

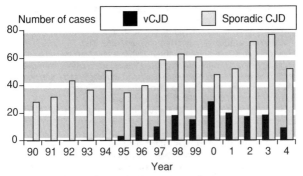

**Figure 3.2.10** Diagnosis of sporadic and new variant Creutzfeldt–Jakob disease in the UK, by year (1990–2004).

## Surveillance

A number of countries have surveillance schemes for various diseases that are by their nature prospective population cohort studies. This may be for communicable diseases, but also for cancer, for example. With internet access, some are available as ongoing projects. One of the best examples is the National Creutzfeldt–Jakob Disease Surveillance Unit (*www.cjd.ed.ac.uk*), set up following bovine spongiform encephalopathy in the UK. The incidence of Creutzfeldt–Jakob disease is monitored in the UK by the National CJD surveillance unit based at the Western General Hospital in Edinburgh, Scotland. The unit brings together a team of clinical neurologists, neuropathologists, and scientists specializing in the investigation of this disease.

Their webpages are a mine of information about CJD and other human spongiform encephalopathies. They also show the ongoing numbers of patients in the UK diagnosed with Creutzfeldt–Jakob disease, and the new variant form associated with the bovine disease (Figure 3.2.10). The number of new variant cases seemed to peak at just over 20 per year per 60 million people (1 in 3 million a year) in 2000, though this does not exclude more cases from a longer incubation period.

## Prevalence, incidence, and health-care planning

Knowing about the prevalence and incidence of disease can help with planning services, especially when new guidance is available or other changes need to be made. An example has been the introduction of TNF-antibodies for rheumatoid arthritis. In the UK the National Institute for Clinical Excellence adopted the British Society of Rheumatology (BSR) guidelines for treatment of rheumatoid arthritis, that anti-TNF agents should be used if the following criteria were met.

- Patients satisfy ACR (American College of Rheumatology) classification for RA.
- Patients have highly active RA.

- Patients have failed treatment on methotrexate and at least one other disease-modifying agent.
- Treated patients are entered on a central register, with drugs, dose, outcomes, and toxicity reported on a quarterly basis.

Treatment costs are presently about £8000 a year, and there is clearly a budgetary impact involved in introducing the agents. But how many patients need to be treated, and how much needs to be budgeted to implement the NICE recommendations and to follow the BSR guidelines? A good study from the West Midlands [9] provides some useful figures.

The West Midlands has 38 consultant rheumatologists in 14 centres serving 5.3 million people. In a 2-week period in summer 2001, 12 centres and 32 consultants reviewed all patients attending outpatient clinics. A standard questionnaire was attached to notes for doctors or nurse specialists to complete. It confirmed that patients had rheumatoid arthritis according to ACR criteria and gave history of response to methotrexate and disease-modifying anti-rheumatic drug (DMARD) use, and any contra-indications to anti-TNF therapy. For those patients failing methotrexate and at least one DMARD and with no contraindications, assessment of disease activity was made using painful and swollen joint counts, patient global assessment of disease activity, and laboratory tests.

Over the 2 weeks, 1441 patients with RA were assessed. Their average age was 58 years and 72% were women. Three of the patients were already using anti-TNF therapy. Table 3.2.2 shows the numbers and percentages of patients who met different criteria for possible anti-TNF use. Thus, 233 patients failed methotrexate therapy because of adverse effects (61%) or lack of efficacy (31%), and 177 had also failed at least one other DMARD. Of this 177, 19 had a contraindication for anti-TNF use and, of the remaining 158, 80 (5.6% of patients assessed) had disease activity above the threshold for anti-TNF use.

There were thus 80 candidates for anti-TNF therapy, but only three patients actually receiving anti-TNF therapy. Use of the additional criteria of failure of methotrexate, and two, three, or more than three failed DMARDs, would reduce the numbers of candidates for anti-TNF therapy, with the most stringent criteria giving only 27 candidates (1.9%).

This is really useful. When new guidelines are introduced, we need a handle on their impact, and this shows how information can be speedily collected. Yes, there is a necessary period of organization, but having a group of clinics collecting information comprehensively over a short period minimizes the duration of a study while maximizing the number of patients studied. It also much reduces the likelihood of patients attending twice and being double counted. Here the participation of 12 of 14 centres, and the inclusion of nurse-led clinics meant that the information was comprehensive.

We can be fairly sure that about 6% of patients with rheumatoid arthritis attending rheumatology outpatient clinics in the UK will be candidates for anti-TNF treatment using NICE guidelines. That may be too much of a budgetary jump at one go, but we know that, even if we restrict access to those who have failed more than three DMARDs, 2% of patients are still candidates. We have a series of bottom lines, each of which can come with budgetary requirements, and can apply it to our own area.

**Table 3.2.2**  Candidate rheumatoid arthritis patients for anti-TNF therapy, according to different criteria

| Patients | Number | % |
|---|---|---|
| RA by ACR criteria | 1441 | 100 |
| Failed methotrexate therapy | 233 | 16.2 |
| Failed further DMARD therapy | 177 | 12.3 |
| No contraindication to anti-TNF therapy | 158 | 11.0 |
| **Disease activity score above threshold for anti-TNF therapy** | **80** | **5.6** |
| **Additional criteria applied** | | |
| Failed methotrexate +2 or more DMARDs | 62 | 4.3 |
| Failed methotrexate +3 or more DMARDs | 40 | 2.8 |
| Failed methotrexate + more than 3 other DMARDs | 27 | 1.9 |

While this study was not designed to produce incidence or prevalence figures, the authors go one step further. Using some literature data and assuming that 80% of patients with rheumatoid arthritis attend hospital outpatient clinics, they arrived at an estimate of 36 patients eligible for anti-TNF therapy per 100,000 population.

## Commentary

Knowing about prevalence and incidence of disease is useful and interesting. There are fairly simple rules to know when we can trust a study of prevalence or incidence, which come down to diagnosis, ascertainment, population, and presentation of the results.

## References

1. Go, A.S. et al. (2001). Prevalence of diagnosed atrial fibrillation in adults. *Journal of the American Medical Association* **285**, 2370–5.
2. Mayers, L.B. et al. (2002). Prevalence of body art (body piercing and tattooing) in university undergraduates and incidence of medical complications. *Mayo Clinic Proceedings* **77**, 29–34.
3. Halbert, R.J. et al. (2003). Interpreting COPD prevalence estimates. What is the true burden of disease? *Chest* **123**, 1684–92.
4. Rothwell, P.M. and Charlton, D. (1998). High incidence and prevalence of multiple sclerosis in south east Scotland: evidence of a genetic predisposition. *Journal of Neurology, Neurosurgery and Psychiatry* **64**, 730–5.
5. van der Mei, I.A.F. et al. (2001). Regional variation in multiple sclerosis prevalence in Australia and its association with ambient ultraviolet radiation. *Neuroepidemiology* **20**, 168–74.
6. Kealey, W.D. et al. (2000). Deprivation, urbanisation and Perthes' disease in Northern Ireland. *Journal of Bone and Joint Surgery* **82B**, 167–71.
7. Margetts, B.M. et al. (2001). The incidence and distribution of Legg–Calvé–Perthes' disease in Liverpool, 1982–95. *Archives of Diseases in Childhood* **84**, 351–4.
8. Twelves, D. et al. (2003). Systematic review of incidence studies in Parkinson's disease. *Movement Disorders* **18**, 19–31.
9. Yee, C.S. et al. (2003). The prevalence of patients with rheumatoid arthritis in the West Midlands fulfilling the BSR criteria for anti-tumour necrosis factor therapy: an out-patient study. *Rheumatology* **42**, 856–9.

# 3.3 Questionnaires/observational studies

There are times when it is important to gain information about people, and patients, and occasionally their carers. This means asking them questions in the form of questionnaires. It is not uncommon that information gathered from questionnaires can be more useful than information gained from clinical trials. What patients want, what patients and carers value, and what they want to do or to have done to them may conflict with evidence. Unless we ask questions we only find this out retrospectively.

### Evidence rules for questionnaires

These are essentially those you would use for cohort studies. Use a comprehensive cohort, or if a selected cohort ensure that selection criteria make sense. Use large numbers, so that random plays of chance are reduced, and any effects from non-responders are minimized. Make sure that the questions asked are valid in the context of the patient demographics or disorder. What constitutes validity is so situation-dependent that no simple rules have yet been devised.

Common sense is the practical, and probably most important way to look at it. Patients themselves will often describe what is most important to them if prompted in a group discussion. Done well, with a little leadership, small group discussions can offer useful examples of questions to be asked of a wider number of people to gauge their importance.

Perhaps the best way of looking at questionnaire or similar studies is to use a few examples that have proved to be useful, mainly from rheumatology and mainly in the community.

### Example 1: knee pain

Most people working in primary care are aware that knee pain is common especially in older people. Much is mild and has little impact on how those affected get on with their lives. But, as with most conditions, there is a gradation in severity so that some have more pain or are disabled, some should be getting specialist advice, and some of those perhaps need a joint replacement. Knowing the numbers would be helpful in planning services, and a Manchester study [1] has provided them using questionnaires.

The survey was conducted in an urban part of Manchester. The population was divided into eight groups defined by age and sex, and about 250 people in each group were sampled in each medical practice with 5600 questionnaires sent initially. This first phase questionnaire asked about musculoskeletal symptoms, pain in various sites for more than 1 week in the past month, demographics, and employment status. It also included a health assessment questionnaire to help define disability.

A second questionnaire was sent to those reporting knee pain only (not multiple pain). This asked about severity, chronicity, and primary care and hospital consultations for knee pain. A sample of responders was invited for examination.

Response rates at all levels of the study were generally good, at about 80% or above. Overall prevalence of knee pain was similar in adult men and women at about 19%, but was higher than this in older persons (Figures 3.3.1

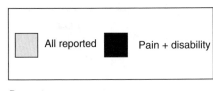

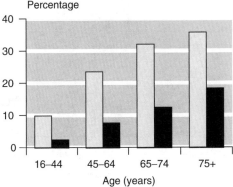

**Figure 3.3.1** Knee pain reported by women, all reported pain, and pain plus disability.

(for women) and 3.3.2 (for men)). Knee pain plus disability, defined as a health assessment questionnaire score of 0.5 or above, was lower at about 6% overall. Knee pain plus disability, defined as work disability in those aged below 65 years, was 2.8%.

Responses to the second questionnaire were similar between women and men and showed the same gradation with age. Overall, 12% of adults had knee pain that was moderate or severe, 9% had knee pain of more than 5 years' duration, and 3.4% had moderate or severe pain and disability.

Predictors of knee pain were sought. Factors associated with increased knee pain were higher BMI (Figure 3.3.3), increasing social deprivation (Figure 3.3.4), and South Asian ethnicity. A significant proportion of knee pain could be ascribed to being overweight or obese. For all knee pain, this was 21%, and for moderate or severe pain with disability up to 37%. Most of this came from being overweight (BMI 25–30), not being obese.

From an analysis of 66 patients seen by a consultant rheumatologist it was estimated that 4.5% of the adult population needed specialist treatment, most (2.8%) for orthopaedics. The unmet need was about twice the level of need currently being met. In a practice population of 10,000 adults, this unmet need amounts to 320 patients.

When planning services, it always helps if you have some idea of what you need to provide. A simple sentence this, but one for which it is often desperately difficult to provide numbers. For knee pain in the community,

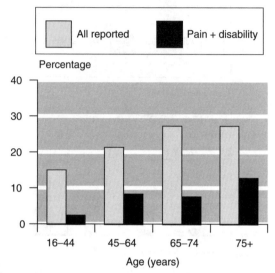

**Figure 3.3.2** Knee pain reported by men, all reported pain, and pain plus disability.

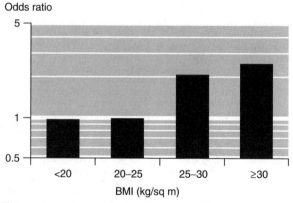

**Figure 3.3.3** Adjusted odds ratio for knee pain and BMI.

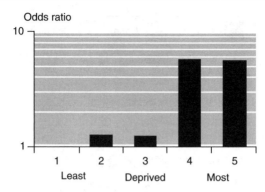

**Figure 3.3.4** Adjusted odds ratio for knee pain and Townsend deprivation index.

we have some numbers to help. Surveys have shown a large unmet need for hip replacements, and the present survey shows another large unmet need for treatment of knee pain, probably including replacement. But it also demonstrates that there is an opportunity to reduce the burden of knee pain, by showing the link with being overweight. Reducing excess weight in the community will have many paybacks, not just in heart disease and cancer, but also in a reduced requirement for specialist services for musculoskeletal conditions.

### Example 2: problems knee patients experience

Patient perspectives of osteoarthritis are not always captured by clinical trials, which use outcomes like WOMAC scales, or pain in the rather contrived setting of walking on a flat surface. Though these are important outcomes, and necessary for proving clinical efficacy, they do not always help the patient or the professional to understand the full benefit of a treatment.

Understanding the patient perspective, and the underlying problems with arthritis should come first. A UK survey of 3127 patients, whose diagnosis of osteoarthritis had been confirmed by a GP, contained results on 18 quality of life indicators [2]. Figure 3.3.5 shows that sleeping, walking, and such everyday activities as bathing and dressing affected people often. It is little wonder that, in chronic diseases, the largest negative impact on quality of life is seen in musculoskeletal disorders of osteoarthritis, rheumatoid arthritis, and back pain.

### Example 3: ranking burden of chronic diseases

A study with about 15,000 patients from Holland used information from a different, standardized questionnaire [3]. This was the SF-36 quality of life form (short-form, with 36 questions in eight main domains). This is one of a number of standard quality of life questionnaires that aim to measure how diseases or conditions impact on quality of life. Such information can help to inform how services might be organized.

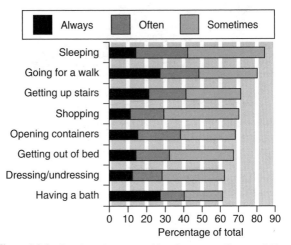

**Figure 3.3.5** Everyday tasks causing problems for patients with osteoarthritis.

All research groups known to examine chronic diseases in the Netherlands were contacted to see what data sets were available. Studies had to use a standardized quality of life instrument, have full coverage of quality of life domains, include a range of chronic diseases, be big (at least 200 patients), have medically confirmed diagnoses, be obtained since 1992, and be geographically broad.

Eight data sets broadly fulfilling these categories were obtained, with information on about 15,000 people. They all used SF-36 or SF-24. These were analysed by quality of life dimension (physical functioning, physical role functioning, bodily pain, general health, vitality, social functioning, and mental health) according to:

- disease clusters (grouping together similar diseases: for instance. musculoskeletal conditions of osteoarthritis, joint complaints, rheumatoid arthritis, and back impairments);
- disease categories (ranking the individual diseases within the cluster);
- patient characteristics (sociodemographic variables like age, sex, education).

The method used was the ranking of mean scores. Thus if three diseases scored (say) 5, 10, and 15 (with 5 the 'best' score), then they would be ranked 1, 2, and 3. This was done for all quality of life domains, and the ranks for individual domains added together. This summed rank produces low scores for the diseases or disease clusters causing the least distress and high scores for those causing the most problems.

The summed rank scores for chronic disease clusters are shown in Figure 3.3.6. Musculoskeletal conditions, renal disease, cerebrovascular/neurological conditions, and gastrointestinal conditions impacted most severely on quality of life.

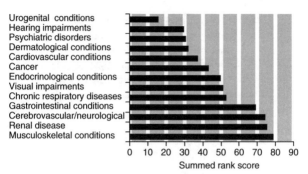

**Figure 3.3.6** Summed rank scores for disease clusters. Higher scores imply poorer quality of life.

In musculoskeletal conditions, osteoarthritis had more adverse impact than back impairments, which scored higher (worse) than rheumatoid arthritis. For neurological conditions, Parkinson's disease or epilepsy, multiple sclerosis, and stroke scored higher than migraine or neuromuscular disease. For psychiatric disorders depression scored worse than anxiety, which in turn was worse than alcohol problems. Patients who were older, female, had a low level of education, were not living with a partner, and/or had at least one co-morbid condition had the poorest quality of life.

There will be limits to how far these data can be subdivided and still give us valid conclusions. So where there is the largest agglomeration of information is where the strongest conclusions lie. For this analysis, this applies to the comparisons across disease categories. Moreover, there are also issues within the quality of life measures that an overall ranking will not highlight, for example, in the difference between mental and physical functioning.

Many professionals will not be overly surprised at the ranking of disease clusters, or the categories within each cluster, or the conclusions regarding patient characteristics. Although this ranking exercise should not be over-interpreted, it does give us a firmer platform on which to base decision-making, and on which to base research efforts.

### Example 4: what migraine patients want

An interesting question this for any therapy area, and one that is so often missed or ignored. A large study [4] that asks useful questions of patients and obtains interesting answers cannot be ignored. Representative American households were identified by random digit survey in 1998. About 5100 were contacted by telephone using a computer-assisted interview to identify people with migraine according to International Headache Society criteria.

Some 688 individuals were identified as having had migraine in the past year, a prevalence of 18% in women and 6% in men. Their mean age was 43 years. About a third had never consulted a doctor. Half did not think their headaches that bad, and the other half had a treatment that worked for

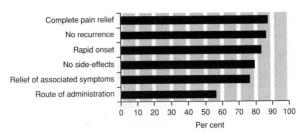

**Figure 3.3.7** What patients want from treatment.

them. Underlying this was the fact that a significant minority (40%) did not think that doctors had any useful remedies or thought that going to the doctor was too inconvenient; about a third thought that seeing a doctor was too expensive (this being the USA).

About a fifth had seen doctors previously, but had not done so in the past year. This was predominantly because treatments were working or the headaches had improved. But about half also thought that their doctor could do nothing for their migraine, could not help them, or was not interested in headache.

Patient satisfaction with their current treatment was predominantly positive. Of the 70% who were not very satisfied, the reasons for dissatisfaction were generally to do with lack of efficacy of treatments rather than adverse effects. When questioned, most people thought that satisfactory pain relief should be achieved within 1 hour, and more than half thought it should be achieved within 30 minutes.

Patients want the headache to go away now, completely, and not come back (Figure 3.3.7). They also want any associated symptoms such as nausea to be relieved. Most want a tablet or rapidly dissolving tablet and are not impressed by subcutaneous or intranasal delivery systems.

The responses to questions about what patients wanted from their doctors produced a constellation of answers, all of which demonstrate clearly that patients see their relationship with their doctor as a partnership. They want questions to be answered and to be educated about controlling their migraines to prevent them happening and how to treat attacks.

This is an absolutely fascinating paper that takes us into the minds of those with migraine. Put simply, they are not interested in fancy methods of drug delivery. They are not wholly satisfied with their current treatment. They want the pain relieved quickly and completely, with a tablet. They want to talk to their doctors about their condition and how to make it easier to control.

## Commentary

Here are just two topics, arthritis and migraine, where a few selected questionnaire studies can show how important the condition is, how negative an impact it has on quality of life, and how related it is to older people, especially those who are overweight and most deprived. With a knowledge of what works and what does not work, this information could help set out new agendas for service planning and delivery.

## References

1. Webb, R. *et al.* (2004). Opportunities for prevention of clinically significant knee pain: results from a population-based cross sectional survey. *Journal of Public Health* **26**, 277–84.
2. Crichton, B. and Green, M. (2002). GP and patient perspectives on treatment with non-steroidal anti-inflammatory drugs for the treatment of pain in osteoarthritis. *Current Medical Research and Opinion* **18**, 92–6.
3. Sprangers, M.A.G. *et al.* (2000). Which chronic conditions are associated with a better or poorer quality of life? *Journal of Clinical Epidemiology* **53**, 895–907.
4. Lipton, R.B. and Stewart, W.F. (1999). Acute migraine therapy: do doctors understand what patients with migraine want from therapy? *Headache* **39**, S20–S26.

# 3.4 Systematic review and meta-analysis of observational studies

Systematic reviews and meta-analyses of observational studies really follow on from what we know about observational studies themselves, except that we do have some guidance to help us, in the form of the MOOSE statement (*www.consort-statement.org*). Although this was concerned primarily with epidemiology, that word has a wide meaning and the statement included many useful thoughts for observational studies in general.

The reporting checklist is shown in Table 3.4.1, and includes a variety of sensible proposals, many of which are often ignored in systematic reviews of observational studies. One of the most important is the definition of the study population of interest, which should be a key point. In reporting of methods, provision of appropriate tables and graphics is stressed. Too often this is ignored, and reviews do not give us access to the information they found in the individual papers that formed the raw material of a review. We have either to accept any analysis presented to us or find the original papers and, in effect, repeat the whole review.

While the MOOSE statement does not provide a guarantee that any review of observational studies that meets its requirements will be without error, the statement and questionnaire help us in making our own evaluations of papers we read. It also helps us if we wish to write a review, and helps journal editors and reviewers in their work.

The MOOSE statement does not encompass all the criteria of quality, validity, and size that are required to make a review of observational studies foolproof. Everything learned so far in this book applies here, especially size. Results founded on a small number of observed events will be subject to the vagaries of random chance as well as systematic and other biases.

Some of the elements of good systematic reviews and occasionally meta-analysis of observational studies are to be found in the following examples.

### Cancer diagnostic assessment centres

It is a curious fact that, while some interventions in medicine are rigorously assessed, others are not. This could refer to the difference between drugs, say, which go through long and exhaustive efficacy and safety trials with complex and detailed regulatory hurdles, and many unconventional therapies that can be sold to patients with little or no testing. But even inside conventional medicine major interventions can be introduced without testing. These are usually top–down management changes, often introduced to improve service delivery and performance where there is some perceived problem.

One such change has been cancer diagnosis, with a move towards one-stop diagnostic assessment (and often treatment) centres in order to better coordinate care by concentrating services, multidisciplinary consultative expertise, patient information resources, and psychosocial support for patients at a difficult time. It would seem blindingly obvious that this is a better idea than any other *ad hoc* arrangement. A systematic review [2] makes uncomfortable reading because of the lack of evidence for any advantage of the one-stop diagnosis centre.

**Table 3.4.1** MOOSE checklist for meta-analysis of observational studies

**Reporting of background should include:**
Problem definition
Hypothesis statement
Description of study outcome(s)
Type of exposure or intervention used
Type of study designs used
Study population

**Reporting of search strategy should include:**
Qualifications of searchers (e.g. librarians and investigators)
Search strategy, including time period included in the synthesis and keywords
Effort to include all available studies, including contact with authors
Databases and registries searched
Search software used, name and version, including special features used (e.g. explosion)
Use of hand searching (e.g. reference lists of obtained articles)
List of citations located and those excluded, including justification
Method of addressing articles published in languages other than English
Method of handling abstracts and unpublished studies
Description of any contact with authors

**Reporting of methods should include:**
Description of relevance or appropriateness of studies assembled for assessing the hypothesis to be tested
Rationale for the selection and coding of data (e.g. sound clinical principles or convenience)
Documentation of how data were classified and coded (e.g. multiple raters, blinding, and interrater reliability)
Assessment of confounding (e.g. comparability of cases and controls in studies where appropriate)
Assessment of study quality, including blinding of quality assessors; stratification or regression on possible predictors of study results
Assessment of heterogeneity
Description of statistical methods (e.g. complete description of fixed or random effects models, justification of whether the chosen models account for predictors of study results, dose–response models, or cumulative meta-analysis) in sufficient detail to be replicated
Provision of appropriate tables and graphics

**Reporting of results should include:**
Graphic summarizing individual study estimates and overall estimate
Table giving descriptive information for each study included
Results of sensitivity testing (e.g. subgroup analysis)
Indication of statistical uncertainty of findings

**Reporting of discussion should include:**
Quantitative assessment of bias (e.g. publication bias)
Justification for exclusion (e.g. exclusion of non-English-language citations)
Assessment of quality of included studies

**Reporting of conclusions should include:**
Consideration of alternative explanations for observed results
Generalization of the conclusions (i.e. appropriate for the data presented and within the domain of the literature review)
Guidelines for future research
Disclosure of funding source

**Table 3.4.2** Major findings in studies of cancer diagnostic and assessment centres

| Cancer | Studies | Patients | Major findings |
|---|---|---|---|
| Breast | 11 total | 4614 | The two randomized trials showed no real difference in anxiety except in first few days |
| | 2 RCTs | 1269 | |
| | 6 prospective cohorts | 1084 | |
| | 2 retrospective cohorts | 1922 | |
| | 1 case-control | 339 | |
| Colorectal | 2 total | 3316 | None |
| | 1 prospective cohort | 3119 | |
| | 1 retrospective cohort | 197 | |
| Head and neck | 5 total | 427 | None |
| | 2 prospective cohorts | 134 | |
| | 3 retrospective cohorts | 293 | |

Multiple databases were searched for English-language articles published between 1985 and end-2002. Randomized trials, case-control studies, and prospective or retrospective cohort studies were sought examining outcomes of one-stop diagnostic centres. Cancer sites involved included breast, lung, prostate, head and neck, and colorectal cancer, and the studies had to involve diagnostic assessment. Only full, published studies were accepted.

There were 20 studies (Table 3.4.2), 11 in breast cancer, three in colorectal cancer, and six in head and neck cancer, with useful information in 18 of the 20 trials. Most were small, and 12 of the 18 reported information on fewer than 500 patients and many on fewer than 150.

Few studies examined quality of care, whether by reporting quality or accuracy of diagnosis, or patients diagnosed in a single visit, or reported clinical or economic outcomes. The two randomized trials in breast cancer hinted that patients treated in diagnostic centres might be less anxious in the first few days, but probably not thereafter.

Systematic reviews that tell us what we do not know can be more useful than those confirming what we do know. Though some work has been done on examining diagnostic assessment units in oncology, no single study has rigorously examined those managerial and clinical characteristics required to deliver a quality service, whether it be observational or controlled trial (difficult, anyway in a management context).

Service changes possibly do not need randomized trials, and this might easily have appeared in a section on management. But even management studies (almost always observational) need to be evaluated, to have quality assessment programmes and checks, to be subject to audit, and even to periodic external review.

## Barrett's oesophagus and colon cancer

Barrett's oesophagus is a complication of long-standing gastro-oesophageal reflux disease (GORD). Prolonged and excessive exposure of the lining of the oesophagus to stomach acid leads to changes in the types of cell that make up the epithelium. Instead of the usual flat, squamous, cells lining the oesophagus, columnar cells take over. This can extend from just a few centimetres from the gastro-oesophageal junction to the full length of the oesophagus. Development of columnar epithelium is associated with an increased risk of oesophageal cancer (about 1 in 50–170 patient-years), and a systematic review [3] demonstrates that patients with Barrett's oesophagus also have an increased risk of colon cancer.

The authors, from South Carolina, did a search to identify papers looking at colon cancer, polyps, neoplasms, or adenomas in Barrett's oesophagus. They extracted data on patients with the disorder and on controls and on the numbers of patients found to have colon cancer or adenomas on colonoscopy.

They found five uncontrolled studies, in which the prevalence of colon cancer in patients with Barrett's oesophagus was 4.6% (8/174). The prevalence of colon adenomas was 27% (36/134). They found nine papers with control groups. In size they varied from 17 to 175 patients and found rates of colon cancer among patients with Barrett's oesophagus of 0 to 14%. Overall, 52 of 685 had colon cancer, an average rate of 7.6%. The prevalence of benign plus malignant colon neoplasms ranged between 18 and 47%. Overall, 176 of 510 had colon cancer, an average rate of 35%.

The authors also created a comparison cohort of 513 patients aged less than 80 years described in studies of colonoscopic screening for colorectal cancer. Of these 513, 8 (1.6%) had colon cancer and 169 (33%) had colon neoplasms, and these were used for comparison with the patients with Barrett's oesophagus (Figure 3.4.1).

The definitions of cancer and neoplasm were as defined in the paper and matter little here, where the conclusion was that, while colon neoplasms

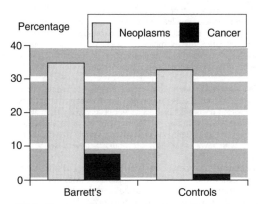

**Figure 3.4.1** Neoplasm and colon cancer in patients with Barrett's oesophagus and controls.

occur at about the same rate in people who have and who do not have Barrett's oesophagus, the risk of developing colon cancer is about five times greater in patients with Barrett's oesophagus. Nearly 8% of them will have colon cancer. This is useful information coming from all of the information available, again from predominantly observational studies, even though there are small numbers of patients, so that results are not robust.

## Effect of stopping smoking in patients with coronary heart disease

Trying to answer this question would ordinarily be quite difficult. No one would suggest for a moment doing a randomized trial of smoking, because the evidence is overwhelming that it is a bad thing. But patients might question whether giving up smoking when the damage is done makes any sense. Fortunately, a meta-analysis of observational studies can help supply an answer—that smokers with coronary heart disease have an extra 1 in 10 chance of dying over 5 years because of their smoking.

A systematic review [4] sought studies of patients diagnosed with previous heart attack or stable or unstable angina and who were smoking at baseline, with smoking status well defined. Prospective cohort studies had to include current smokers at baseline, with smoking status measured at end point to find who had quit smoking, in which the follow-up was at least 2 years, and with all-cause mortality as an outcome measure. The search strategy was extensive, examining nine electronic databases, and studies were not restricted by language.

There were 20 included studies with 12, 600 patients, mostly using data collected in the 1960s and 1970s. Most cases were men (80%) and the average cessation rate was 45%. Follow-up ranged from 2 to 26 years, though most studies reported follow-up of 3–7 years, with a mean of 5 years. Most studies involved follow-up hospital case series, and reporting of smoking status was usually at some follow-up appointment, though it was not validated, for example, by biochemical measurement, in most studies. Most studies had a clear definition of the cardiac event. Loss to follow-up was usually small. Size varied from under 100 to over 4000 patients.

There were fewer deaths in quitters (18%) than in people who continued to smoke (27%) and the degree of reduction was consistent across all death rates reported (Figure 3.4.2). Results were broadly similar in all studies and in six higher-quality studies with about two-thirds of all patients (Table 3.4.3). Higher quality here was defined by a sample size of 500 smokers at baseline, with fewer than 15% drop-outs, and with adequate or good control of confounding.

A secondary outcome was nonfatal reinfarction, and while this was a less frequent event, the same degree of reduction was seen (Table 3.4.3). Relative risk was reduced by about 30%, and the absolute risk by about 9% for mortality, translating into a number needed to treat of about 12 for one additional non-smoking patient to be alive at 5 years, and a number needed to treat of about 28 for one non-smoking patient to avoid a nonfatal reinfarction.

Mortality (%) in quitters

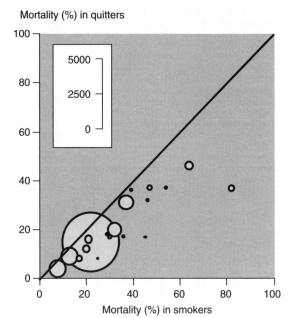

**Figure 3.4.2** Death rates in patients with CHD who continued smoking, or who quit.

**Table 3.4.3** NNTs to prevent one death or reinfarction over 5 years through CHD patients quitting smoking compared with continuing to smoke

| Event | Number events/total (%) | | Relative risk (95% CI) | NNT (95% CI) |
|---|---|---|---|---|
| | Quitters | Smokers | | |
| Death (all studies) | 1044/5649 (18) | 1884/6944 (27) | 0.64 (0.58–0.72) | 12 (10–14) |
| Death (better studies) | 645/3371 (19) | 1294/5027 (26) | 0.71 (0.65–0.77) | 15 (12–21) |
| Nonfatal reinfarction (all studies) | 263/2467 (11) | 516/3622 (14) | 0.68 (0.57–0.82) | 28 (19–52) |

As with controlled trials, size matters. If we plot the death rates in patients with CHD who have stopped smoking against the number of patients in a particular study, we find that most of the variability is in the small studies (Figure 3.4.3). While the overall death rate in quitters was 18%, studies of only a few hundred patients and below had rates up to 50%. This is probably a feature both of clinical heterogeneity of populations studied, and the random play of chance in small samples.

This review gives the consistent and unequivocal answer that smoking remains harmful after a coronary event. Carrying on smoking carries a 5-year risk of 1 in 10 of dying because you smoke. By contrast, the risk of dying on the roads over 5 years would be more like 1 in 4000. Smoking in those circumstances is 400 times more dangerous than driving. Smoking while driving is even more dangerous.

Also interesting in the review is the discussion about limitations and how limitations may affect the result. Most limitations make the results more

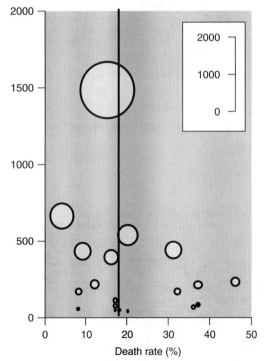

**Figure 3.4.3**  Size and mortality in patients with CHD who gave up smoking.

conservative. For instance, if people who said they had stopped smoking were lying, the quitter results would be worse than they should be, and the benefits of stopping smoking underestimated.

### Gastrointestinal bleeding with NSAIDs

A systematic review of observational studies was a seminal paper in helping us accept the key risk factors for NSAID-associated gastrointestinal (GI) bleeding. It collected together epidemiological studies associating NSAID use and upper GI problems published in the 1990s [5] to give a much clearer picture of risks. To be included studies had to:

- be case control or cohort studies of non-aspirin NSAIDs;
- include data on bleeding, perforation, or other serious upper gastro-intestinal tract event resulting in hospital admission or referral to a specialist;
- have data to calculate relative risk.

Eighteen studies were found. All had specific definitions of exposure and outcome and similar ascertainment for comparison groups. All but two attempted to control for potential confounding factors such as age, sex, history of ulcer, or concomitant medicines.

The main result was that, compared with non-users, NSAID users had a higher risk of upper GI bleed (UGIB) when they were current NSAID users and used a higher dose. The duration of use was unimportant, but different NSAIDs had different risks, with ibuprofen (especially doses below 2400 mg a day) being least harmful.

The analysis also provided important insights into the effect of ulcer history and age, as shown in Figures 3.4.4 and 3.4.5. People with a history of ulcer or with a previous bleed who took NSAIDs were at much greater risk than those with no history of ulcer who took NSAIDs. Older people who

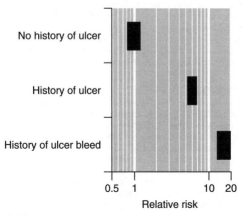

**Figure 3.4.4** Effect of history of ulcer in users of NSAIDs.

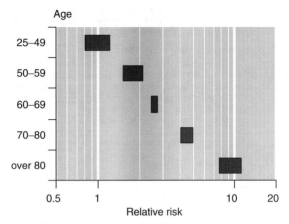

**Figure 3.4.5** Effect of age in users of NSAIDs.

took NSAIDs were at greater risk than those aged less than 50 years who took NSAIDs.

In this set of high-quality studies, there was a clear effect of size of study on the relative risk of upper gastrointestinal bleed with NSAID. The pooled estimate was 3.8 (3.6 to 4.1). In studies with fewer than 1000 cases, results were highly variable (Figure 3.4.6). With fewer than 200 cases of upper gastrointestinal bleeding, the measured relative risk varied from as high as a relative risk of almost 8 to one of 0.8, which suggested that NSAIDs protected against gastrointestinal bleeding. That was a 10-fold variation in the estimate of the risk.

There are many lessons to be learned from this very important study. A systematic review and meta-analysis of well-conducted and relatively large observational studies told us a great deal about which patients are most at risk, according to dose, drug, age, and medical history. Now that is useful.

## Commentary

Systematic reviews and meta-analyses of observational studies are really useful, or can be if they follow standard rules of including studies of good quality, making sure that what is measured is valid, and paying appropriate attention to size. Two examples here, smoking and coronary heart disease and NSAIDs and gastrointestinal bleeding, make the same point—with small numbers of patients or events the variability in results is great but when we have large numbers the variability is low.

That lesson is even more important when all we have available is a single study, or when we try to extrapolate from small numbers of patients or events. The possibility of being wrong is large in that circumstance. It is the same lesson that we found for randomized trials—with small numbers of events a result can be just plain wrong, even if everything else is right.

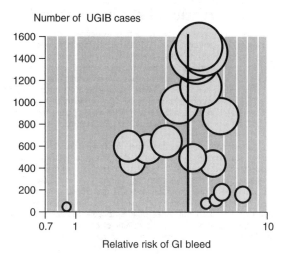

**Figure 3.4.6** Effect of size of study in determining overall relative risk of GI bleed for NSAID users compared with non-users (vertical line shows overall point estimate of a relative risk of 3.8).

## References

1. Stroup, D.F. *et al.* (2000). Meta-analysis of observational studies in epidemiology: a proposal for reporting. *Journal of the American Medical Association* **283**, 2008–12.
2. Gagliardi, A. *et al.* (2004). Evaluation of diagnostic assessment units in oncology: a systematic review. *Journal of Clinical Oncology* **22**, 1126–35.
3. Howden, C.W. and Hornung, C.A. (1995). A systematic review of the association between Barrett's esophagus and colon neoplasms. *American Journal of Gastroenterology* **90**, 1814–19.
4. Critchley, J.A. and Capewell, S. (2003). Mortality risk reduction associated with smoking cessation in patients with coronary heart disease. A systematic review. *Journal of the American Medical Association* **290**, 86–97.
5. Hernández-Diaz, S. and García Rodriguez, L.A. (2000). Association between nonsteroidal anti-inflammatory drugs and upper gastrointestinal tract bleeding and perforation: an overview of epidemiological studies published in the 1990s. *Archives of Internal Medicine* **160**, 2093–9.

## 3.5    Observational studies versus RCTs

It has become received wisdom to dismiss evidence from observational studies by saying something like, 'Of course, that's just an observational study.' A supercilious tone helps convey just the right amount of contempt that anyone might even consider using evidence from observational studies. This has come about for two main reasons. We know that non-randomized studies can (and often do) overestimate the benefits of treatment. We also know of cases where observational studies gave answers that were overturned by subsequent randomized trials [1]. However, before throwing this particular baby out with the bathwater, let's just step back for a moment and think.

Take non-randomized trials for a start. What we were doing there was comparing randomized comparative studies from the past with non-randomized comparative studies from the past. This form of medical archaeology tells us a great deal, but it tells us principally about the past. Clinical trials have improved immeasurably over the past 30–40 years, even over the past 15 years. Trials used to be small, sometimes of poor design and reporting quality, used outcomes of questionable relevance, and often were of short duration. Before the advent of coxibs in the mid to late 1990s, our data on NSAIDs had been characterized as small in number, inadequate in outcomes, and short in duration [2]. Only coxib trials rescued us from this lack of knowledge. Modern observational studies are not just the non-randomized comparisons of yesteryear.

As was pointed out earlier in this section, 'observational studies propose, RCTs dispose' [1]. There is little doubt that observational studies and RCTs can give different results, even in meta-analyses. For hormone replacement therapy and coronary heart disease, for instance, an early systematic review of observational data [3] was highly suggestive of a protective effect of HRT. A later meta-analysis of RCTs came to the opposite conclusion, and was able to look at other risks as well [4].

There were over 20,000 women in the randomized trials, followed up for an average of almost 5 years. For coronary heart disease there were almost 700 events, and for stroke almost 500. The relative risks for HRT use were 1.1 (0.96–1.3) and 1.3 (1.06–1.5), respectively. How could the observational studies have got it wrong, reporting a strong protective effect? Perhaps the answer comes from another systematic review of observational studies [5], published at about the same time as the meta-analysis of RCTs. Using almost the same data set as previously, but excluding studies of dubious quality, it found no significant association for past, ever, or any use of HRT and cardiovascular disease or coronary artery disease death. Neither did HRT reduce the incidence of heart disease, actually suggesting a small increased risk. The problem turned out not to be the observational studies *per se*; rather it was including poor observational studies in a meta-analysis.

We have been here before, with randomized trials, where a meta-analysis of randomized trials did not agree with a later large randomized trial [6]. This case, of magnesium in acute myocardial infarction, can more easily be explained by the fact that the trials included in the meta-analysis were trivially small to detect any effect and should never have been

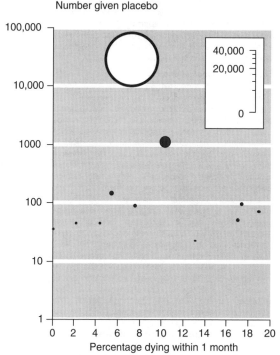

**Figure 3.5.1** Size and baseline risk in trials included in a meta-analysis of magnesium in acute myocardial infarction (dark symbols) and a large randomized trial (light symbol).

included in the meta-analysis in the first place (Figure 3.5.1). Randomized trials can disagree with randomized trials because of issues of quality, validity, or size, so we should not be too surprised when the same thing happens with observational and randomized trials.

#### From the general to particular

Perhaps finding examples of where observational studies and randomized trials disagree is a bit sterile. What is better is to try and find the conditions within which we could be sure that these different study architectures are likely to produce the same answer. If we knew that, then we would have rules that would allow us to trust the evidence before us, and we would know when to move forward based on evidence, and when to be cautious based on insufficient evidence.

We can be pretty sure that size will be important, and that will mean meta-analyses, as individual studies will often be too small to trust. Studies will also need to be of decent reporting quality and be valid in whatever way they have to be designed for any particular case. So what follows are a series of examples where there is agreement or disagreement, to examine how quality, validity, and size measure up.

### TNF-alpha for rheumatoid arthritis

A NICE review [7] had information on about 1000 patients given etanercept, and about 630 given infliximab in a meta-analysis of randomized trials. That formed the best available form of evidence we had at that time, but an observational study was also available. In the University Hospital of Lund in southern Sweden, a clinical treatment protocol was adapted to monitor new treatments in rheumatoid arthritis [8]. Six non-teaching hospitals also used the protocol, so that coverage of patients with rheumatoid arthritis in southern Sweden was complete. For etanercept, infliximab, and leflunomide, initial doses were according to licence, with changes as necessary. Assessments were mandated before treatment started, and at 3, 6, and 12 months, and every 3–6 months thereafter.

There were strict eligibility criteria, including a proper diagnosis of rheumatoid arthritis and failure to respond to or tolerate at least two disease-modifying drugs, including methotrexate. Though not approved by the European Medicines Agency at the time (1999–2000), Swedish law allowed use of several treatments on an individual patient basis.

Of 369 patients treated, 166 were on etanercept, 135 on infliximab, and 103 on leflunomide. Some (33) tried two treatments and one all three. Patients on the TNF-antagonists etanercept and infliximab were similar, but those on leflunomide were older, had more severe joint damage, were more often treated with monotherapy, and had somewhat lower inflammatory activity as judged by ESR values.

After 12 months of treatment with etanercept, about 60% of patients had an ACR20 response, 40% an ACR50 response, and about 18% an ACR70 response. Figure 3.5.2 shows that these results were similar to those of a trial of the licensed dose at 6 months. After 20 months, 79% of patients who began treatment were still using it.

After 12 months of treatment with infliximab, about 60% of patients had an ACR20 response, 40% an ACR50 response, and about 18% an ACR70 response. Figure 3.5.3 shows that these results were similar to those of trials of similar doses and dose intervals at about 6 months. After 20 months, 75% of patients who began treatment were still using it.

This real-world study provided significant information about treating patients with rheumatoid arthritis using new therapies. The amount of information in terms of patient numbers multiplied by duration of treatment was, for the TNF-antagonists, about equal or more than that from the clinical trials in the meta-analysis then available. Both trials and the observational study involved a high-quality of design, with sensible inclusion criteria, evaluation, and outcomes. Both architectures fulfilled criteria of quality, validity, and size. Results on efficacy were similar to those of clinical trials.

This shows that high-quality monitoring of new treatments can be done without the intervention of manufacturers, who may be biased. There was no industrial sponsorship for the Swedish observational study. There is no

Percentage with ACR criteria

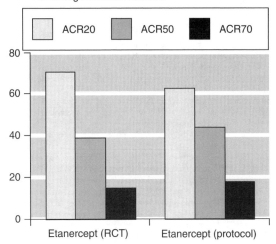

**Figure 3.5.2** Etanercept results from RCT and protocol.

Percentage with ACR criteria

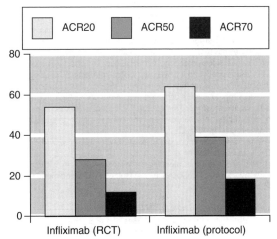

**Figure 3.5.3** Infliximab results from RCT and protocol.

reason why similar schemes could not be put in place for most new interventions.

### Gastrointestinal bleeding with coxibs versus NSAIDs

The era of coxibs has provided us with a wealth of information of all sorts: randomized trials, meta-analyses, and observational studies. Randomized trials alone have included well over 100,000 patients in the period up to 2005. This has provided us with much useful information on many important clinical issues, but it is also a testing ground for methodological issues with modern trials and observational studies.

For instance, compared with NSAIDs, coxibs are designed to produce less gastrointestinal bleeding. This was tested first in small trials, then in large trials designed to detect a difference if one were present, and then in observational studies in the real world, rather than in the special circumstance of clinical trials.

Small trials were not designed to measure a difference in gastrointestinal bleeding, though most had prospective data collection and independent adjudication of bleeding events. These trials, when combined in meta-analysis, demonstrated a reduction in bleeding events with coxibs compared with NSAIDs (Table 3.5.1). The problem for most of the early meta-analyses was that there were few bleeding events, between 10 and 38, even though up to 11,000 patients were included in individual meta-analyses.

Large trials designed to look for a difference generally found one. These trials were large, and usually up to 1 year in length, though the average duration was about 9 months. Here the number of events was larger, a product both of larger size and longer duration, so that 50 to 120 events were obtained (Table 3.5.1). These trials also demonstrated a reduction in bleeding events with coxibs compared with NSAIDs.

Observational studies were different. Whereas randomized trials ensured similarity in patients given a coxib and those given an NSAID, in the observational studies patients given coxibs tended to be sicker and more likely to have risk factors for bleeding. Patients given coxibs were at higher baseline risk of bleeding. Yet here, too, in cohort and case control studies, coxibs produced a lower rate of gastrointestinal bleeding. Despite looking at very large numbers of patients, the number of events could be very small. Only 17 events occurred in patients on NSAIDs in one study in Canada, where most were on coxibs. Only four events occurred in a UK study in patients on coxibs, where the overwhelming preponderance of information was on NSAIDs.

Despite these differences between study architectures, and despite the relatively low number of events in some of them, there was a general consistent agreement that bleeding events were less likely with coxibs than NSAIDs, by about a half. Observational studies, RCTs, and meta-analyses of RCTs all agreed.

### Circumcision for preventing urinary tract infection

A systematic review [9] sought all studies of any architecture on the effect of male circumcision on urinary tract infection, without any restriction on age of boys. Diagnosis of urinary tract infection was the only outcome sought. There were 12 available studies; one randomized study, four cohort studies, and seven case-control studies. Table 3.5.2 shows the results.

**Table 3.5.1** Studies of gastrointestinal bleeding comparing coxibs and NSAIDS

| Study | Number of subjects | Relative risk (95% CI) | Number of events |
|---|---|---|---|
| **Meta-analyses of RCTs** | | | |
| Langman, M.J. et al. (1999). *Journal of the American Medical Association* **282**, 1924–38. | 5435 | 0.5 (0.3–1.0) | 38 events; meta-analysis of small trials |
| Goldstein, J.L. et al. (2000). *American Journal of Gastroenterology* **95**, 1681–91. | 11,008 | 0.1 (0.02–0.5) | 11 events; meta-analysis of small trials |
| Edwards, J.E. et al. (2004). *BMC Anaesthesiology* **4**, 3. | 4579 | 0.4 (0.2–1.2) | 10 events; meta-analysis of small trials |
| Moore, R.A. et al. (2005). *Arthritis Research and Therapy* **7**, R644–R665. | 31,171 | 0.6 (0.4–0.8) | 173 events; meta-analysis of all trials |
| **RCTs powered to detect a difference** | | | |
| Bombardier, C. et al. (2000). *New England Journal of Medicine* **343**, 1520–8. | 8076 | 0.4 (0.2–0.8) | 53 complicated events |
| Silverstein, F.E. et al. (2000). *Journal of the American Medical Association* **284**, 1247–55. | 8059 | 0.6 (0.4–0.98) | 83 complicated events |
| Schnitzer, T.J. et al. (2004). *Lancet* **364**, 665–74. | 18,325 | 0.3 (0.2–0.5) | 114 ulcer complications |
| **Observational studies** | | | |
| Mamdani, M. et al. (2002). *British Medical Journal* **325**, 624. | 14,5000 | 0.4 (0.3–0.7) | 187 events, but only 17 with NSAIDs |
| MacDonald, T.M. et al. (2003). *Gut* **52**, 1265–70. | 1,300,000 | 0.6 (0.2–1.5) | 8,526 events, but only 4 with coxibs |
| Nørgard, B. et al. (2004). *Alimentary Pharmacology and Therapeutics* **19**, 817–25. | 3696 | 0.5 (0.3–0.7) | 780 cases, 114 recent users of coxib or NSAID |

**Table 3.5.2** Results for UTI reduction in circumcised versus uncircumcised boys, according to study design

| Study design | Number of | | | Relative risk (95% CI) |
| --- | --- | --- | --- | --- |
| | Studies | Boys | UTI episodes | |
| RCT | 1 | 70 | 3 | 0.17 (0.01–3.3) |
| Cohort | 4 | 400,700 | 1590 | 0.13 (0.12–0.14) |
| Case-control | 7 | 2138 | 324 | 0.16 (0.11–0.23) |

There was incredible disparity between the number of boys and urinary tract episodes in the different study types. The one randomized trial had only three episodes of urinary tract infection, while the four cohort studies had almost 1600. And yet there was a remarkable degree of consistency in relative risk between all three different study designs.

Overall, 1.4% of boys who were not circumcised had a urinary tract infection, compared with 0.1% who were circumcised. The difference amounts to a number needed to treat of about 81 (95% confidence interval, 76–85). As we have seen before, the variability between studies came in the small studies, where without circumcision urinary tract infection rates of up

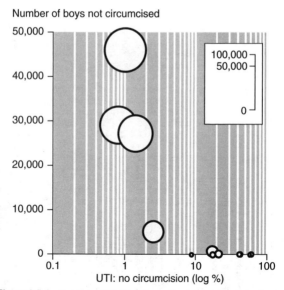

Number of boys not circumcised

**Figure 3.5.4** Variation of UTI rate in boys without circumcision according to study size.

to 60% were seen (Figure 3.5.4). Yet the large cohort studies all had rates of 0.8–2.5%.

In this example, the agreement between the randomized and the observational studies was serendipitous. With only 70 boys and three events, to come up with same answer as over 400,000 boys and nearly 2000 events is lucky indeed.

### Pneumococcal polysaccharide vaccines

This is tiger country, where there are bitter arguments about the effectiveness of vaccines. This stems from the problem that randomized trials have tended not to demonstrate effectiveness, except in some older trials in very different circumstances from those in most developed countries (New Guinea highlanders, South African gold workers). Systematic reviews [10, for example] also concluded that pneumococcal vaccines were ineffective for most outcomes in most people.

A problem, though, is that some outcomes in the trials, such as bacteraemia or death from pneumococcal pneumonia, are rare (usually affecting less than 1%) so, despite conducting large studies, there are few actual events. Of course, if the events are that rare or the difference between vaccine and placebo that small, the chance of a difference in clinically relevant outcomes will also be small. But the trials may have missed something important, and the more important outcomes have tended to be those that were most infrequent, where there was little chance of finding a difference. For pneumococcal bacteraemia, for instance, only 9000 patients provided data in three trials [10], with a rate of only about 1%. Although the proportion affected with vaccine was lower (0.8%) than for those not vaccinated (1.4%), the relative risk of 0.5 did not achieve statistical significance with these small numbers. It may just be that the randomized trials were not measuring enough useful outcomes.

A systematic review of observational studies [11] was able to include 13 studies. For invasive disease, the observational studies had 4984 events, with a significant reduction for vaccination, with an odds ratio of 0.5 (0.4–0.55). The study also chose to look at randomized studies, in which there were only 62 events of invasive disease, but with a non-significant odds ratio of 0.6 (0.4–1.04).

While in general there was a tendency to agree between randomized trials and observational studies, this was across all patient groups. In elderly patients with chronic disease, randomized trials showed no effect, while observational studies found a significant reduction in invasive disease in vaccinated patients.

There remains genuine uncertainty, though observational studies have so many more events that it might be difficult to bet against them. There will genuinely be times when the call for 'more research' is the correct response. This also asks an important question, for which right now there is no easy answer likely to be right every time. Which is more important, the number of events or the study architecture? When does this cross over? It is likely that there will be circumstances where good observational studies with large numbers of relevant events will be better than small randomized trials with few events.

### Systematic examination of randomized trials and observational studies

There are at least two systematic attempts to evaluate observational studies and randomized trials [12, 13].

Benson and Hartz [12] searched for observational studies comparing two different interventions for the same condition, and then sought the randomized trials comparing those same interventions for that same condition. There were 136 reports in 19 treatments. In 17/19, treatment pairings gave the same magnitude of effect, and in only 2/19 were there small differences outside the 95% confidence interval. The main problem was that these were small data sets to which no criteria of quality, validity, or size had been applied.

By contrast Concato and colleagues [13] examined meta-analyses of RCTs compared with meta-analyses of observational studies for the same topics published in five major medical journals. For five clinical topics and 99 reports, RCTs and observational meta-analyses gave the same result. They concluded that *well-designed* observational studies do *not* overestimate effects of treatment compared with randomized trials, and here certain quality and validity criteria were used.

Both of these articles have attracted considerable correspondence, and not everyone was happy with the results, but this section should at least provide some backing to both these findings. There will be times when even the best of trials or observational studies might disagree, but if they fulfil the required criteria of quality, are valid, and have sufficient events, then that is not likely.

### Commentary

Observational studies and randomized trials (or meta-analyses of them) will tend to agree when they fulfil criteria of quality, validity, and size. This is important, because it begins to set the rules for how we investigate difficult areas of care, where randomized trials may be difficult to impossible, or where ethical considerations overrule doing them. If we are careful, observational studies can give the same result as a randomized trial.

### References

1. Davey Smith, G. and Ebrahim, S. (2002). Data dredging, bias, or confounding. They can all get you into the British Medical Journal and the Friday papers. *British Medical Journal* **325**, 1437–8.
2. Gøtzsche, P.C. (2001). Reporting of outcomes in arthritis trials measured on ordinal and interval scales is inadequate in relation to meta-analysis. *Annals of the Rheumatic Diseases* **59**, 407–8.
3. Stampfer, M.J. and Colditz, G.A. (1991). Estrogen replacement therapy and coronary heart disease: a quantitative assessment of the epidemiological evidence. *Preventive Medicine* **20**, 47–63.
4. Beral, V. *et al.* (2002). Evidence from randomised trials on the long-term effects of hormone replacement therapy. *Lancet* **360**, 942–4.
5. Humphrey, L.L. *et al.* (2002). Postmenopausal hormone replacement therapy and the primary prevention of cardiovascular disease. *Annals of Internal Medicine* **137**, 273–84.
6. Egger, M. and Davey Smith, G. (1995). Misleading meta-analysis. Lessons from 'an effective, safe, simple' intervention that wasn't. *British Medical Journal* **310**, 752–4.

7. Jobanputra, P. *et al.* (2002). The clinical effectiveness and cost-effectiveness of new drug treatments for rheumatoid arthritis: etanercept and infliximab. NICE 2002, (*www.nice.org.uk/Docref.asp?d=29675*).

8. Geborek, P. *et al.* (2002). Etanercept, infliximab, and leflunomide in established rheumatoid arthritis: clinical experience using a structured follow up programme in southern Sweden. *Annals of the Rheumatic Diseases* **61**, 793–8.

9. Singh-Grewal, D. *et al.* (2005). Circumcision for the prevention of urinary tract infection in boys: a systematic review of randomised trials and observational studies. *Archives of Diseases of Childhood* **90**, 853–8.

10. Moore, R.A. *et al.* (2000). Are the pneumococcal polysaccharide vaccines effective? Meta-analysis of the prospective trials. *BMC Family Practice* **1**,1. (*http://www.biomedcentral.com/1471–2296/1/1*).

11. Conaty, S. *et al.* (2004). The effectiveness of pneumococcal polysaccharide vaccines in adults: a systematic review of observational studies and comparison with results from randomised controlled studies. *Vaccine* **22**, 3214–24.

12. Benson, K. and Hartz, A.J. (2000). A comparison of observational studies and randomized controlled trials. *New England Journal of Medicine* **342**, 1878–86.

13. Concato, J. *et al.* (2000). Randomized, controlled trials, observational studies, and the hierarchy of research designs. *New England Journal of Medicine* **342**, 1887–92.

# Section 4
# Diagnostic testing

# 4.1 Diagnostic testing: fundamentals

For many readers of this book, a section on diagnostics may not seem all that interesting, because their focus will be on clinical trials or observational studies where there is so much concentration in medical matters. Yet if one sits and thinks for a minute, it becomes clear that any clinical trial or observational study is only as good as the diagnostic criteria used to categorize people as having a disease or condition in the first place. Without good diagnosis, all else fails.

Yet, for the casual reader who has got just this far, there is a disturbing bottom line: most evidence concerning diagnostic tests is at best poor, and at worst rubbish. It makes one think. Below is what might be regarded as a typical example of studies that get done, and to make it obvious we will use a slightly inflammatory example.

Imagine that someone comes along and says that they have a test that can tell White people from Black people. When you ask for more details, you are told that the test was tested on 10 Celtic types (red hair, freckles, skin so fair that it goes salmon-pink in a nanosecond of exposure to the sun) and 10 people from the most pigmented of all in the world. The test performed perfectly, showing all Whites to be White and all Blacks to be Black. If you have any neurons firing at all, you will be outraged, not at the idea of the test in the first place, but rather about all the millions of people with different skin types and colours in whom the test has not been tested.

Change skin colour for a medical condition, where a test is tested in people without a condition and with those with the most severe symptoms or stage of the condition, and you have a pretty typical design used in studying diagnostic tests. Those diagnostic tests can be laboratory, or clinical, or signs and symptoms, or imaging. The take-home bottom lines are therefore these.

- Most diagnostic tests are evaluated using study designs subject to immense bias.
- Few systematic reviews of diagnostic tests are useful, because they just summarize wrong results.
- For many tests there is too little information about how to use them, and when that has been examined it demonstrates massive lack of agreement.
- In most circumstances we need to start afresh with new, better, and more directed research.
- There are great paradigms for us in the Ottawa ankle and knee rules and the CARE study.
- Diagnostic testing is a source of major economic waste in health services.

Health-care systems avoid tackling the problems at their peril. Accurate and fast diagnosis is the key to accurate, fast, and cost-effective treatment. Major research investment cannot be avoided, but diagnostic research can cement relationships and be a driver for better use of knowledge and evidence. This chapter will look at some of the fundamentals, using some good and some bad examples to help navigate through difficult waters.

### Good tests can make a difference

This should not be seen as a counsel of despair, though. There are quite a few examples where a test and a treatment come together to make a difference. Examples include:

- Testing for *Helicobacter pylori* and effective treatments to eradicate ulcers.
- Using gene amplification methods for *Chlamydia* combined with azithromycin in screening.
- Measuring HIV viral load and treating with protease inhibitors to make a real difference.

There are probably many more, but the problem is finding them. The evidence base for effective diagnostics or diagnosis remains rather thin.

### How doctors use tests

An important study [1] asked groups of about 50 physicians and surgeons how they used diagnostic tests. The results were that very few knew or used Bayesian methods, or ROC curves, or likelihood ratios. So the formal ways we have of explaining diagnostic test results, including sensitivity and specificity, are just not understood or used by the people who use the tests.

Yale researchers used a stratified random sample of physicians in six specialties with direct patient care (at least 40% of time with patients) across the USA. The physicians were contacted by letter and telephone, in order to perform a 10 minute telephone survey about their attitudes to formal methods of test use. They were told that interviewers were not necessarily advocates of the use of formal methods. There were 10 questions. An example of a question (question 4) was: 'Do you use test sensitivity and specificity values when you order tests or interpret test results?'

There were 300 physicians in the final sample, 50 in each specialty. They had a mean age of 46 years, 80% were men, and they spent a median of 90% of their professional time providing direct patient care. They worked in a variety of settings. The main result was that few of them used formal methods of assessing test accuracy (Table 4.1.1). Bayesian methods were used by 3%, and ROC and likelihood ratio data by 1% each.

This points to another important question when tests are being used. How should a result be reported? How does one use the result? What is a result anyway? The Yale example demonstrates that almost all doctors use tests in an informal way, and that there is an immense gulf between them

**Table 4.1.1** Percentage use of methods of assessing test accuracy ($n = 300$)

| | Bayesian method | ROC curve | Likelihood ratios |
|---|---|---|---|
| Specialist physician | 5 | 1 | 1 |
| Generalist physician | 2 | 0 | 1 |
| Paediatrician | 1 | 1 | 0 |
| General surgeon | 0 | 1 | 0 |
| Family practice | 0 | 0 | 0 |
| Obstetrics/gynaecology | 0 | 0 | 0 |
| Overall percentage | 3% | 1% | 1% |

and the academics producing 'evidence' about diagnostic tests and their accuracy. Few of them know how to define sensitivity, specificity, or a likelihood ratio. Don't panic, definitions follow. But even definitions do not necessarily make it any easier. To even begin to get a grip on diagnostic testing evidence, we need to have a nodding acquaintance with some technical terms.

### Test performance: the pointy-head bit

Here are some technical terms to begin with, which are made easier by following the calculations in Table 4.1.2.

#### Sensitivity

Proportion of people with the target disorder who have a positive test, usually presented as a percentage rather than a proportion. When a sign/test/symptom has a high sensitivity, a negative result rules out the diagnosis. For example, the sensitivity of a history of ankle swelling for diagnosing ascites is 93%; if a person does not have a history of ankle swelling, it is highly unlikely that the person has ascites.

#### Specificity

Proportion of people without the target disorder who have a negative test, usually presented as a percentage rather than a proportion. When a sign/test/symptom has a high specificity, a positive result rules in the diagnosis. For example, the specificity of a fluid wave for diagnosing ascites is 92%; therefore if a person does have a fluid wave, it rules in the diagnosis of ascites.

#### Positive predictive value

Proportion of people with a positive test who have the target disorder, usually presented as a percentage rather than a proportion.

#### Negative predictive value

Proportion of people with a negative test who are free of the target disorder, usually presented as a percentage rather than a proportion.

#### Likelihood ratio

The likelihood that a given test result would be expected in a patient with the target disorder compared with the likelihood that the same result

**Table 4.1.2** Calculating terms for diagnostic accuracy

| Diagnostic test result | Target disorder | |
|---|---|---|
| | Present | Absent |
| Positive | $a$ | $b$ |
| Negative | $c$ | $d$ |

Sensitivity = $a/(a + c)$
Specificity = $d/(b + d)$
Positive predictive value = $a/(a + b)$
Negative predictive value = $d/(c + d)$
Positive likelihood ratio = $(1 - \text{sensitivity})/\text{specificity}$
Negative likelihood ratio = $\text{sensitivity}/(1 - \text{specificity})$

would be expected in a patient without the target disorder. Likelihood ratios can be calculated for positive and negative test results, as shown in Table 4.1.2.

### A worked example [2]

Five hundred consecutive in- and outpatients (those with known thyroid disease being excluded) at Flinders Medical Centre had case notes examined for:

- thyroid function test (TFT) results;
- clinical signs and symptoms noted by the clinician during the consultation from which the referral for TFT was made;
- subsequent clinical diagnosis of thyroid status. The degree of clinical suspicion from signs and symptoms from a generally accepted list (Table 4.1.3) was correlated with final outcome.

Of the 500 patients, 21 (4.2%) were found to have thyroid dysfunction needing treatment (Table 4.1.4). In the 23 patients with five or more clinical signs or symptoms in whom the degree of clinical suspicion was high, the majority (18, 78%) had a thyroid disorder needing treatment. Using final diagnosis as the gold standard, the likelihood ratio for having a high degree of clinical suspicion was 82. This meant that from a pre-test probability of 4.2%, the post-test probability was over 80%.

In those with high or intermediate degree of clinical suspicion, 19 (33%) had a thyroid disorder needing treatment. Using final diagnosis as the gold standard, the likelihood ratio for having a high or intermediate degree of clinical suspicion was 11. This meant that from a pre-test probability of 4.2% the post-test probability approached 40%.

In those with low degree of clinical suspicion, 2 of 442 patients (0.45%) had thyroid disorder needing treatment. Using final diagnosis as the gold

**Table 4.1.3** Signs and symptoms of thyroid dysfunction

| **Signs, symptoms, and clinical suspicion of thyroid dysfunction** | | |
|---|---|---|
| 1 | Thyroid | Goitre, thyroid bruit, fine tremor, weight loss, increased appetite lid lag, sweating, heat intolerance, family history, lethargy, weight gain, hoarseness, dry skin, hair loss, cold intolerance, delayed reflex, constipation, short stature |
| 2 | Cardiovascular | Recent myocardial infarction, chronic cardiac failure, coronary artery disease, arrhythmias, pulse > 90/min, hypertension |
| 3 | Others | Pneumonia, asthma, diabetes |

| **Degree of clinical suspicion** | |
|---|---|
| High | Patient presenting with 5 or more signs/symptoms listed in groups 1 and 2 |
| Intermediate | Patient presenting with 3 or 4 signs/symptoms listed in groups 1 and 2 |
| Low | Patient presenting with 1 or 2 signs/symptoms listed in groups 1, 2, and 3 |

**Table 4.1.4** Results according to degree of suspicion

| Degree of suspicion | Total number of patients | Patients with thyroid disease | |
| --- | --- | --- | --- |
| | | Number | Per cent |
| High | 23 | 18 | 78 |
| Intermediate | 35 | 1 | 2.9 |
| Low | 442 | 2 | 0.45 |
| Total | 500 | 21 | 4.2 |

standard, the likelihood ratio for having a low degree of clinical suspicion was 0.1 (calculated as the likelihood ratio of a negative test). This meant that from a pre-test probability of 4.2% the post-test probability was less than 1%.

How this works for calculating sensitivity, specificity, and other methods of assessing test performance can be seen in Tables 4.1.5 and 4.1.6, where high plus intermediate suspicion has been contrasted with low suspicion, or high suspicion has been contrasted with intermediate plus low suspicion. Though the numbers change by just a few, there are large differences, especially in likelihood ratios.

## Using likelihood ratios

To use a likelihood ratio, it is easiest to use a likelihood ratio nomogram, as in Figure 4.1.1. The nomogram has three vertical lines, with one for the likelihood ratio sandwiched between a pre-test and a post-test probability. To start, we need to find the pre-test probability of thyroid disease in our population.

The incidence of thyroid disease in the general population is the of order of 1% or so. In the population in the paper [2] some selection has already

**Table 4.1.5** Worked calculation for thyroid function (higher + intermediate vs low)

| Degree of suspicion | Thyroid disease | | |
| --- | --- | --- | --- |
| | Present | Absent | Total |
| High + intermediate | 19 | 39 | 58 |
| Low | 2 | 440 | 442 |
| Total | 21 | 479 | 500 |

Sensitivity of +ve test = $19/(19 + 2) = 0.90 = 90\%$
Specificity of −ve test = $440/(39 + 440) = 0.92 = 92\%$
Positive predictive value = $19/(19 + 39) = 0.33 = 33\%$
Negative predictive value = $440/(2 + 440)$
= $0.995 = 99.5\%$
LR+ = $0.90/(1 − 0.92) = 1.0/0.08 = 12.5$
LR− = $(1 − 0.90)/0.92 = 0.1/0.92 = 0.11$

LR, Likelihood ratio.

**Table 4.1.6** Worked calculation for thyroid function (higher versus intermediate + low)

| Degree of suspicion | Thyroid disease | | |
| --- | --- | --- | --- |
| | Present | Absent | Total |
| High | 18 | 5 | 23 |
| Low + intermediate | 3 | 474 | 477 |
| Total | 21 | 479 | 500 |

Sensitivity of +ve test = 18/(18 + 3) = 0.86 = 86%
Specificity of −ve test = 474/(5 + 474) = 0.99 = 99%
Positive predictive value = 18/(18 + 5) = 0.78 = 78%
Negative predictive value = 474/(3 + 474)
=0.994 = 99.4%
LR+ = 0.86/(1 − 0.99) = 0.86/0.01 =86
LR− = (1 − 0.86)/0.99 = 0.14/0.99 = 0.14

LR, Likelihood ratio.

gone on to create a 4.2% incidence (21 of 500) in the population in the paper. No matter, let's use 2% as a pre-test probability, for no better reason than 2% being clearly marked on the pre-test probability axis. To find the post-test probability of a patient with a positive test having thyroid disease, lines simply join the starting point with the likelihood ratio of a positive test and extrapolate through to the post-test probability line. To find the post-test probability of a patient with a negative test having thyroid disease, we do the same thing for the negative likelihood ratio. For our two examples, the results are shown in Figures 4.1.2 and 4.1.3.

The utility of high plus intermediate (Figure 4.1.2) as a cut-off point for clinical suspicion is limited, because the best post-test probability we get is improved only to about 22%, though a negative test gives a useful low post-test likelihood of 0.3%. A higher cut-off point (Figure 4.1.3) gives both a high post-test probability of disease (70%) and a low post-test probability for a negative disease (0.4%).

Especially with signs and symptoms some knowledge of how tests behave is useful, because they can be used as simple paradigms that lead to action. It may be easier to think about this with reference to Figure 4.1.4. At some points on either end of the probability spectrum, the possibility of the disorder is so remote that neither tests nor treatment are appropriate, or the possibility of the disorder is so high that tests are not appropriate, but treatment is. In the middle we test until we get to one or other of the extreme zones.

### Using natural frequencies

Another method of looking at test results is to use natural frequencies to try and determine action levels. An example with antenatal screening for Down's syndrome might be useful [3]. For those who want an in-depth look at natural frequencies, Bandolier recommends reading a very useful book [4].

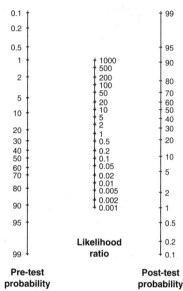

**Likelihood ratio nomogram
signs & symptoms
of thyroid disease**

**Figure 4.1.1** Likelihood ratio nomogram.

The population was 46, 193 pregnant women in 14 London hospitals over 5 years, in which the quadruple test (alphafetoprotein, unconjugated oestriol, human chorionic gonadotrophin, and inhibin-A measured in maternal blood) was applied to serum samples between 14 and 22 weeks of pregnancy. A test was deemed positive if the computed risk of an affected foetus was 1 in 300 or greater (where greater risk means lower numerical values, 1 in 200, 1 in 100, etc.). Gestational age was determined by ultrasound in 80% of women.

There were 88 affected pregnancies, giving an overall risk in this population of 1 in 525, not taking age into account. With the quadruple test there were 3271 positive tests that detected 71 affected fetuses. Just under 98% of all positive tests were false-positives. The paper also tells us that the uptake of amniocentesis rose with increasing risk, from 43% of women with risks between 1 in 250 to 1 in 300 to 74% in those with risks higher than 1 in 50. Of women who tested positive and had an affected pregnancy, 62 of 71 had amniocentesis, and 59 of the 62 had a termination. Twenty children were born with Down's syndrome.

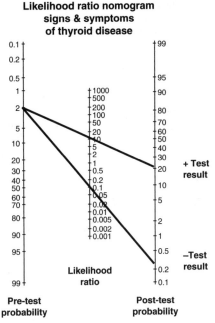

**Likelihood ratio nomogram
signs & symptoms
of thyroid disease**

**Figure 4.1.2** Likelihood ratio nomogram for data from Table 4.1.5.

Sensitivity, specificity, and likelihood ratios are shown in Table 4.1.7, which also gives the results of the natural frequency calculations in terms of chance or odds. Using the quadruple test, the chance of an affected fetus following a positive test was 1 in 46, and with a negative test was 1 in 2525.

By comparison, maternal age alone, using 35 years or older as a cut-off, would have detected 45 affected fetuses had all 6659 women proceeded to amniocentesis. The chance of an affected fetus using age over 35 alone was 1 in 148, but was 1 in 850 with a negative test.

Natural frequencies for the quadruple test and maternal age are shown in Figure 4.1.5, and the calculations below. To calculate the chance of an affected fetus with a positive test, the 71 actual cases detected are divided into the sum of all positive tests, in the case of the quadruple test:

$(3200 + 71)/71 = 46$ (1 chance in 46).

To calculate the chance of an affected fetus with a negative test, the 17 cases not detected are divided into the sum of all negative tests, in the case of the quadruple test:

$(42, 905 + 17)/17 = 2525$ (1 chance in 2525).

The result is that, using a large amount of real-life information and a screening test with a particular set of cut-offs, we have some useful

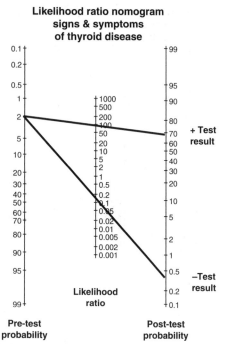

**Figure 4.1.3** Likelihood ratio nomogram for data from Table 4.1.6.

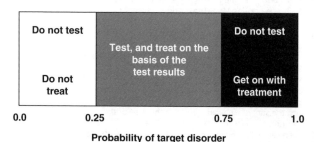

**Figure 4.1.4** Using tests.

**Table 4.1.7** Results of Down's syndrome screening using the quadruple test and maternal age

| Scenario | Sensitivity | Specificity | Likelihood ratio Positive | Negative | Chance of an affected fetus with test Positive | Negative |
|---|---|---|---|---|---|---|
| Quadruple test | 0.81 | 0.93 | 11.6 | 0.21 | 1 in 46 | 1 in 2525 |
| Maternal age 35 or older | 0.51 | 0.79 | 2.5 | 0.62 | 1 in 148 | 1 in 850 |

Outcomes predicted from a cohort of 46, 193 women tested over 5 years at London hospitals. The risk of an affected fetus overall was 1 in 525.

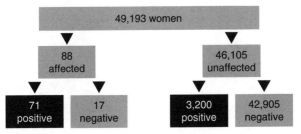

Quadruple test with risk worse than 1 in 300

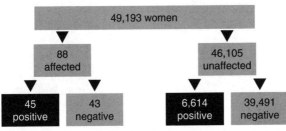

Maternal age 35 years or older

**Figure 4.1.5** Screening for Down's syndrome using natural frequencies for the quadruple test and maternal age.

assessment of risks. That assessment is easily used by professional and patient.

## Commentary

Diagnostic testing is not easy or straightforward, and is made less easy by the fact that most of the terms used to describe test results (how they are performing, not just a number or opinion) are arcane and useless to almost all of us. Some others, such as likelihood ratios or natural frequencies, produce results as chances, which most of us can handle reasonably well. For some diagnostic situations, chances could be calculated once and used by many. In others it will be more difficult. For sure, though, diagnostic testing, however important, will be a closed book unless more work is done to remove obfuscations. A later section will examine how well some diagnostic tests actually work.

## References

1. Reid, M.C. *et al.* (1998). Academic calculations versus clinical judgements: practicing physicians' use of quantitative measures of test accuracy. *American Journal of Medicine* **104**, 374–80.
2. White, G.H. and Walmsley, R.N. (1978). Can the initial clinical assessment of thyroid function be improved? *Lancet* **ii**, 933–5.
3. Wald, N.J. *et al.* (2003). Antenatal screening for Down's syndrome with the quadruple test. *Lancet* **361**, 835–6.
4. Gigerenzer, G. (2002). *Reckoning with risk*. Penguin Books Ltd, London.

# 4.2 Evidence and bias in diagnostic testing

Various levels of evidence have been devised for treatments, and this has also been done in a number of other areas, including diagnostics. The aim is to try to help us to use the best available evidence in making our decisions. One of the best places to see some thoughtful stuff is at the Centre for Evidence-Based Medicine. Usually at the top level is a systematic review of qualitatively good studies. But there are problems with this, because we may not always be able to recognize what constitutes a good study. Another set of levels of evidence in diagnostic testing uses criteria set out for individual studies of diagnostic tests (Table 4.2.1).

The top level is taken up by studies of independent, blinded comparisons of the test with a reference standard, using consecutive patients. The important aspect of this level of evidence is that it excludes studies testing a test on selected patients; rather it looks at all the patients who might reasonably be expected to be targets for the test, with all the complications that brings. It is a real test of the test.

Other study architectures are given a lower level of evidence. Level 2 is the same as level 1, but using non-consecutive patients, for instance, testing the test on a group of people with the disease and a group of people without the disease, the most common study architecture. The problem for us is that we do not always recognize how big this difference is, and whether lower levels of evidence are so low as to mean that we can, or should, ignore studies like that because they will mislead us. We are not told, and this is perhaps the biggest problem with using levels of evidence. We might make incorrect decisions because implicit in levels of evidence is that, while one study type might be better than another, that other is still OK to use if it is the only one available to us. It may not be.

A review from Holland [1] provides an important insight into the size of the gap between level 1 and level 2 studies. It searched for and found 26 systematic reviews of diagnostic tests with at least five included studies. Only 11 could be used in the analysis, because 15 were either not system-

**Table 4.2.1** Levels of evidence for studies of diagnostic methods

| Level | Criteria |
|-------|----------|
| 1 | An independent, masked comparison with reference standard among an appropriate population of consecutive patients |
| 2 | An independent, masked comparison with reference standard among non-consecutive patients or confined to a narrow population of study patients |
| 3 | An independent, masked comparison with an appropriate population of patients, but reference standard not applied to all study patients |
| 4 | Reference standard not applied independently or masked |
| 5 | Expert opinion with no explicit critical appraisal, based on physiology, bench research, or first principles |

**Table 4.2.2** Effect of different quality criteria on relative diagnostic odds ratios

| Study characteristic | Relative diagnostic odds ratio (95% CI) | Description |
|---|---|---|
| Case–control | 3.0 (2.0–4.5) | A group of patients already known to have the disease compared with a separate group of normal patients |
| Different reference tests | 2.2 (1.5–3.3) | Different reference tests used for patients with and without the disease |
| Not blinded | 1.3 (1.0–1.9) | Interpretation of test and reference is not blinded to outcomes |
| No description of test | 1.7 (1.1–1.7) | Test not properly described |
| No description of population | 1.4 (1.1–1.7) | Population under investigation not properly described |
| No description reference | 0.7 (0.6–0.9) | Reference standard not properly described |

atic in their searching or did not report any sensitivity or specificity. Data from the remainder were subjected to mathematical analysis, to investigate whether the presence or absence of some item of proposed study quality made a difference to the perceived value of the test. There were 218 studies, only 15 of which satisfied all eight criteria of quality used in the analysis. Thirty per cent fulfilled at least six of eight criteria.

The relative diagnostic odds ratio used as the output indicates the diagnostic performance of a test in studies failing to satisfy the methodological criterion relative to its performance in studies with the corresponding feature. For our purposes relative diagnostic odds ratio is roughly equivalent to the odds ratio in clinical trials, but not worth spending time in learning about here. Overestimation of effectiveness (positive bias) of a diagnostic test was shown by a lower confidence interval for the relative diagnostic odds ratio of more than 1 (Table 4.2.2).

The size of the bias is rather large, and tells us that, if we use studies that compare people with the disease with those who do not have it (our level 2 evidence), the results we get will be wrong. They will massively overestimate the effectiveness of the test. That effectiveness will also be overestimated by a range of other architectural problems.

Not only do diagnostic test studies often have inadequate study architecture, but they are often poorly reported. A study by Read and colleagues in 1995 [2] examined issues of quality of reporting of diagnostic tests. It described seven quality criteria, and then explored how those criteria were met in papers on diagnostic testing published by the four major English-language medical journals. The results were not encouraging: few told us anything useful about the patients being tested, and only a quarter told us how reliable and reproducible the test was (Table 4.2.3).

**Table 4.2.3** Standards of reporting quality for studies of diagnostic tests

| Reporting standard | Background | Criteria | % meeting standard |
|---|---|---|---|
| Spectrum composition | The sensitivity and specificity of a test depend on the characteristics of the population studied. Change the population and you change these indices. Since most diagnostic tests are evaluated on populations with more severe disease, the reported values for sensitivity and specificity may not be applicable to other populations with less severe disease in which the test will be used | For this standard to be met the report had to contain information on any three of these four criteria: age distribution, sex distribution, summary of presenting clinical symptoms and/or disease stage, and eligibility criteria for study subjects | 27 |
| Pertinent subgroups | Sensitivity and specificity may represent average values for a population. Unless the condition for which a test is to be used is narrowly defined, then the indices may vary in different medical subgroups. For successful use of the test, separate indices of accuracy are needed for pertinent individual subgroups within the spectrum of tested patients | This standard is met when results for indices of accuracy were reported for any pertinent demographic or clinical subgroup (for example symptomatic versus asymptomatic patients) | 9 |
| Avoidance of work-up bias | This form of bias can occur when patients with positive or negative diagnostic test results are preferentially referred to receive verification of diagnosis by the gold standard procedure | For this standard to be met in cohort studies, all subjects had to be assigned to receive both the diagnostic test and the gold standard verification either by direct procedure or by clinical follow up. In case-control studies credit depended on whether the diagnostic test preceded or followed the gold standard procedure. If it preceded, credit was given if disease verification was obtained for a consecutive series of study subjects regardless of their diagnostic test result. If the diagnostic test followed, credit was given if test results were stratified according to the clinical factors that evoked the gold standard procedure | 51 |

(contd.)

**Table 4.2.3** (contd.)

| Reporting standard | Background | Criteria | % meeting standard |
|---|---|---|---|
| Avoidance of review bias | This form of bias can be introduced if the diagnostic test or the gold standard is appraised without precautions to achieve objectivity in their sequential interpretation—like blinding in clinical trials of a treatment. It can be avoided if the test and gold standard are interpreted separately by persons unaware of the results of the other | For this standard to be met in either prospective cohort studies or case-control studies, a statement was required regarding the independent evaluation of the two tests | 43 |
| Precision of results for test accuracy | The reliability of sensitivity and specificity depends on how many patients have been evaluated. Like many other measures, the point estimate should have confidence intervals around it, which are easily calculated | For this standard to be met, confidence intervals or standard errors must be quoted, regardless of magnitude | 12 |
| Presentation of indeterminate test results | Not all tests come out with a black or white, yes/no answer. Sometimes they are equivocal, or indeterminate. The frequency of indeterminate results will limit a test's applicability, or make it cost more because further diagnostic procedures are needed. The frequency of indeterminate results and how they are used in calculations of test performance represent critically important information about the test's clinical effectiveness | For this standard to be met a study had to report all of the appropriate positive, negative or indeterminate results generated during the evaluation and whether indeterminate results had been included or excluded when indices of accuracy were calculated | 26 |
| Test reproducibility | Tests may not always give the same result—for a whole variety of reasons of test variability or observer interpretation. The reasons for this, and its extent, should be investigated | For this standard to be met in tests requiring observer interpretation, at least some of the tests should have been evaluated for a summary measure of observer variability. For tests without observer interpretation, credit was given for a summary measure of instrument variability | 26 |

It is clear that for diagnostic testing the building blocks of evidence, individual studies, have many flaws. These flaws will frequently be so great that it makes any information they contain suspect and probably unsound. Unless we have the best possible studies, we should be very, very careful about using information from studies of diagnostic tests.

Systematic reviews of diagnostic tests face these problems as well. We would hesitate to base major decisions on trials of treatment that were known to have massively biased results, and yet for diagnostic testing that's usually all we have. For some major areas of medicine one can start with several thousand papers on diagnostic tests, and end up with fewer than a handful that might be included in a review.

### Size and diagnostic tests

This is an issue that has probably not been addressed sufficiently. To explain how important size is, let's take the example of sperm counts [3, 4]. Everyone knows that sperm counts are falling, and the reasons might include tight underpants, or oestrogens in the water supply, or even feminism. The evidence comes from a review of sperm count studies [4]. This showed that sperm counts earlier in the century were higher than sperm counts later in the century (Table 4.2.4), which can be seen by eye in Figure 4.2.1.

The problem is that the early data came from a few studies with small numbers of men. If we re-plot the data with the symbols properly related to the size of the individual study, we get a very different picture. The overall sperm count in the review, weighted by study size, was 77 million per mL. Only large studies with at least 1000 men came close to measuring it accurately, and small studies had values with averages from 30 to 140 million per mL (Figure 4.2.1).

And this is before we get to the point about how to measure sperm, what is a sperm, and what quality control between laboratories looks like. There is some suggestion in the literature that individual laboratories vary widely in the results they give to the same sample, and that the accuracy of sperm counts is considered a major problem for infertility practice. This is not good evidence that sperm counts are falling. All the large (and good) studies give the same result.

**Table 4.2.4**   Sperm counts in USA and other countries from 1930 to 1990

| Period | United States | | Rest of the world | |
| --- | --- | --- | --- | --- |
| | Number of men | Weighted mean sperm count (million/mL) | Number of men | Weighted mean sperm count (million/mL) |
| 1930–50 | 496 | 119 | 100 | 95 |
| 1951–70 | 1184 | 107 | 0 | No data |
| 1971–80 | 1868 | 72 | 427 | 73 |
| 1981–90 | 4868 | 67 | 6004 | 77 |

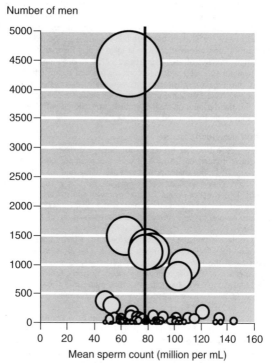

**Figure 4.2.1** Sperm counts in individual studies.

## Commentary

What we have is a major problem. Most study architectures that have been used to measure test accuracy or performance have been flawed, probably fatally so. The only one we can probably trust is where we have fully masked comparisons with consecutive populations within a particular clinical situation. For instance, using PSA as a measure of possible prostate cancer will have different results when it is used as a screen for all men of a certain age irrespective of whether or not they have urinary problems, or whether it is used in primary care as a test where there is suspicion, or whether it is used in secondary care to distinguish between prostate cancer and benign prostatic hyperplasia, alongside other tests.

## References

1. Lijmer, J.G. et al. (1999). Empirical evidence of design-related bias in studies of diagnostic tests. Journal of the American Medical Association 282, 1061–6.

2. Read, M.C. *et al.* (1995). Use of methodological standards in diagnostic test research: getting better but still not good. *Journal of the American Medical Association* **274**, 645–51.

3. Becker, S. and Birhane, K. (1997). A meta-analysis of 61 sperm count studies revisited. *Fertility and Sterility* **67**, 1103–8.

4. Carlsen, E. *et al.* (1992). Evidence for decreasing quality of semen during past 50 years. *British Medical Journal* **305**, 609–13.

# 4.3 Systematic reviews of diagnostic tests

Systematic reviews of diagnostic tests are uncommon, and most are not helpful, either because they include studies of no value because those studies are biased, or because the results of the reviews are unhelpful to the ordinary reader. What constitutes good reporting of diagnostic test papers has been established, at least in part, and it is a useful reference [1] when looking at diagnostic test studies.

The checklist is in Table 4.3.1. It includes items such as identification of study populations and their recruitment, reference standards and their blind application, as well as other methodologically important issues. Like any checklist, there will be circumstances where it will not apply, but it is a useful *aide-mémoire* to have when reading and evaluating any study of diagnostic accuracy, and systematic reviews of them.

## An unhelpful systematic review

A systematic review of hysteroscopy for endometrial cancer and hyperplasia [2] offers an opportunity to examine some of these issues again. The review focused on observational studies in which hysteroscopy was compared with results of the reference standard of endometrial histology. Verification of hysteroscopy diagnosis was followed either at the same time or after a short delay. The outcome was the accuracy of endometrial cancer and hyperplasia diagnosis.

Searching involved MEDLINE and EMBASE to the end of 2001, as well as the Cochrane Library, and without language restriction. Studies retrieved were assessed for methodological quality using a five-item hierarchy (Table 4.3.2). Studies in levels 1–3 were considered to be high quality, and 4 and 5 low quality. Technical failure in hysteroscopy so that no diagnosis was made was categorized as a failed procedure. Information from the studies was collected on setting and pre- or postmenopausal status.

There were 65 primary studies involving 26, 346 women. Of these studies, only 12 (18%) were of high quality (Table 4.3.2). Only one study was of the ideal quality, that is, an independent, blind comparison with reference standard among an appropriate population of consecutive patients. One more was at level 2, but most had lower levels of quality.

In 35 studies failure rates were reported, with an overall failure to make a diagnosis with hysteroscopy of 3.6%. Potentially severe uterine complications were reported in eight cases, but only 19 studies with 9413 procedures explicitly stated an intention to report them. A worst-case risk of a serious complication would then be 1 in 1177 cases.

### Endometrial cancer

For endometrial cancer there were 56 unique studies with 61 sets of data, only 11 of which were deemed of high quality. The post-test probability of endometrial cancer with positive hysteroscopy and with a prevalence of 3.9% is shown in Figure 4.3.1. There was considerable variability according to high versus low quality, by different settings, and by menopausal status.

In high-quality studies the likelihood ratio for a positive test was reported as 35, giving a post-test probability of endometrial cancer of 59%. The

**Table 4.3.1** STARD checklist for the reporting of diagnostic accuracy[*]

| | Item # | | On page # |
|---|---|---|---|
| **Title/abstract/ keywords** | 1 | Identify the article as a study of diagnostic accuracy (recommend MeSH heading 'sensitivity and specificity') | |
| **Introduction** | 2 | State the research questions or study aims, such as estimating diagnostic accuracy or comparing accuracy between tests or across participant groups | |
| **Methods** Participants | 3 | Describe the study population: The inclusion and exclusion criteria, setting and locations where the data were collected | |
| | 4 | Describe participant recruitment: Was recruitment based on presenting symptoms, results from previous tests, or the fact that the participants had received the index tests or the reference standard? | |
| | 5 | Describe participant sampling: Was the study population a consecutive series of participants defined by the selection criteria in items 3 and 4? If not, specify how participants were further selected | |
| | 6 | Describe data collection: Was data collection planned before the index test and reference standard were performed (prospective study) or after (retrospective study)? | |
| Test methods | 7 | Describe the reference standard and its rationale | |
| | 8 | Describe technical specifications of material and methods involved including how and when measurements were taken, and/or cite references for index tests and reference standard | |
| | 9 | Describe definition of and rationale for the units, cut-offs, and/or categories of the results of the index tests and the reference standard | |
| | 10 | Describe the number, training, and expertise of the persons executing and reading the index tests and the reference standard | |
| | 11 | Describe whether or not the readers of the index tests and reference standard were blind (masked) to the results of the other test and describe any other clinical information available to the readers | |
| Statistical methods | 12 | Describe methods for calculating or comparing measures of diagnostic accuracy, and the statistical methods used to quantify uncertainty (e.g. 95% confidence intervals) | |

(contd.)

**Table 4.3.1** (contd.)

| | Item # | | On page # |
|---|---|---|---|
| | 13 | Describe methods for calculating test reproducibility, if done | |

**Results**

| Participants | 14 | Report when study was done, including beginning and ending dates of recruitment | |
|---|---|---|---|
| | 15 | Report clinical and demographic characteristics of the study population (e.g. age, sex, spectrum of presenting symptoms, co-morbidity, current treatments, recruitment centres) | |
| | 16 | Report the number of participants satisfying the criteria for inclusion who did or did not undergo the index tests and/or the reference standard; describe why participants failed to receive either test (a flow diagram is strongly recommended) | |
| Test results | 17 | Report time interval from the index tests to the reference standard, and any treatment administered between | |
| | 18 | Report distribution of severity of disease (define criteria) in those with the target condition; other diagnoses in participants without the target condition | |
| | 19 | Report a cross-tabulation of the results of the index tests (including indeterminate and missing results) by the results of the reference standard; for continuous results, the distribution of the test results by the results of the reference standard | |
| | 20 | Report any adverse events from performing the index tests or the reference standard | |
| Estimates | 21 | Report estimates of diagnostic accuracy and measures of statistical uncertainty (e.g. 95% confidence intervals) | |
| | 22 | Report how indeterminate results, missing responses, and outliers of the index tests were handled | |
| | 23 | Report estimates of variability of diagnostic accuracy between subgroups of participants, readers, or centres, if done | |
| | 24 | Report estimates of test reproducibility, if done | |
| **Discussion** | 25 | Discuss the clinical applicability of the study findings | |

[*] First official version, January 2003.

**Table 4.3.2** Definitions of quality criteria for study and number of studies with particular quality scores

| Quality | Definition | Number |
|---|---|---|
| 1 | An independent, blind comparison with reference standard among an appropriate population of consecutive patients | 1 |
| 2 | An independent, blind comparison with reference standard among an appropriate population of non-consecutive patients or confined to a narrow population of study patients | 1 |
| 3 | An independent, non-blind comparison with reference standard among an appropriate population of consecutive patients | 10 |
| 4 | An independent, non-blind comparison with reference standard among an appropriate population of non-consecutive patients or confined to a narrow population of study patients | 42 |
| 5 | An independent, blind comparison among an appropriate population of patients, but reference standard not applied to all patients | 11 |

likelihood ratio for a negative test was reported as 0.2, giving a post-test probability of endometrial cancer of 0.8%.

*Endometrial disease*

Endometrial disease was defined as endometrial cancer, hyperplasia, or both. For endometrial disease there were 41 unique studies with 71 sets of data, only 12 of which were deemed of high quality. The post-test probability of endometrial disease with positive hysteroscopy and with a prevalence of 10.6% is shown in Figure 4.3.2. There was considerable variability according to high versus low quality, different settings, and menopausal status.

In high-quality studies the likelihood ratio for a positive test was reported as 5.5, giving a post-test probability of endometrial disease of 39%. The likelihood ratio for a negative test was reported as 0.3, giving a post-test probability of endometrial disease of 3.5%.

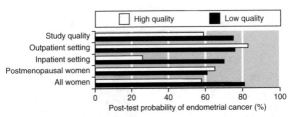

**Figure 4.3.1** Post-test probability of endometrial cancer, by quality, setting, and menopausal status.

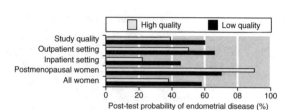

**Figure 4.3.2** Post-test probability of endometrial disease, by quality, setting, and menopausal status.

The definition of high-quality studies in this review was probably justified. Certainly those in grades 4 and 5 are studies known to be associated with bias. There may still be a question mark over whether non-blind comparisons are subject to bias and, if they were, then 10 out of the 12 studies rated high quality would also be subject to possible bias. That would leave only two studies, not much grist for the mill of meta-analysis.

Why then bother to perform an analysis using studies known to have potential faults? Perhaps because there's no further information. Good

**Endometrial cancer and hysteroscopy**

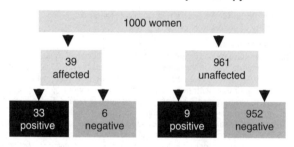

**Endometrial disease and hysteroscopy**

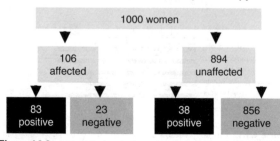

**Figure 4.3.3** Natural frequencies for endometrial cancer and endometrial disease in cohorts of 1000 women.

studies of diagnostic tests are exceptional, as this review proves. So, even if we included studies of poor design, what was the result?

One way of looking at it for cohorts of 1000 theoretical women is shown in Figure 4.3.3, using frequency analysis.

- Women with a positive test for endometrial cancer have an 8 out of 10 chance of actually having endometrial cancer and those with a negative test have only a 1 in 200 chance of having endometrial cancer.
- Women with a positive test for endometrial disease have a 7 out of 10 chance of actually having endometrial disease and those with a negative test have only a 1 in 40 chance of having endometrial disease.

But these results may just be the figments of the imagination of biased trials. To know how good hysteroscopy actually is we have to wait for new studies. We also need reassurance that the gold standard, of histopathology, really is gold and not some shiny but otherwise base metal. Agreement in histopathology is not always high, and the quality of histopathology will have a major impact on the results.

## A helpful systematic review

Anyone wanting to study how diagnostic tests are developed, assessed, and evaluated should look at the Ottawa ankle rules as an example of how good clinical diagnostic tests can be developed. The rules have been evaluated in numerous studies, and we even have a meta-analysis [3].

The review used a systematic search for studies of the Ottawa ankle and foot rules, using several databases and without language restriction. For each study information was sought on methodological issues, such as whether enrolment was consecutive, whether radiologists were blinded, and whether radiography was used in all patients. Pooled assessment was made for sensitivity, but not specificity, and negative likelihood ratios calculated, with sensitivity analyses.

In total 32 studies were found, some looking at the ankle rules, some at the foot rules, some at both and, while most were in adults, some were in children. In 27 studies with data for a pooled analysis, out of 15, 581 patients, 27 (0.3%) had a false-negative result where the Ottawa test was negative, but where they actually had a fracture.

Overall, the pooled sensitivity (percentage with a fracture testing positive and correctly classified as such) was 98%, and most studies achieved very high levels of sensitivity. Specificity (the percentage without a fracture who tested negative) was highly variable, some studies being as low as about 10%, with most at about 40%, and some as high as 70%. The likelihood ratio for a negative test was about 0.1, meaning that with a fracture prevalence of about 10%, the chance of there actually being a fracture was about 1 in 100.

The Ottawa ankle and foot rules were designed to minimize the number of radiographs needed. Specificity was the key to this. Table 4.3.3 shows the calculations for a cohort of 1000 persons, in whom there were 100 actual fractures, applied to the best, average, and worse specificity values found in the review, as well as the chances found applying those sensitivity and specificity values to natural frequencies. As specificity declines, many more positive tests, most of them false, would be found, requiring more radiographs. As specificity declines, the reason for the clinical diagnostic

**Table 4.3.3** Results of studies of Ottawa ankle and foot rules, using an ideal scenario, and best, average, and worst specificities from systematic review

| Scenario | Sensitivity | Specificity | Number of tests | | Chance of a fracture in test | |
|---|---|---|---|---|---|---|
| | | | Positive | Negative | Positive | Negative |
| Ideal specificity | 0.98 | 0.9 | 198 | 802 | 1 in 2 | 1 in 400 |
| Best specificity | 0.98 | 0.7 | 348 | 652 | 1 in 4 | 1 in 326 |
| Average specificity | 0.98 | 0.4 | 648 | 352 | 1 in 7 | 1 in 176 |
| Worst specificity | 0.98 | 0.1 | 898 | 102 | 1 in 9 | 1 in 51 |

Outcomes predicted from a cohort of 1000 people presenting with possible fractured ankle, in which 100 (10%) actually have a broken ankle.

test diminishes. The ideal specificity of about 0.9 would yield only about 200 tests out of 1000 people. The actual results required between 350 and 900.

With the best specificity, the probability of a fracture with a negative test was 1 in 330, and with a positive test was 1 in 4. High probabilities are best with a negative test, and low probability best for a positive test. The ideal result would mean that 1 in 2 people with a positive test would actually have a fracture, and only 1 in 400 with a negative test.

Figure 4.3.4 shows how this looks for the example of the best specificity found in the review, using natural frequencies. It allows the calculation of these probabilities rather easily. It also makes us aware of how the utility of the test would degrade as the specificity declined, meaning that vigilance would be required in the application of the test to make it worthwhile using it. The review can form a basis on which to make decisions about management practices for ankle and foot injuries in an emergency room setting.

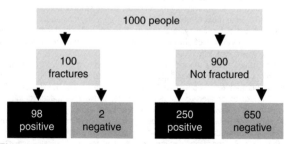

**Figure 4.3.4** Ottawa ankle and foot rules using natural frequencies and 'best' results for specificity from systematic review.

## Commentary

Systematic reviews of diagnostic tests are few and far between. Those that have been able both to review good primary studies and to give us an intelligible result are even more rare. There is every chance that things will get better, but how long we have to wait is another question. History is against much improvement. Diagnostic testing is very much the poor relation of therapeutic interventions, even though knowing anything about therapeutic intervention depends on knowing about initial and final diagnosis.

## References

1. Bossuyt, P.M. *et al.* (2003). Towards complete and accurate reporting of studies of diagnostic accuracy: The STARD initiative. *Clinical Chemistry* **49**, 1–6.
2. Clark, T.J. *et al.* (2002). Accuracy of hysteroscopy in the diagnosis of endometrial cancer and hyperplasia. A systematic quantitative review. *Journal of the American Medical Association* **288**, 1610–21.
3. Bachmann, L.M. *et al.* (2003). Accuracy of Ottawa ankle rules to exclude fractures of the ankle and mid-foot: a systematic review. *British Medical Journal* **326**, 417–23.

## 4.4 Diagnostic testing: examples

Because evidence in diagnostic testing is of a somewhat different nature than that in therapy or epidemiology, this section contains some examples of good studies in diagnostics that nevertheless demonstrate the problems that can occur.

### Blunders

A dictionary definition of a blunder is 'a gross mistake'. As a verb it is also defined as 'to mismanage'. Because we live in an imperfect world, we expect blunders to occur. How we feel about them depends—if we make them they are less of blunder than if someone else makes them. If the battery in our new car fails on a trip to the supermarket we might be less cross than if it fails in torrential rain in the middle of one of those empty bits of Wales or Scotland, or on a bad day on the M25.

Most of us would accept that, while blunders do occur, we should take every reasonable step to see that they do not. Bandolier was speaking with a group of GPs about diagnostic tests, and was surprised to learn that none of them were aware of blunder rates in tests, which in the past have been said to occur at about 1%. So we thought we would see what the literature said about blunders, and found some interesting papers in clinical biochemistry.

#### Defining a blunder

You know one when you see one, so here are some true-life examples:

- A high drug level is reported in Mrs X. But Mrs X isn't taking that drug and didn't have a blood sample taken! It is discovered that actually the sample was from Mr Y, but that the wrong labels were used on sample and request form.
- An imaging report says there is an abdominal mass in a patient sent for a head and neck scan, but the report refers to a different patient than the one sent for the scan.
- Five patients are all reported to have very high prolactin levels. It turns out that they were all analysed together, and that the first had so much prolactin that it resulted in significant carry-over into the next four specimens.
- A new computer system is installed that fails to recognize results with three integers—only those with two. Thus a result of 123 is reported as 23.

These examples point out the areas where blunders can occur—in ordering tests, in the analysis stage, and in transcribing and misreporting errors. Errors may be picked up by the laboratory, or by those receiving the results, or, importantly, by external quality control schemes.

#### Analytical errors

A study of 220, 000 individual clinical chemistry results obtained in methods comparison studies in the USA compared each result with its replicate [1]. It found 98 examples where replicates were ≥ 7 standard deviations from the expected value and an additional 360 in which the difference was 4 to 6 standard deviations from the expected value.

This gives a crude error rate of 0.045% at the 7 SD level and 0.081% at the 4 SD level. That is, less than 1 analytical blunder per 1000 analyses. Of these, however, only nine results were sufficiently different to be judged as likely to influence patient care.

An influential Scottish study [2] came to similar conclusions for analytical blunders. In a study over three time periods involving almost 300,000 results, the analytical blunder rate was 0.034%. But the total blunder rate, including ward, sample handling, reporting, and clerical errors produced a total blunder rate 10 times higher at 0.3%. The blunder rate for external quality assessment samples was 0.2%.

Similar results (an overall rate of about 0.3% of results) were found in an English study of two clinical biochemistry laboratories over 1 year, involving 248, 000 samples and 997,000 results [3]. The two laboratories had blunder rates for external quality assessment samples of 0.5% and 0.2% per analyte and 1.7% and 0.7% per sample, respectively [4].

### An Australian perspective

In 1994 14 laboratories from all over Australia participated in a study to examine laboratory errors [5]. Each randomly selected 100 hand-written pathology request forms, and they scored the number of transcription errors, defined as any instance where the data on individual request forms were not identical to the data entered into the laboratory's computer system. Laboratories also scored the total number of quality assurance samples analysed and the proportion of results that lay outside the allowable limits of error of the program.

Transcription errors varied widely. While most laboratories clustered around median error rates of 1% to 3%, at least two laboratories were more than 2 standard deviations above the mean error rate, as Table 4.4.1 shows.

Analytical errors from one cycle of analysis in 1993 and 1994 occurred in up to 26% of analytical results, and were above 10% in eight of the 14 laboratories.

The combined error rates (transcription plus analytical) were calculated as being up to 46% in the worst performing laboratory. One laboratory had more than 95% of error-free results, while six of the 14 laboratories had better than 80% of error-free results.

### The primary care perspective

All of the above, of course, examines the problem of blunders in laboratory testing principally from the laboratory perspective. But what about the consumers—do they see blunders? In the USA 124 primary care physicians

**Table 4.4.1** Transcription error rates on pathology request forms [5]

| Details | Error rate (%) | | |
| --- | --- | --- | --- |
| | Best laboratory | Median laboratory | Worst laboratory |
| Patient identification | 0 | 1.0 | 9 |
| Patient sex and age | 0 | 2.0 | 17 |
| Patient ward or address | 0 | 2.5 | 9 |
| Tests requested | 0 | 2.5 | 15 |
| Requesting doctor identification | 0 | 1.5 | 17 |

in 49 practices participated in a prospective study in which they reported problems over a 6-month period [6].

They reported 180 problems, of which just over a quarter were judged to have an effect on patient care. The crude result was 1.1 problems per 1000 patient visits (or about 0.1%). But not all patient visits result in a sample being taken for analysis. An estimated one-third of all visits to these practices resulted in a blood sample being taken for laboratory analysis. So the best estimate of problems with laboratory testing in primary care in the USA is 3.4 per 1000 visits, or 0.34%—a figure remarkably similar to these found in the two UK laboratory studies. Analytical errors were only about 10% of the total, at 0.044%.

Lest any of Bandolier's clinical biochemistry friends think that we are picking on them specifically, it is worth pointing out that clinical biochemistry has long been in the vanguard of quality assessment and quality improvement. That is why we have so much data!

There is some consistency in the findings. Overall, the rate of blunders seems to be pretty constant at about 0.3% of results (3 per 1000), and the analytical error is perhaps 0.04% (less than 1 per 1000; Table 4.4.2). Blunders do happen in the best-regulated systems so, if a result looks wrong, it is probably worth checking. There will be blunders that never get picked up. If Mrs A's sample for thyroxine is mixed up with Mrs B's, and both are normal, who could tell?

The Khoury study [5] sticks out like a sore thumb, and it is hard to understand how such high rates of analytical error are allowed in quality assurance schemes (though perhaps Bandolier is missing something). Perhaps, as the paper comments, the fact that there is no minimum standard of performance that laboratories are required to maintain is an important negative influence on overall performance. In the UK there are mechanisms whereby poorly performing laboratories are given help and counselling. This means that no laboratory can perform consistently poorly on one or many tests.

Even so there is a clear message from this important study. In the same circumstances some laboratories do brilliantly, while some are awful. The equipment, the funding, and people probably don't differ by much. But management and leadership can make a huge difference to quality of service.

**Table 4.4.2** Survey data about blunder rates in laboratories (QA here means quality assurance, a process in laboratories for checking that they give clinicians the correct answer)

| | Blunder rates (% of results or samples) | | |
|---|---|---|---|
| **Reference** | **Analytical** | **Overall** | **Comment** |
| Witte et al. [1] | 0.05 | NA | Results |
| Chambers et al. [2] | 0.04 | 0.30 | Results |
| Lapworth and Teal [3,4] | 0.35 | 0.30 | Analytical on QA samples |
| Khoury et al. [5] | 11.40 | NA | QA samples outside limits |
| Nutting et al. [6] | 0.04 | 0.34 | Samples |

NA, Not applicable.

Blunders occur in several different types of laboratory, as a systematic review [7] has shown. Blunders in molecular genetics testing occurred at a rate of 0.33%, very similar to the rate in biochemistry laboratories. Transfusion errors of various sorts were also identified, resulting in death in 1 in 29,000 transfusions in one study, though errors on checking wristbands were as high as 2.7%.

Errors of various types occur throughout medicine [8]. They will inevitably occur in diagnostic testing, though the possibility is often ignored, despite the fact that very frequent use of diagnostic tests makes rare events common.

## How good is a test?

### Pathology

Pathologists often have to recognize one set of visual impressions as being cancer or not. Histopathology has long been regarded as providing a 'gold standard' diagnosis against which all others have to be measured. The trouble with gold standards is to know (rather than to guess) that the standards are gold, and making sure that our comparisons are with the best available. Testing the best to make sure it is the best should be fundamental to this. There are two main weaknesses—both pretty fundamental— interobserver variability and the lack of statistically based predictive power of the 'diagnoses'.

Interobserver variability (how different pathologists interpret a slide) has to be distinguished from intra-observer variability (how the same pathologist interprets the same slide at different times). Even if the same specimen is shown to the same observer there is not always perfect agreement between the two opinions.

The main problem is the variability between observers. When any paper assesses the accuracy of a diagnostic test that depends upon an individual's perception, on their vision or hearing, or on some subjective decision-making process, it is essential to ensure that the study includes an assessment of the degree of interobserver variability. Any such paper should be using a statistical technique, of which the kappa is the most widely used, to assess the degree of the interobserver variability.

Techniques such as kappa allow for agreement by chance, taking into account the prevalence of the condition being assessed, so the degree of agreement in those areas where agreement or disagreement matters can be assessed. Kappa (or κ) has values between 0 (a random effect) and 1

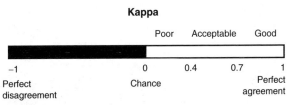

**Figure 4.4.1**  Kappa scores.

(perfect agreement; Figure 4.4.1). In practice, a kappa score of greater than 0.4 is taken to indicate that agreement is becoming reasonable, while 0.6 or above is good agreement.

An editorial in the *Journal of Pathology* [9] pointed out that, apart from grouping lesions into broad categories (benign versus malignant), poor agreement is not infrequent. Some examples from the literature (albeit generally with small numbers of pathologists, but with perhaps more attention given than is the norm in clinical practice) quoted in the editorial are reproduced in Table 4.4.3.

### Diagnosis of melanoma

As part of the National Institutes of Health consensus conferences on the diagnosis and treatment of early melanoma, a study was conducted to review pathology specimens and measure interpathologist agreement [10]. A panel of eight pathologists expert in melanoma diagnosis was selected. Each submitted five cases (slide plus clinical history and eventual diagnosis), which they considered 'classic' cases of melanomas or melanocytic naevi that shared histological features with melanomas.

From these 37 cases were selected and anonymized. Slides with histories (but not eventual diagnosis) were then randomized independently of the organizing group. The slides were sent to each panel member in turn, so that each panel member used the same glass slides. Each case was to be scored as benign, malignant, or indeterminate. Any description other than this had to be defined.

All 37 cases were reviewed, without loss or breakage. Eight benign cases and five malignant cases were agreed unanimously. Lack of unanimous agreement occurred in 24 cases (62%). Two or more discordant diagnoses were made in 14 cases (38%) and discordance was three or more in 8 cases (22%). The kappa was 0.5, indicating only moderate agreement.

It is illuminating to look at the extremes. One expert (and these were all experts in melanoma, don't forget) thought 21 cases were malignant and 16 were benign. Another thought 10 were malignant, 26 benign, and one

**Table 4.4.3** Results of studies on agreement between histopathologists

| Organ feature | Agreement (%) | Kappa |
|---|---|---|
| Liver—piecemeal necrosis | 47 | 0.2 |
| Rectal cancer—grading | 50–69 | 0.1–0.5 |
| Lymph node—Hodgkin's classification | 56 | 0.4 |
| Cervical intra-epithelial neoplasia | No data | 0.01–0.5 |
| Grading anal intra-epithelial neoplasm | No data | 0.1–0.6 |
| Liver transplant acute rejection | No data | 0.3–0.5 |
| Breast cancer classification | 73 | 0.4 |
| Breast cancer grade | | 0.3 |
| Breast cancer invasive subtype | | 0–0.3 |
| Breast cancer atypical hyperplasia | | 0.2 |

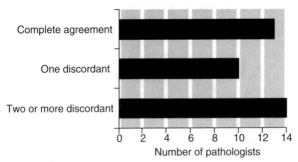

**Figure 4.4.2** Discordant results between melanoma experts.

indeterminate. Between them, these two pathologists disagreed on 12 out of 37 cases, and in 11 cases one pathologist identified a case as malignant while the other identified the same case as benign (Figure 4.4.2).

An accompanying editorial [11] speaks of 'shattered illusions'. It comments that 'the conclusions of the article ... should be chilling not only to physicians, but to patients, and sobering to lawyers for plaintiffs.' This is scary stuff, but these were difficult cases. It is instructive to consider how to improve results.

The CRC Melanoma Pathology Panel studied 95 sections from pigmented lesions, including equal proportions of benign naevi and primary malignant melanoma, of which half were selected with Breslow thickness < 0.76 mm [12]. These were sent to a panel of seven pathologists with a major interest in melanoma plus a dermatopathologist also with a major interest in melanoma.

Slides were sent to panel members before and particularly after a series of meetings to clarify the understanding and use of terms used in making a diagnosis. A series of carefully worded definitions were made for severe nuclear atypia, intraepidermal architectural atypia, an invasive component of radial growth phase, a vertical growth phase or component, mitotic count, regression, and established regression.

In a detailed paper with many results the highlights were these.
- The level of agreement improved after discussion and re-definition of criteria of several features.
- A high level of agreement was obtained for an overall benign or malignant diagnosis (kappa = 0.77).
- Use of more specific diagnostic terms with three or four levels of diagnosis resulted in lower levels of agreement.
- The agreement for individual pathologists reviewing the same slide at different times was high at over 80% for any one, and over 90% on average.

One hundred and forty-eight UK pathologists participated in two circulations. In the first circulation of 20 slides no standardized diagnostic criteria were used and the kappa was 0.45 for three categories—benign naevi with no atypia, benign naevi with atypia, and melanoma. The same panel as in the CRC study had a kappa of 0.75.

A second survey [13] used 25 slides (19 from the first circulation and six new ones) and used diagnostic criteria of benign, melanocytic intraepidermal neoplasia with or without microinvasion, and melanoma with vertical growth phase. Using these criteria the agreement for pathologists and the panel was the same with a kappa of 0.68.

Both these important papers demonstrate that good agreement can be obtained by the use of standardized criteria. But with melanoma there are always going to be difficult cases where even the experts have problems in making a diagnosis, and where they may disagree.

The main lesson is that discussion and quality assessment is not just for special occasions but ongoing. The Dutch now have a system where pathologists faced with a difficult case can refer it to one of three experts, who can then refer to two more if the first expert also finds difficulty in making the diagnosis. In a stimulating and thoughtful editorial [14], Mark Cook speaks of the difficulties in continuous quality improvement and in providing the best possible diagnostic service for melanoma. He points out that it will be difficult and expensive (though how much more expensive than making the wrong diagnosis is not dwelt upon). Just because something is difficult doesn't mean it shouldn't be attempted, and to make things better one needs evidence about how bad they are in the first place. That (showing how bad things are) is what quality control is all about. Most of medicine has much to learn from what has happened in laboratories over the past 30–40 years.

### Dementia diagnosis

A detailed study of systems of diagnosing dementia has shown a 10-fold variation in prevalence in 1879 subjects, from 3.1% to 29% [15], depending upon which of a number of internationally recognized clinical diagnostic schemes were used.

A Canadian study of health and ageing surveyed 10, 263 people aged 16 years or over, of whom 1879 had a full clinical examination, including a neuropsychological examination. A neurologist, a neuropsychologist, and a nurse examined records independently to agree whether each patient met criteria included in each of a number of different diagnostic systems, and to make a clinical consensus. Diagnostic schemes used were:

- *Diagnostic and statistical manual of mental disorder* (DSM)-III;
- DSM-III-R;
- DSM-IV;
- International Classification of Disease (ICD)-9;
- ICD-10;
- Cambridge Examination for Mental Disorders of the Elderly (CAMDEX).

The mean age of the 1879 included in the study was 80 years, and two-thirds lived in the community. The results for the different schemes in this population are shown in Figure 4.4.3. The lowest prevalence was 3.1% with ICD-10, and the highest was DSM-III with 29.1%. Clinical consensus in the Canadian study was 20.9%. Only 20 people were given a diagnosis of dementia by all six systems.

### Diagnosing obstructive airway disease

Any prize for the most important contribution to the evidence base of diagnosis would certainly go to the CARE group investigating the diagnosis of obstructive airway disease [16]. When an innovative method using

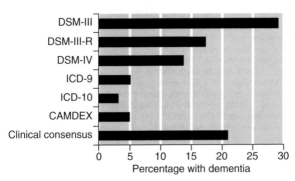

**Figure 4.4.3** Prevalence of dementia according to system of diagnosis in 1879 people.

clinicians around the world collaborating through the Internet comes up with the right stuff it is as welcome as a cold glass of water in the desert.

The study [17] derived from a systematic review of diagnostic criteria for obstructive airways disease (OAD). The review sought physical signs for differentiating between patients with OAD and those with normal pulmonary function in papers and textbooks. Many criteria were mentioned, but no single sign was found in more than a third of studies. For each of the four most commonly used physical signs, the range of diagnostic accuracy from the literature was huge. Positive likelihood ratios spanned the range from about 1 to over 10: from useless to highly predictive.

The review also examined the quantity and quality of evidence from systematic reviews for a variety of signs for different conditions. There were few high-quality studies, and those few were small. The bottom line was that we had little or no objective proof of the quality of diagnostic accuracy of the clinical examination for OAD.

Investigators from around the world were recruited via the CARE Internet site (*www.carestudy.com*) and the evidence-based email discussion group. Participating groups had at least one physician and one spirometrist and enrolled at least four consecutive patients from each of three categories:

- patients known to have chronic OAD. This was defined as prior pulmonary function test results less than fifth percentile, patient self-report of chronic OAD, bronchitis or emphysema, or use of bronchodilators or steroids;
- patients suspected of having OAD who did not fulfil criteria of known OAD but were referred for suspected OAD or the physician thought that OAD was a diagnostic possibility;
- patients neither known nor suspected of having OAD.

There were various exclusions, such as reversible airway obstruction like asthma and those with terminal illnesses or concomitant serious medical conditions. All patients underwent clinical examination and independent blinded spirometry. Diagnostic criteria chosen for examination, based on the earlier systematic review and consensus, were:

- self reported-history of chronic OAD;
- smoking history;
- laryngeal height (distance between the top of the thyroid cartilage and the suprasternal notch: At end-expiration with the patient sitting up, looking straight ahead, and with hands relaxed in his/her lap, palpate the top of the thyroid cartilage which is readily identified by the notch on its superior edge. Hook your index finger over the thyroid cartilage and using the rest of your fingers, measure the distance from the top of the thyroid cartilage to the sternal notch in finger-breadths. Convert these finger-breadths to centimetres and record this distance). (www.carestudy. com/CareStudy/PREOP1/manoeuvre1.asp);
- laryngeal descent (maximum laryngeal height was measured at end of inspiration and minimum laryngeal height at end of expiration);
- wheezing.

Each patient underwent a standard protocol for spirometry within 30 minutes of the clinical examination. The gold standard definition of OAD was $FEV_1$ and $FEV_1/FVC$ ratio less than the fifth percentile.

Twenty-five investigator groups in 13 countries recruited 322 patients in 1 month. After excluding some with asthma the final sample size was 309. Likelihood ratios were calculated for all patients, and for those without known chronic OAD. The key indicators were self-reported history of chronic OAD, smoking history of more than 40 pack years, age 45 or more, maximum laryngeal height 4 cm or less.

For all patients, if all four factors were present, the likelihood ratio was a massive 221 (Table 4.4.4). Given a population in which the prior likelihood of OAD was 10%, the post-test probability would be 96%. This would essentially rule in OAD. When all four factors were absent, the post-test probability would be about 1%, essentially ruling out the diagnosis. Where there was no prior history, the three remaining factors achieved much the same result.

**Table 4.4.4** Likelihood ratios for the four important diagnostic criteria for chronic obstructive airways disease

| | Likelihood ratios | | | |
| | All 309 patients | | 233 patients without known chronic OAD | |
| Diagnostic element | Factor present | Factor absent | Factor present | Factor absent |
|---|---|---|---|---|
| Self-reported history of OAD | 7.3 | 0.5 | | |
| Smoked more than 40 pack-years | 8.3 | 0.8 | 11.6 | 0.9 |
| 45 years or more | 1.3 | 0.4 | 1.4 | 0.5 |
| Maximum laryngeal height 4 cm or less | 2.8 | 0.8 | 3.6 | 0.7 |
| All factors | 221 | 0.13 | 59 | 0.32 |

This study tripled the number of patients and increased the number of clinicians 10-fold over the previous rigorous examination of diagnosis of chronic OAD. It demonstrates that exemplary information about diagnosis can be achieved quickly by use of the Internet. Investigators were involved from Argentina, Australia, Canada, Chile, Colombia, England, Italy, New Zealand, Romania, Spain, Saudi Arabia, United Arab Emirates, and the United States. It is a model for diagnostic testing research and shows that a number of different issues can quickly be resolved with a bit of thought. Just imagine what could be done if real resources were put into sorting out diagnostic testing.

### Right patient, right treatment

In his groundbreaking classic book on evidence-based health-care [18], Muir Gray has a chapter entitled 'Doing the right things right'. It is always worth re-reading, and it is also worth extending, perhaps to whether we do the right things, to the right patients, at the right time, and in the right way. In this chapter, emphasis has been laid on the importance of diagnosis as the foundation of treatment, though without much evidence in support. A major reason is that people usually don't do that sort of research, and examples are hard to come by, however obvious the proposition. A study from Norway suggests that treating the right patient right can have real benefits [19].

Actually there were two studies in one. The main study looked at different levels of intervention for people off sick from work with musculoskeletal problems for more than 8 weeks. The subsidiary study examined the effectiveness of treatment depending on an initial prognosis determined by a screening instrument. The setting was the area around Bergen, with a population of 270,000. Participants were recruited from sickness insurance records if they were off work for 8 weeks or more. The total approached was 1988 (0.74% of the total population). Because some people did not accept the invitation to participate, the final sample was 654 individuals (33% of the total approached).

The screening instrument consisted of a questionnaire and a structured examination by a physiotherapist. The details are too many to explain here, but in a fairly simple process participants were graded as having a good, medium, or poor prognosis for return to work.

A properly randomized open study involved three treatments.

1. Ordinary treatment involved referral back to a general practitioner.
2. Light multidisciplinary treatment and follow-up comprised a lecture on exercise and lifestyle and fear avoidance advice, with information and feedback. Patients were encouraged gradually to increase their activity level. Patients received individual exercise programmes. Some were referred to physiotherapists. Over a year each patient received an average of three individual follow-ups.
3. Extensive multidisciplinary treatment and follow-up involved a more intensive treatment programme lasting for 4 weeks, with six hour-long sessions 5 days a week. It involved cognitive-behavioural modification, education, exercise, and occasional workplace interventions. Patients were encouraged to take responsibility for their own health and lifestyle. Follow-up was over 1 year with individual pain management programmes.

**Table 4.4.5** Return to work and initial prognosis

| Initial prognosis | % in work at 1 year |
| --- | --- |
| Good | 61 |
| Medium | 57 |
| Poor | 44 |

The outcome was return to work by 1 year after the intervention, which took place about 2 months after screening. A cost–benefit analysis was also carried out for the light and extensive multidisciplinary treatments. Economic returns were measured in terms of productivity gain when patients returned to work minus the costs of the treatment programmes.

At baseline the three treatment groups were well matched. The mean age was 44 years, about two-thirds were women, and three-quarters of patients had back pain or neck or shoulder pain. About half were considered to have a medium prognosis for return to work, 22% had a good prognosis, and 28% a poor prognosis. More patients had returned to work at 1 year with a good prognosis or medium prognosis than with a poor prognosis (Table 4.4.5).

Ordinary treatment led to fewer patients at work at 1 year (50%) than for either the light or extensive multidisciplinary treatments (60%).
- For patients with a good prognosis, there was no difference between treatments.
- For patients with a medium prognosis there was no additional effect of extensive over light multidisciplinary treatment. Ordinary treatment for these patients gave poor results (Table 4.4.6).
- For patients with poor prognosis extensive multidisciplinary treatment was superior to ordinary or light multidisciplinary treatment (Table 4.4.6).

Most patients returned to work if they were given treatment appropriate to their screening category (Figure 4.4.4). Between 55% and 64% returned to work when given the right treatment.

If screening results rather than randomization had been the determining factor for the type of treatment, then productivity gains would have outweighed the cost of treatment by US $800 per treated patient. What we have here is a demonstration from a randomized trial that doing the right thing for the right patient pays dividends. The patients benefit because they get back to work, and society benefits because the productivity gains

**Table 4.4.6** Results of different treatment strategies with medium and poor prognosis

| Initial prognosis | % in work at 1 year | | |
| --- | --- | --- | --- |
| | Ordinary treatment | Light multidisciplinary | Extensive multidisciplinary |
| Medium | 48 | 63 | 62 |
| Poor | 37 | 44 | 55 |

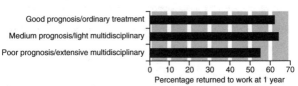

**Figure 4.4.4** Treating the right patients right.

outweigh the costs of getting people back to work. Right people could be treated right because a right diagnosis was made.

## Commentary

By now the point that evidence about diagnosis or diagnostics is pretty thin should have been made. In one sense, it possibly sounds worse than it is. Biochemistry laboratories were world leaders in initiating and developing internal and external quality control schemes some 40 years ago. It is why a cortisol level measured in Aberdeen would have had the same result if it were measured in Exeter. Laboratories in the 21st century are leaders in information technology systems, with much attention paid to avoiding blunders, and getting the right result on the right patient to the right professional as quickly as possible. Laboratories looked at their systems and found them wanting, so made them better.

What has been lacking anywhere in the world has been any academic attention for diagnostics and diagnosis. There have been isolated exceptions, but most academic centres of laboratory medicine have busied themselves with looking in detail at specific things, rather than the broad business of diagnosis, if we may think of it like that. Because there were no academic brownie points for doing it, nothing happened.

A consequence has been inattention and the inevitable repetition of mistakes made, lessons learned and forgotten. It is truly disheartening to write about the missing evidence for diagnosis and diagnostics.

## References

1. Witte, D.L. *et al.* (1997). Errors, mistakes, blunders, outliers, or unacceptable results: how many? *Clinical Chemistry* **43**, 1352–6.
2. Chambers, A.M. *et al.* (1986). The blunder-rate in a clinical biochemistry service. *Annals of Clinical Biochemistry* **23**, 470–3.
3. Lapworth, R. and Teal, T.K. (1994). Laboratory blunders revisited. *Annals of Clinical Biochemistry* **31**, 391.
4. Lapworth, R. and Teal, T.K. (1994). Laboratory blunders revisited. *Annals of Clinical Biochemistry* **31**, 78–84.
5. Khoury, M. *et al.* (1996). Error rates in Australian chemical pathology laboratories. *Medical Journal of Australia* **165**, 128–30.
6. Nutting, P.A. *et al.* (1996). Problems in laboratory testing in primary care. *Journal of the American Medical Association* **275**, 635–9.
7. Bonini, P. *et al.* (2002). Errors in laboratory medicine. *Clinical Chemistry* **48**, 691–8.
8. Kalra, J. *et al.* (2004). Medical errors: impact on clinical laboratories and other critical areas. *Clinical Biochemistry* **37**, 1052–62.
9. Fleming, K.A. (1996). Evidence-based pathology. *Journal of Pathology* **179**, 127–8.
10. Farmer, E.R. *et al.* (1996). Discordance in the histopathologic diagnosis of melanoma and melanocytic nevi between expert pathologists. *Human Pathology* **27**, 528–31.

11. Ackerman, A.B. (1996). Discordance among expert pathologists in diagnosis of melanocytic neoplasms. *Human Pathology* **27**, 1115–16.

12. Cook, M.G. *et al.* (1996). The evaluation of diagnostic and prognostic criteria and the terminology of thin cutaneous malignant melanoma by the CRC Melanoma Pathology Panel. *Histopathology* **28**, 497–512.

13. Cook, M.G. *et al.* (1997). A nationwide survey of observer variation in the diagnosis of thin cutaneous malignant melanoma including the MIN terminology. *Journal of Clinical Pathology* **50**, 202–5.

14. Cook, M.G. (1997). Diagnostic discord with melanoma. *Journal of Pathology* **182**, 247–9.

15. Erikinjuntti, T. *et al.* (1997). The effect of different diagnostic criteria on the prevalence of dementia. *New England Journal of Medicine* **337**, 1667–74.

16. Straus, S.E. *et al.* (2000). The accuracy of patient history, wheezing, and laryngeal measurements in diagnosing obstructive airway disease. *Journal of the American Medical Association* **283**, 1853–7.

17. McAlister, F.A. *et al.* (1999). Why we need large, simple studies of the clinical examination: the problem and a proposed solution. *Lancet* **354**, 1721–4.

18. Muir Gray, J.A. (1997). *Evidence-based healthcare*. Churchill Livingstone, Edinburgh.

19. Haland Haldorsen, E.M. *et al.* (2002). Is there a right treatment for a particular patient group? Comparison of ordinary treatment, light multidisciplinary treatment, and extensive multidisciplinary treatment for long-term sick-listed employees with musculoskeletal pain. *Pain* **95**, 49–63.

# 5.1 Adverse events: thinking and definitions

### Introduction and definitions

Adverse events are complicated beasts. There is a whole series of nomenclature around adverse events, starting with whether it is an adverse event or an adverse effect. The trouble is that the latter implies causation and, for the sake of simplicity, we will use the generic term adverse event throughout this chapter and the book. Another warning is that, whatever definitions are put forward for adverse events, many, perhaps most, reports use the Red Queen defence: words mean what you want them to mean. How adverse event terms are used is often *ad hoc*. In practice people use many definitions and words interchangeably. It all causes not a little confusion, so understanding the evidence around adverse events is understandably difficult.

Some common terms and their definitions are in Table 5.1.1 (from [1]). These are now tending to be used with greater regularity, at least in clinical trials conducted in the last decade. Clinical trials, and especially metaanalyses of clinical trials of adverse events, tend to respect the terms, especially when the trials have been performed by pharmaceutical companies for drug registration. The simple reason is that registration authorities demand consistent good quality data collection and reporting of adverse events, and they get it.

### Dimensions of adverse events

Adverse events have many dimensions (Figure 5.1.1), all of which are important in their own way.

#### Common or rare

The frequency with which adverse events can occur varies from substantial minorities of patients (tens of per cents), to one in perhaps 100,000 (or more) people receiving the intervention. Descriptors of how common or rare an adverse event may be have been proposed and evaluated. The EU has guideline descriptors for the frequency of an adverse event, but four studies involving more than 750 people demonstrate that people invariably overestimate frequency from them [2]. Results from 200 undergraduates who were asked to estimate the probability of having a sideeffect given the EU descriptors are shown in Table 5.1.2. For the very rare adverse events, the undergraduates overestimated the likelihood by at least 400-fold.

#### Reversible or irreversible

This is obvious, and important to patients, but rarely discussed. Constipation may occur with opioids, but bowel habit returns to normal when treatment is stopped. Most common adverse events are reversible by stopping treatment, though some may take time. Other adverse events are not reversible. For instance, gastrointestinal bleeding with NSAIDs can be catastrophic and lead to disability or death. Rare adverse events are often irreversible.

**Table 5.1.1** Definitions of adverse event terms

| | |
|---|---|
| Adverse event | An unfavourable outcome that occurs during or after the use of a drug or other intervention but is not necessarily caused by it. It can be defined as 'any abnormal sign, symptom, or laboratory test, or any syndromic combination of such abnormalities, any untoward or unplanned occurrence (e.g. an accident or unplanned pregnancy), or any unexpected worsening or improvement in a concurrent illness' (Aronson J.K. and Ferner R.E. (2005). *Drug Safety* **28**, 851–70. |
| Adverse effect | An adverse event for which the causal relation between the drug/intervention and the event is at least a reasonable possibility. This term applies to all interventions |
| Adverse drug reaction (ADR) | This term is used only with drugs. The terms ADR and adverse effect are otherwise used interchangeably (Edwards, I.R. and Aronson, J.K. (2000). *Lancet* **356**, 1255–9). Seriousness and intensity (often confused with seriousness, severity is better termed 'intensity'. The WHO severity) of the adverse effect terminology differentiates between the terms 'serious' and 'severe' in this way: 'serious' refers to adverse effects that have significant *medical* consequences, e.g. lead to death, permanent disability, prolonged hospitalization. Some reports use other definitions, which may include effects that the patient considers serious. In contrast, 'severe' refers to the intensity of a particular adverse effect. For example, a non-serious adverse effect, such as headache, may be severe in intensity (as opposed to mild or moderate) |
| Side-effect | Any unintended effect of a pharmaceutical product that occurs at doses normally used for therapeutic purposes in man and is related to the pharmacological properties of the drug. While some side-effects may be harmful (adverse effects), there are also side-effects that are beneficial |
| Safety | This word usually refers to (the relative lack of) serious adverse reactions, such as those that threaten life, require or prolong hospitalization, result in permanent disability, or cause birth defects. But, serious, indirect adverse effects, such as traffic accidents, violence, and damaging consequences of mood change, can also be categorized by this term |
| Tolerability | The term is usually used to refer to medically less important (without serious or permanent sequelae), but unpleasant, adverse effects of drugs. These include symptoms such as dry mouth, tiredness, etc. that can affect a person's quality of life and willingness to continue the treatment |

*Mild or severe*

Adverse events are often classified as mild, moderate, or severe (Table 5.1.1), especially in clinical trials. Definitions sometimes used are: mild (causing no limitation of usual activities), moderate (causing some limitation of usual activities), or severe (causing inability to carry out usual activities).

*Serious or minor*

A serious adverse event is described as one causing significant hazard, contraindication, side-effect, or precaution, including any event that is

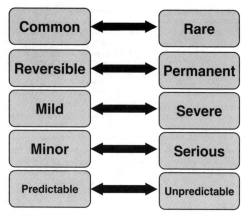

**Figure 5.1.1** Dimensions of adverse events.

fatal, life-threatening, causes significant incapacity or disability, causes or prolongs inpatient hospitalization, causes a congenital anomaly or birth defect, or is an important medical event. Adverse events can be severe without being serious (a severe headache, for instance). Serious adverse events are probably always severe.

*Predictable or unpredictable*

Many classes of drug, for instance, have predictable adverse events. Examples would be nausea, dizziness, or constipation with opioids, or dry mouth with tricyclic antidepressants. Predictability is a function of dose (the more you give, the more frequent or severe the adverse event), time, or susceptibility (older people have reduced renal function, for instance)[3]. Some adverse events are idiosyncratic (an abnormal susceptibility to some drug or other agent, peculiar to the individual) and these are not normally predictable, though cases of apparently unpredictable adverse events discovered through yellow card reporting have been found to have *post-hoc*

**Table 5.1.2** Evaluation of EU descriptor of adverse events

| Qualitative descriptor | EU assigned frequency (%) | Mean frequency estimated by participants (%) |
|---|---|---|
| Very common | >10 | 65 |
| Common | 1–10 | 45 |
| Uncommon | 0.1–1 | 18 |
| Rare | 0.01–0.1 | 8 |
| Very rare | 0.01 | 4 |

predictability because altered genotypes have altered drug metabolism and susceptibility [4].

One might recognize that common adverse events are often reversible, mild, not serious, and predictable. Anything that is irreversible, serious, and to a degree unpredictable is likely to be rare because otherwise drugs would not have obtained regulatory approval.

### Adverse events reported in studies

There are certain categories of adverse events that are commonly reported in clinical trials and clinical practice, and have a general utility, if only because they are often the only sort of adverse event information available to us. They include:

- patients experiencing at least one adverse event. It is not uncommon for some patients to have several adverse events from a treatment, but summing all the adverse events is not always helpful. What we want is information about patients at least minimally affected (those with at least one adverse event) and those not affected (the remainder). This is a simple dichotomous outcome that is readily understandable.
- discontinuations because of adverse events. This is a higher hurdle, where at least one adverse event must be sufficiently troublesome that patients would rather discontinue the treatment.
- discontinuations because of lack of efficacy. Strictly speaking, lack of efficacy is not an adverse event. The argument that it should be classified in this way depends on understanding that discontinuation of treatment can have major practical implications for patients.
- patients experiencing particular adverse events. We want to know how many patients have each of several possible or actual adverse events.

Other forms of adverse events reported in studies include abnormal laboratory findings, whether or not they have any physical impact on patients.

### Other reports of adverse events

Adverse events can be reported or examined in other ways. For instance, several countries have established spontaneous reporting systems (yellow card system), where rare (in practice mostly rare, though they need not just be rare) adverse events noticed or suspected by professionals can be reported to a central authority. Case reports are another way in which rare events can be reported [5].

### Is it safe?

Estimating the risk of harm is a critical part of clinical decisions. Systematic reviews should report adverse events as well as efficacy, and consider the issue of rare but important adverse events. Large RCTs apart, most trials study limited patient numbers. New medicines may be launched after trials on only 1500 patients [6], potentially missing these rare but important adverse events. The rule of three is important here. If a particular serious event does not occur in 1500 patients given the treatment, we can be 95% confident that the chance of it occurring is at most 1 in 500 (1500/3) [7].

Put more formally, if you observe $n$ patients, and none of these patients have an adverse event, then we can be 95% confident that it will occur in no more than $n/3$ patients.

The subject of adverse events is not easy, and is one that causes considerable problems over sources and meaning of evidence. We can have situations where systematic reviews of randomized trials can provide little useful information on an important aspect of potential harm, while a well-done case report can be the most important evidence we have. It all depends. The hard bit is working out when to trust and distrust the evidence before us.

## A sideways look at adverse events

When placebo is used in clinical trials and adverse events occur, all sorts of convoluted discussions take place about placebo 'causing' adverse events. What we really need is some information about adverse event frequency in people not taking part in a trial and not on any drugs, as a background to inform our discussions and thinking. Only two studies [8, 9] seem to have measured adverse events in a population not in a trial and not on any drugs.

Both studies were retrospective questionnaires about the presence of symptoms often listed as adverse events of drugs. The first was conducted in medical and non-medical people in Philadelphia in the late 1960s, and the second reproduced the study in medical students in Magdeburg 30 years later. In both studies, subjects initially recruited were screened for any diseases or medicines being taken, and only those without disease and taking no medicines were asked to complete the symptom questionnaire. The exception was that oral contraceptives were allowed in the German study. Subjects were asked to record whether they had any of the listed symptoms in the 3 days before questioning.

Most people in the surveys were young and in their 20s. Symptom reporting was common, and the list of symptoms and the frequency with which they were reported are shown in Table 5.1.3. Fatigue was the most common symptom noted in 40% or more, with nasal congestion, sleepiness, irritability, headaches and pain in muscles and joints occurring in 10% or more (Table 5.1.3). There were no major differences between medical and non-medical subjects, nor between studies conducted 30 years apart.

Over the 544 subjects in all three groups, 83% reported at least one symptom over the preceding 3 days, and only 17% reported none of these symptoms. Large percentages of subjects reported multiple symptoms (Figure 5.1.2).

What are we to make of this high level of symptom (adverse event) reporting in young, healthy individuals? The results were consistent, but both studies used retrospective rather than prospective questioning. It might be conservative, since people taking analgesics or medicines for allergies were omitted.

Certainly it makes us look in a new light at clinical trial results with high levels of reported adverse events, but no difference between active and placebo. It is what we should expect, and not necessarily related to being in a trial. We might also wish to speculate about the results we would find in older, but fit populations, or populations that include people who do have disorders being treated.

Many conditions or symptoms commonly recorded as adverse events are common in the population at large, without any intervention, as the studies on young people above showed. But take something like

**Table 5.1.3** Presence of symptoms often listed as adverse events over previous 3 days in healthy, young, individuals in USA and Germany, 30 years apart

| Symptom | % with symptom | | |
|---|---|---|---|
| | US medical (n = 239) | US non-medical (n = 175) | German medical students (n = 130) |
| Fatigue | 41 | 37 | 65 |
| Nasal congestion | 31 | 13 | 30 |
| Inability to concentrate | 25 | 27 | 13 |
| Excessive sleepiness | 23 | 23 | 8 |
| Bleeding from gums after brushing teeth | 21 | 20 | 15 |
| Irritability | 20 | 17 | 9 |
| Headaches | 15 | 13 | 25 |
| Pain in muscles | 10 | 11 | 13 |
| Pain in joints | 9 | 5 | 12 |
| Skin rash | 8 | 3 | 4 |
| Bad dreams | 8 | 3 | 4 |
| Insomnia | 7 | 10 | 8 |
| Faintness or dizziness when first standing up | 5 | 5 | 7 |
| Urticaria | 5 | 3 | 3 |
| Dry mouth | 5 | 3 | 5 |
| Diarrhoea | 5 | 2 | 2 |
| Constipation | 4 | 3 | 3 |
| Loss of appetite | 3 | 6 | 5 |
| Palpitations | 3 | 3 | 5 |
| Bleeding or bruising | 3 | 3 | No data |
| Nausea | 3 | 2 | 1 |
| Fever | 3 | 1 | 2 |
| Giddiness or weakness | 2 | 3 | 4 |
| Excessive bleeding from gums after brushing teeth | 1 | 1 | No data |
| Vomiting | 0 | 0 | 2 |

constipation, often associated with drug treatment. A systematic review of constipation prevalence in the US [10] shows both how common it is, and how complex, varying with age, sex, race, and method of ascertainment.

The overall average percentage of people with constipation was about 15% (1 in 7 adults). The range was 1.9–27%, depending to some extent on how constipation was ascertained. Most reports were in the range 12–19%,

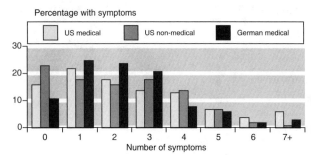

**Figure 5.1.2** Frequency of reported symptoms.

with some self-reported prevalence being higher, and two face-to-face questioning reports below 4%. There was a distinctly higher prevalence in women compared with men in almost every study, irrespective of method of ascertainment. Prevalence of constipation in women was on average about twice as high as in men. There was also a consistent finding of higher constipation prevalence in non-Caucasian people, by a factor of about 1.4 to 1, though non-white racial groups were not subdivided.

Other trends were for decreased prevalence in people with the highest income and highest educational attainment or years of education, though these may well be measuring different aspects of the same phenomenon. Older age, especially age over 70 years, was also associated with higher constipation rates. Because different age ranges were reported the results were not consistent between studies, but an example from a study using face-to-face questioning is shown in Figure 5.1.3.

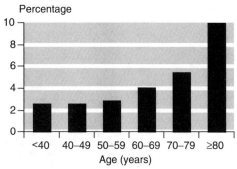

**Figure 5.1.3** Constipation frequency by age in US adults.

## Commentary

Common symptoms may be reported as adverse events in clinical trials, though their rates should be balanced out by the process of randomization, given sufficient size. If there is no additional effect from an intervention, then there should be no difference between different treatment groups. Where there is an additional effect from an intervention, if it is large enough then statistical difference should result.

The crucial take-home message is that adverse events are important and complex. They deserve more attention than the footnote they often get in reports of trials and in systematic reviews.

## References

1. Loke, Y.K. *et al.* (2005). Including adverse effects. In *Cochrane handbook for systematic reviews of interventions 4.2.5* (ed. J.P.T. Higgins and S. Green), updated May 2005, Appendix 6b. *http://www.cochrane.org/resources/handbook/hbook.htm* (accessed 15th Aug 2005).
2. Berry, D.C. *et al.* (2002). Provision of information about drug side effects to patients. *Lancet* **359**, 853–4.
3. Aronson, J.K. and Ferner, R.E. (2003). Joining the DoTS: new approach to classifying adverse drug reactions. *British Medical Journal* **327**, 1222–5.
4. Ford, G.A. *et al.* (2000). CYP2D6 and CYP2C19 genotypes of patients with terodiline cardiotoxicity identified through the yellow card system. *British Journal of Clinical Pharmacology* **50**, 77–80.
5. Aronsen, J.K. (2005). Unity from diversity: the evidential use of anecdotal reports of adverse drug reactions and interactions. *Journal of Evaluation in Clinical Practice* **11**, 195–208.
6. Moore, T.J. (1995). *Deadly medicine*. Simon and Schuster, New York.
7. Eypasch, E. *et al.* (1995). Probability of adverse events that have not yet occurred: a statistical reminder. *British Medical Journal* **311**, 619–20.
8. Reidenberg, M.M. and Lowenthal, D.T. (1968). Adverse nondrug reactions. *New England Journal of Medicine* **279**, 678–9.
9. Meyer, F.P. *et al.* (1996). Adverse nondrug reactions: an update. *Clinical Pharmacology and Therapeutics* **60**, 347–52.
10. Higgins, P.D. and Johanson, J.F. (2004). Epidemiology of constipation in North America: a systematic review. *American Journal of Gastroenterology* **99**, 750–9.

# 5.2  Case reports of adverse events

Anecdotal reports form an important source of information about adverse drug reactions, or complications occurring with any procedure. Anecdotal, or case reports of the efficacy of an intervention have been denigrated as being low down on the levels of evidence that we will trust or believe. Case reports about adverse events may, however, be very valuable. Case reports are often, but not always, about adverse events but, whether they are or not, the key is good reporting. A well-reported case can be a valuable source of information. One that is poorly reported is not. Case reports of possible adverse reactions are rarely confirmed by subsequent research [1], which makes distinguishing between genuine alerts and false alarms difficult.

The key reference [2] is a brilliant exposition of how and why anecdotal reports of adverse drug reactions are helpful whether alone, in narrative, or in systematic review. Reasons for publishing case reports include the following:

- to describe a newly recognized adverse reaction or interaction;
- to describe a new disease;
- to recognize rare manifestations of disease;
- to generate hypotheses;
- to test hypotheses;
- to demonstrate diagnostic techniques;
- to elucidate mechanisms;
- to elucidate methods of clinical management;
- to remind or educate.

Here we will consider only the first of these. The study design best suited to examining suspected events depends on the frequency of the event itself, and the background frequency of the event in a group of patients (Table 5.2.1). If the event is common with the intervention, and it occurs rarely in background, then it will be picked up by clinical observation, in randomized trials, or meta-analyses of randomized trials. By contrast, the most difficult circumstance is when an event caused by a drug or intervention is rare, but the event it causes is relatively common. Here case reports can be very useful.

Aspartame is a dipeptide sweetener of phenylalanine and aspartic acid widely used in the food industry, especially in diet products to reduce sugar

**Table 5.2.1**  Study designs useful for proving associations for adverse events

| Incidence of event | Background incidence | Ease of proving the association |
| --- | --- | --- |
| Common | Rare | Easy—direct clinical observation |
| Rare | Rare | Difficult—observational study |
| Common | Common | Difficult—large trial |
| Uncommon | Moderately common | Very difficult—large observational study |
| Rare | Common | Almost impossible (perhaps n-of-1 trial) |

content; many substances that are sugar-free contain aspartame. The idea that aspartame caused headache and migraine has been around for some years, and it is mentioned as a possible trigger for migraine, though there is little evidence. High doses of aspartame were not differentiated from placebo in small trials in patients claiming aspartame-triggered headache.

A case report confirmed that, for some patients, aspartame may be a trigger [3]. Two patients had migraines shown by exclusion diets to be associated with aspartame. Their migraines were well controlled with standard therapies including oral rizatriptan. For reasons of convenience, they asked to have the wafer melt formulation of rizatriptan. The wafer formulation consistently made headaches worse, not better, but oral rizatriptan still worked as well as before. It turned out that these melt formulations contain 4 mg aspartame—about a tenth of that in a packet of sweetener.

This was an example of the importance of case reports in contributing important information. We know that headache and migraine are common, and we have no evidence that migraines caused by aspartame are anything other than very rare. Even in these circumstances, a detailed case report can demonstrate that, for a very few, the effect is real.

## Quality standards for case reports

There is a series of items that should appear in case reports to provide a degree of assurance of quality and validity. The 21 items that might be looked for are shown in Table 5.2.2. It might not be realistic to find all of these items in a case report, and the reality is that most case reports probably have fewer than half of them [4].

Case reports have a valuable place in evidence acquisition about adverse events. A well-written case report is much more than the poor relation of randomized trials and meta-analysis. Case reports are often correct,

**Table 5.2.2**   Quality and validity items in case reports

| Details for inclusion in reports of adverse drug reactions and interactions | |
|---|---|
| Age | Sex |
| Weight | Ethnicity |
| Diagnosis | Allergies |
| Family history | Social history |
| Intensity (severity) | Time-course |
| Effect of withdrawal | Effect of rechallenge |
| Diagnostic tests | Plasma drug concentrations |
| Animal/*in vitro* evidence | Possible mechanisms |
| Treatment | Outcome |
| Assessment of likelihood | Assessment of classification |
| Drug treatment (current/past), including dosage regimens | |

especially about adverse events, and we now have several helpful guides about how to write them well, and evaluate them [2, 4, 5].

## Yellow card reporting scheme

In the UK doctors and other professionals are asked to report all suspected adverse reactions for new medicines and serious adverse reactions for established medicines. These are reported using the Yellow Card reporting scheme. This is a specialist form of case report, and information collected can be used to identify unexpected adverse effects, to indicate that known adverse events are more common than previously believed, or to show that some people have special susceptibility to adverse reactions.

A number of other countries operate similar schemes, with 76 member countries and 12 associate member countries participating in a WHO International Drug Monitoring Programme in July 2005. Information from the programme is used to identify adverse reactions to drugs on an international basis, and for a variety of other purposes. Yellow card reporting can provide really important insights. Three examples illuminate this.

In the UK, eight patients surviving ventricular tachycardia or torsades de pointes suspected to be due to terodiline had blood samples taken for investigation of genotypes of drug-metabolizing enzymes [6]. Analysis showed that being a poor debrisoquine metabolizer was not primarily responsible for terodiline cardiotoxicity, and pointed instead to a particular allele of a particular enzyme.

In Spain, yellow card reporting of adverse events to drugs in children over 10 years involved 1419 reports [7]. Analysis showed the most commonly involved organs to be skin, digestive tract, and nervous system (63% of total), and the most common drug classes to be antibiotics, respiratory medicines, and vaccines (69% of total). Few (less than 5%) involved life-threatening reactions.

These analyses show just two benefits of yellow card reporting: directing new research and knowledge for safer drugs or prescribing, and examining quality control of current prescribing to make it better in future. Yellow card reporting of adverse reactions is important. A further example [8], also from Spain, examined problems with agranulocytosis, and demonstrates just how much information can be gained from yellow card reporting schemes.

## Drug-induced agranulocytosis

Agranulocytosis (abnormally low levels of some white cells in the blood) can occur when drugs cause injury to the bone marrow. It is a serious condition, and about 1 in 10 cases can result in death. Drug-induced agranulocytosis is rare, perhaps affecting a few people per million of population per year. Because it is rare, agranulocytosis rates are difficult to measure, and it is difficult to know whether certain drugs cause agranulocytosis, and what the risk is.

The population of Barcelona (about four million people) was observed from 1980 to 2001 for cases of agranulocytosis. All potential cases were found through weekly calls to 17 haematology units, and using prespecified definitions for agranulocytosis based on laboratory results. These included blood count results and, usually, a bone marrow aspirate.

Exclusions included children under 2 years and patients receiving treatments (like chemotherapy or immunosuppressants) known to interfere with bone marrow function or with conditions (like leukaemia or AIDS) known to involve impaired bone marrow function. Patients also had to be able to participate in interviews relating to drug use.

For each case four controls were selected randomly, and personnel unaware of their status, using a structured questionnaire, interviewed cases and controls. Details of drug use within the previous 6 months were obtained. Drug exposure was defined as use in the week before an index day, defined as the day when the first symptom of agranulocytosis occurred.

There were 79 million person-years of observation, during which there were 396 cases of agranulocytosis, with 273 admitted to hospital because of agranulocytosis (community cases) and 123 cases in which agranulocytosis developed during an admission. The overall incidence was 5 cases per million per year, with 3.5 per million per year for community cases. Incidence was similar in men and women, but increased with age (Figure 5.2.1), and more than half the community cases were older than 64 years.

Overall fatality in the 4 weeks after diagnosis was 9.1%, and 7% for community cases. Fatality was also age-related, and was much higher in those older than 64 years (Figure 5.2.2).

Drugs significantly associated with agranulocytosis in 177 community cases are shown in Table 5.2.3, together with the attributable incidence. These drugs accounted for about two-thirds of cases. For some of these there were few case and control patients receiving the drugs, with 10 or fewer for calcium dobesilate, spironolactone, and carbamazepine. No drug had an attributable incidence of more than one case per million population per year.

In this study agranulocytosis was defined according to sensible criteria, comprehensively identified and followed up, in a large defined population with a universal free health-care service of high quality, for over 20 years. Few cases were likely to be missed. These are great strengths of the study. Weaknesses were that for some drugs there were very few events, and

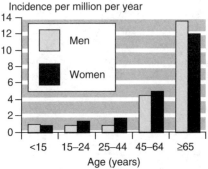

Incidence per million per year

**Figure 5.2.1** Agranulocytosis incidence by sex and age.

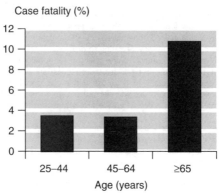

**Figure 5.2.2**   Case fatality rate for agranulocytosis by age, over 20 years.

some of the drugs significantly associated with agranulocytosis are not commonly used around the world, and some not now in Spain.

The study helps in several ways. It highlights those drugs that are likely to be associated with increased risk of agranulocytosis, helping to make sure cases are not missed. It tells us to keep a special look on older people on these drugs. And it also informs us of a lack of association with agranulocytosis for the many drugs used in a typical population.

Many questions remain unanswered. A *Lancet* editorial [9] has examined issues around agranulocytosis with dipyrone. Part of the problem is low

**Table 5.2.3**   Drug-related agranulocytosis for those with a statistically significant association, giving numbers of patients using the drug in cases and controls, odds ratios, and attributable incidence

| Drug | Numbers cases (n = 177)/ controls (n = 586) | Odds ratio (95% CI) | Attributable incidence (per million per year) |
|---|---|---|---|
| Ticlopidine hydrochloride | 20/1 | 103 (13–840) | 0.39 |
| Calcium dobesilate | 9/1 | 78 (4.5–1300) | 0.17 |
| Antithyroid drugs | 13/1 | 53 (5.8–480) | 0.25 |
| Dipyrone | 30/9 | 26 (8.4–79) | 0.56 |
| Spironolactone | 6/4 | 20 (2.3–180) | 0.11 |
| Carbamazepine | 5/1 | 11 (1.2–100) | 0.09 |
| Sulphonamides | 11/5 | 8.0 (2.1–31) | 0.19 |
| β-lactam antibiotics | 27/17 | 4.7 (1.7–13) | 0.42 |
| Diclofenac sodium | 10/11 | 3.9 (1.0–15) | 0.14 |

numbers of events, and part is apparently varying rates associated with drugs in different parts of the world. There is still much to be learned, but yellow card reporting schemes can be enormously helpful in understanding issues around rare adverse events.

## Commentary

Case reports are not to be ignored. They can play a really important part of understanding adverse events. Their reporting needs to follow clear rules, and guidance has been provided. For some rare adverse events, case reports will be the only way we are likely to find out about them.

## References

1. Loke Y.K. *et al.* (2006). Case reports of suspected adverse drug reactions—systematic literature survey and follow-up. *British Medical Journal* **332**, 335–9.
2. Aronson, J.K. (2005). Unity from diversity: the evidential use of anecdotal reports of adverse drug reactions and interactions. *Journal of Evaluation in Clinical Practice* **11**, 195–208.
3. Newman, L.C. and Lipton, R.B. (2001). Migraine MLT-down: an unusual presentation of migraine in patients with aspartame-triggered headaches. *Headache* **41**, 899–901.
4. Aronson, J.K. (2003). Anecdotes as evidence. *British Medical Journal* **326**, 1346.
5. Vandenbroucke, J.P. (2001). In defense of case reports and case series. *Annals of Internal Medicine* **134**, 330–4.
6. Ford, G.A. *et al.* (2000). CYP2D6 and CYP2D19 genotypes of patients with terodiline cardiotoxicity identified through the yellow card system. *British Journal of Clinical Pharmacology* **50**, 77–80.
7. Morales-Olivas, F.J. *et al.* (2000). Adverse drug reactions in children reported by means of the yellow card in Spain. *Journal of Clinical Epidemiology* **53**, 1076–80.
8. Ibáñez, L. *et al.* (2005). Population-based drug-induced agranulocytosis. *Archives of Internal Medicine* **165**, 869–74.
9. Edwards, J.E. and McQuay, H.J. (2002). Dipyrone and agranulocytosis: what is the risk? *Lancet* **360**, 1438.

# 5.3 Adverse events in randomized trials

Randomized controlled trials minimize bias. Trials are usually of a size that will allow a statistical difference for a chosen outcome to be detected most of the time, if a real difference of the expected size exists. Chosen outcomes are usually efficacy outcomes, and few trials will be done for safety purposes. Trials are usually of limited duration. Trials will therefore be most useful for examining information about adverse events that are relatively common; they are unlikely to measure accurately rare but serious adverse events, or those occurring with a significant time delay.

## Collecting adverse event information

Just think for a moment that you are contemplating performing a randomized trial. It is highly probable that the main thrust of that trial will be for measuring efficacy. You anticipate that there may be some adverse events. How do you propose to capture any information on adverse events?

- You might ask patients to report any adverse events spontaneously—without any prompting from investigators.
- At specific investigator/patient interactions, investigators could ask a specific question about adverse events in general, something like 'Have you experienced any unexpected or unusual symptoms?'.
- At specific investigator/patient interactions, investigators could ask a specific question about specific adverse events, something like 'Have you experienced any unexpected or unusual headache, nausea, gastrointestinal problems, …?'
- You could give each patient a diary, which might ask either general questions about adverse events or ask specific questions about whether he/she was experiencing any of a long list of potential adverse events.

But of course, you may not trust the patient to answer questions like these sensibly, so you might just ask the investigator to note the presence of any adverse symptoms, perhaps while measuring vital signs, or taking blood.

There are many other ways of approaching the issue of collecting information on adverse events in clinical trials, over and above the obvious clinical events like death, MI, or bleeding that might just be noticed both by patient and investigator. The point, though, is that we need to think about how adverse event information is collected.

### Are methods of collection reported?

The answer seems to be 'not often'. A systematic review [1] examined reporting of adverse drug reactions in randomized trials. In 185 trials published in seven eminent medical journals in 1997, 25 (14%) made no mention of adverse events at all. In 60 trials (32%) reporting was so poor that the authors of the review were unable to perform any analyses. In general, only 6% of a paper was used to report and discuss adverse events.

Results for 104 trials where an analysis was possible are shown in Table 5.3.1. It shows that, for a variety of adverse drug reactions identified by investigative tests, as targeted clinical assessments, or spontaneous reports of patient symptoms, most trials did not specify the methods used to collect data on adverse events.

**Table 5.3.1** Availability of information on the methods used in recording adverse drug reactions categorized by type of adverse drug reaction

| Types of ADR | Number of trials | Number (%) | |
|---|---|---|---|
| | | Specific details on how ADR was recorded | Did not specify methods |
| Investigative tests | 68 | 37 (55) | 31 (45) |
| Clinical events | 95 | 14 (15) | 81 (85) |
| Patient symptoms | 104 | 18 (17) | 86 (83) |

Investigative tests include vital signs and laboratory tests; clinical events were specific targeted clinical assessment; patient symptoms were spontaneous reports.

Information on common, minor, reversible adverse events might be present in clinical trial reports, but is frequently of secondary importance to efficacy, and consequently is poorly reported [1, 2]. In a review of adverse event reporting in 192 randomized trials in seven clinical areas, the number of discontinuations was most commonly reported in 75% of trials, though the reason for discontinuation was reported in only 46% [2]. Inadequate reporting was found in a full half of all the randomized trials (Table 5.3.2) [3].

A similar picture can be seen in acute pain trials from systematic reviews of paracetamol and ibuprofen [3]. Table 5.3.3 shows that full details on frequency and type of adverse events was seen in just over a half of all trials.

**Table 5.3.2** Adequacy of reporting of adverse events in 192 randomized trials

| Reporting of safety | % of trials | Range* |
|---|---|---|
| **Discontinuations because of harm** | | |
| Number per group given | 75 | 30–100 |
| Reasons per group given | 46 | 20–68 |
| **Clinical adverse events** | | |
| Adequate reporting | 39 | 0–62 |
| Partially adequate reporting | 11 | 0–20 |
| Inadequate reporting | 50 | 22–100 |
| **Laboratory defined toxicity** | | |
| Adequate reporting | 29 | 0–62 |
| Partially adequate reporting | 8 | 0–20 |
| Inadequate reporting | 63 | 25–100 |

*Range refers to the limits found in each of seven clinical areas.

Adverse events can be collected in systematic reviews, and some systematic reviews do this, though many unfortunately ignore adverse events of treatment. Because reporting is commonly not done in any standard way in clinical trials, we usually make do with one of several ways of reporting adverse events.

- Patients' reports of any adverse event: this collects information on all patients who had any complaint, of any severity.
- Particular adverse events: this collects patient information about specific (hopefully well defined) adverse events.
- Severe adverse events: if there is a definition of an adverse event that has a clinically evident severe consequence.

If reported, information can be dealt with in the same way as with efficacy, using L'Abbé plots, statistical tests, numbers needed to harm, and finally percentage of patients with the event. The biggest problem is that adverse events often occur less frequently than do efficacy outcomes, and that means amounts of information available are often inadequate for a sensible answer. Adverse events are more complicated to assess and analyse because there may be several different types of adverse events with different severity. The importance of an adverse event also depends on the patient (cannot possibly tolerate a dry mouth or inability to drive a car) and his/her condition (constipation after bowel surgery). How should all these different measures be taken into account? In addition, different methods of collecting common adverse events produce different results, and right now we just don't have a clue whether any one method is better than any other [3].

The method of assessment (spontaneous report, checklist, patient diary) and data provided by the informed consent form affect the incidence of adverse events, and that complicates the comparison of results across trials. This was shown by Edwards [3] who sought and analysed for adverse events all randomized controlled trials of single oral doses of paracetamol and ibuprofen in postoperative pain. In 55 trials, 33% used patient diaries, 13% spontaneous reporting, and 11% direct questioning, but a third didn't mention the method used (Table 5.3.3). This was important, because for both paracetamol and ibuprofen patient diaries were more sensitive in reporting adverse events than either spontaneous reporting or direct questioning. Adverse event rates were very similar in the active and control (placebo) groups indicating that most 'adverse events' were probably not due to the analgesic itself but could have been caused by the intervention or anaesthesia given. This makes it difficult to identify an adverse event that is solely due to the analgesic used because there is so much background noise.

## Dose-response of adverse events

It is almost universally known, but seldom acknowledged, that both the efficacy and harm of drugs are functions of the dose given. Clinical trials occasionally use more than one dose of a drug, but seldom with sufficient numbers of patients to make sense of complex adverse event information. Making sense of dose-response and adverse events usually requires meta-analysis (to be dealt with later). A matter of major importance is that dose-response curves for efficacy and harm may not be the same, emphasizing the importance of dose when making statements about harm.

**Table 5.3.3**  Adverse event assessment and reporting methods in 55 paracetamol and ibuprofen acute pain trials

| | Trials | |
|---|---|---|
| | Number | Per cent |
| **Method of assessment** | | |
| Spontaneous | 7 | 13 |
| Patient diaries | 18 | 33 |
| Direct questioning | 6 | 11 |
| Not stated | 19 | 35 |
| Adverse effects not reported | 2 | 4 |
| **Reporting of adverse events** | | |
| Adverse effect information not reported | 2 | 4 |
| No adverse effects occurred | 6 | 11 |
| No difference as only mention | 2 | 4 |
| No details on frequency and type | 8 | 15 |
| Full details on frequency and type | 34 | 62 |

### Trial situations

Adverse event rates can vary considerably between similar clinical trials. Cause of variation can be as simple as the random play of chance, as for efficacy outcomes, or any of the complex issues of adverse event definition and method of collection. Adverse event rates can also be affected by the type of patient being studied, their age, sex, severity of disease, or race, or cultural context. One example of the latter was a comparison of two implantable contraceptives (Norplant and Implanon) in young women [4]. Clinical trials had rates for women experiencing any adverse event from about 5% to about 90% (Figure 5.3.1). The large trial with low adverse events was performed in East Asia, while those with high adverse event rates were performed in Europe, which may simply be because East Asian women don't complain about adverse events that are found unacceptable by European women.

### Commentary

There is much to be learned still about adverse events in clinical trials. It is not a topic that has received an overabundance of attention, but fortunately it is a subject of increasing interest.

### References

1. Loke, Y.K. and Derry, S. (2001). Reporting of adverse drug reactions in randomised controlled trials—a systematic survey. *BMC Clinical Pharmacology* **1**, 3.
2. Ioannidis, J.P.A. and Lau, J. (2001). Completeness of safety reporting in randomized trials: an evaluation of 7 medical areas. *Journal of the American Medical Association* **285**, 437–43.

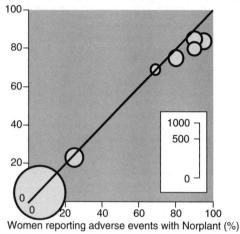

**Figure 5.3.1** Reported adverse event rates for implantable contraceptives in young women.

3. Edwards, J.E. et al. (1999). Reporting of adverse effects in clinical trials should be improved. Lessons from acute postoperative pain. *Journal of Pain Symptom Management* **81**, 289–97.
4. Edwards, J.E. and Moore, A. (1999). Implanon: a review of clinical studies. *British Journal of Family Planning* **4**, 3–16.

# 5.4 Observational studies of adverse events

Observational studies are our best available study architecture for evaluating rare but (usually) serious adverse events. Everything said about observational studies in Section 3 holds true here, but the most important thing is to remind ourselves of the criteria for causation (Table 5.4.1), which apply particularly for adverse events, as there can often be real problems of confounding by indication—using particular therapies only on ill people.

Observational studies are also useful for evaluating adverse events that are not immediately apparent with a therapy, but where there is a delayed onset (e.g. carcinogens). Clinical trials, which almost always have a finite duration that is often short in comparison with sometimes lifetime use of therapy, may not adequately address the problem of delayed onset. Observational studies may also be the only ones that address problems occurring when medicines are stopped.

A series of examples of good observational studies concerning adverse events illustrates their utility.

## Polyneuropathy and statins

Myopathy is a recognized risk associated with the use of statins. In general practice in the UK the incidence of myopathy in users of lipid-lowering drugs is 2.3 per 10,000 person-years, with a relative risk compared with non-users of 42 for fibrates and 8 for statins [2]. A case-control study [3] tells us that polyneuropathy is also likely to be a problem, and that it needs looking at.

The study was conducted in a county of Denmark with a population of 465,000. Residents have a civil registration number that is used in discharge prescription registries, so that it is possible to find all residents with a particular disorder, and find out what drugs they have been prescribed.

In a 5-year period to the end of 1998, all patients with a discharge diagnosis of polyneuropathy were examined. Some lived elsewhere, some were diagnosed before the study period, some had predisposing conditions (renal failure, diabetes, thyroid), and others had no proper diagnosis or were wrongly diagnosed. Clinical diagnostic features were distal symmetric sensory symptoms, or symmetric motor symptoms and no upper motor neuron signs, or both. Neurophysiological criteria were abnormal conduction in two or more peripheral nerves, with at least one being a leg nerve.

A diagnosis of peripheral neuropathy was accepted only if both clinical and nerve conduction criteria were compatible with the diagnosis. Several levels of confidence were defined for idiopathic polyneuropathy (Table 5.4.2). For each case, 25 control subjects of the same sex and age were randomly chosen from the remaining population.

There were 166 cases of first-time diagnosis of polyneuropathy in the 5 years, of which 35 were definite, 54 probable, and 77 possible. Of these, nine (5.4%) had a previous exposure to statins (eight current users), with a median duration of 2.8 years. There were 4150 controls, of whom 66 (1.6%) had exposure to statins (49 current users).

**Table 5.4.1** Reminder of Bradford-Hill criteria for causation [1]

| Feature | Comment |
| --- | --- |
| Consistency and unbiasedness of findings | Confirmation of the association by different investigators, in different populations, using different methods |
| Strength of association | Two aspects: the frequency with which the factor is found in the disease, and the frequency with which it occurs in the absence of the disease. The larger the relative risk, the more the hypothesis is strengthened |
| Temporal sequence | Obviously, exposure to the factor must occur before onset of the disease. In addition, if it is possible to show a temporal relationship, as between exposure to the factor in the population and frequency of the disease, the case is strengthened |
| Biological gradient (dose–response relationship) | Finding a quantitative relationship between the factor and the frequency of the disease. The intensity or duration of exposure may be measured |
| Specificity | If the determinant being studied can be isolated from others and shown to produce changes in the incidence of the disease, e.g. if thyroid cancer can be shown to have a higher incidence specifically associated with fluoride, this is convincing evidence of causation |
| Coherence with biological background and previous knowledge | The evidence must fit the facts that are thought to be related, e.g. the rising incidence of dental fluorosis and the rising consumption of fluoride are coherent |
| Biological plausibility | The statistically significant association fits well with previously existing knowledge |
| Reasoning by analogy | Common sense, especially when you have other similar examples for types of intervention and outcome |
| Experimental evidence | This aspect focuses on what happens when the suspected offending agent is removed. Is there improvement? The evidence of remission—or even resolution of significant medical symptoms—following explantation obviously would strengthen the case. It is unethical to do an experiment that exposes people to the risk of illness, but it is permissible and indeed desirable to conduct an experimental, i.e. a randomized controlled trial, on control measures. If fluoride is suspected of causing thyroid dysfunction, for example, the experiment of eliminating or reducing occupational exposure to the toxin and conducting detailed endocrine tests on the workers could help to confirm or refute the suspicion |

**Table 5.4.2** Definition of diagnosis of polyneuropathy

| Description | Definition |
|---|---|
| Definite | Adequate work-up and tested for exclusion diagnoses and conditions, and no apparent cause of neuropathy established |
| Probable | Only sufficient information to rule out alcohol overuse, diabetes, and renal insufficiency |
| Possible | Information not sufficient to ascertain presence or absence of any exclusion diagnosis |

The odds ratio of polyneuropathy for current users was 4.6 (2.1–10) for all cases with current use, and 16 (5.7–45) for definite cases with current use (Table 5.4.3). Odds ratios were higher for more than 2 years of use compared with less than 2 years, and for larger numbers of doses than smaller numbers.

The number needed to harm (NNH) based on all patients was calculated as 5500 (2200–18,500). In those over 50, the incidence of polyneuropathy in the background population was 1.7 per 10,000 person-years, with an excess rate of 4.5 per 10,000 person-years among those exposed to statins. That is roughly one excess case of polyneuropathy for every 2200 (880–7300) person-years of statin use.

In 1998 about 1% of the Danish population used a statin. If a population with 100,000 inhabitants had 1% taking statins, a case of polyneuropathy might be expected every second year. That's twice as frequent as a case of myopathy.

### Rhabdomyolysis with statins

Rhabdomyolysis is another example of muscle problems occurring with statins and other lipid-lowering drugs. While some people seem unable to take statins because of muscle soreness or weakness, the vast majority are unaffected. There is a biological progression, from muscle soreness, through more severe muscle weakness or discomfort, to increased levels of creatinine kinase enzymes, to rhabdomyolysis, and even death from rhabdomyolysis (in about 1 in 15 cases of rhabdomyolysis).

Most of the spontaneous reports of rhabdomyolysis to the FDA were associated with cerivastatin, now withdrawn [4]. The problem with

**Table 5.4.3** Statin exposure in all cases and definite cases of polyneuropathy

| Statin exposure | Cases | Controls | Odds ratio (95% CI) |
|---|---|---|---|
| **All cases** | | | |
| Never use | 157 | 4084 | 1 |
| Current use | 8 | 49 | 4.6 (2.1–10) |
| **Definite cases** | | | |
| Never use | 27 | 854 | 1 |
| Current use | 7 | 17 | 16 (5.7–45) |

spontaneous reporting is that, while it may identify cases, there is always uncertainty about denominators, so rates of adverse events are imprecise. Randomized trials are poor at finding rare but serious adverse events, because the events do not occur in sufficient numbers. Only 12 cases of rhabdomyolysis were reported in 16,000 patients in the 30 randomized trials reviewed [4].

One way of overcoming both these problems is by using large cohort studies, where people prescribed a drug (statins in this case) are enrolled in good databases that can identify cases of the adverse events examined. Such a cohort study on statins and rhabdomyolysis [5] is informative. This was a retrospective cohort study of patients in 11 US health plans providing pharmacy benefits, and with automated claims files covering prescription drugs, outpatient visits, and hospital admissions. Patients with a first prescription of statin or fibrate were entered, as long as there was no such prescription in the previous 6 months.

Potential cases of hospital admission for rhabdomyolysis were identified from records of members of the cohort using coded discharge diagnoses. Also used were claims for measurement of creatinine kinase within 7 days of admission or discharge, or a discharge diagnosis of renal failure plus a creatinine kinase measurement. Three assessors, blind to statin or fibrate exposure status, reviewed abstracts of medical records. Rhabdomyolysis was defined as severe muscle injury present at admission, plus a diagnosis of rhabdomyolysis or creatinine kinase more than 10 times the upper limit of normal. Severe rhabdomyolysis was defined as a serum creatinine kinase above 10,000 IU/L or more than 50 times the upper limit of normal.

The cohort included a quarter of a million people with 225,000 person-years of monotherapy for statin or fibrate, and 7300 person-years of combined therapy of statin plus fibrate. There was little information for fluvastatin or lovastatin, and these drugs were ignored in favour of the bulk of statin information on atorvastatin, pravastatin, and simvastatin. Fibrate information was much lower than that for statins, and included gemfibrozil and fenofibrate. Within the cohort there were 77,000 person-years not exposed to lipid-lowering drugs, during which no cases of rhabdomyolysis were reported.

Thirty-one patients met the inclusion criteria for rhabdomyolysis. Seven were excluded because rhabdomyolysis occurred during a period when the prescription records showed that they were not exposed to a lipid-lowering drug, although in each case their hospital records showed that they were taking a statin at the time of the event.

Of the 24 events remaining, there were 13 events on statin monotherapy, three on fibrate monotherapy, and eight cases with combined therapy with both statin and a fibrate. Various doses of each statin and each fibrate were being used for monotherapy and combined therapy. Three-quarters of the events were defined as severe rhabdomyolysis. Hospital stay was 1–11 days (average 6). Two patients underwent haemodialysis, and one died.

### Monotherapy

There was no difference in rate of hospital admission for rhabdomyolysis between atorvastatin, pravastatin, and simvastatin. The combined event rate was 0.44 per 10,000 person-years of exposure (Table 5.4.4), and the

**Table 5.4.4** Rhabdomyolysis cases, rate, and NNH for different lipid-lowering treatments

| Lipid-lowering drug | Patients | Person-years | Rhabdo-myolysis cases | Rate per 10,000 patient-years (95% CI) | 1-year NNH |
|---|---|---|---|---|---|
| Atorvastatin, pravastatin, simvastatin | 213,377 | 203,456 | 9 | 0.44 (0.2–0.8) | 22,727 |
| Cerivastatin | 12,695 | 7486 | 4 | 5.3 (1.5–14) | 1873 |
| Gemfibrozil, fenofibrate | 20,485 | 10,631 | 3 | 2.8 (0.6–8.2) | 3546 |

1-year number needed to harm (NNH) was 22,700. For cerivastatin, the rate was about 10 times higher, with an NNH of 1870. For fibrates the NNH was 3550. Age over 65 years and having diabetes increased the risk of rhabdomyolysis with statin monotherapy, but duration of use made no difference to the event rate.

*Combined therapy*

Combined use of statin and fibrate increased the risk of rhabdomyolysis. With atorvastatin or simvastatin plus a fibrate the incidence rate was between 17 and 23 per 10,000 person-years, about 40 times higher than with statins alone. The NNH for 1 year of therapy with atorvastatin, pravastatin, or simvastatin plus a fibrate to produce one case of hospital admission for rhabdomyolysis was 1670. For a patient aged 65 years or older with diabetes treated with both a statin and a fibrate the NNH was 480.

Combined use of cerivastatin plus gemfibrozil produced a rate of about 1000 per 10,000 person years, with an NNH of about 10.

The problems researchers face over rare but serious adverse events are clear here. Start with a quarter of a million patients and end up with only 24 actual events. Those 24 events include several drugs, at several doses, and given either separately or in combination. And, while this is probably the best study of rhabdomyolysis with statins we have, even this has a problem. Seven cases occurred when patients were not on statins according to the prescription analysis, but were on statins according to the hospital records. Fortunately, including or excluding the results made no difference.

Despite all these concerns we have some reasonably clear results. Rhabdomyolysis did not occur in the cohort when they were not taking statins or fibrates, as best we can judge. Rhabdomyolysis did occur when they were taking statins or fibrates. We have a reasonable estimate of how frequently the events occurred, both in single and combined use (Figure 5.4.1). This allows an estimate of risk of rhabdomyolysis, which is really extremely rare in people taking the most commonly prescribed statins.

With fibrates, or combined therapy, or people more at risk, or with certain combinations (now impossible because one of the drugs has been withdrawn), the risks are higher. What we also know is that the risk of dying was very small. In the 225,000 person-years of therapy, even including

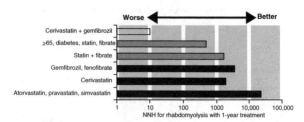

**Figure 5.4.1** NNH for rhabdomyolysis for different treatments, combinations, and conditions.

the withdrawn cerivastatin, only 31 cases occurred, and only 3 of those died. As 10 of the cases were associated with cerivastatin, it would be reasonable to estimate that risk of death with statin, fibrate, or combination with drugs commonly prescribed is of the order of 1 per 100, 000 per year, and is probably less common than that.

### Antipsychotics and sudden cardiac death

Sudden cardiac death has been reported with the use of antipsychotics since the 1960s, though there have been few studies, and those we have were small and took little account of potential confounding factors. The evidence was therefore weak. A large case-control study from a high-quality database with full patient information [6] provides more information.

A large Dutch electronic database of about half a million patients in 150 general practices provided the information. The records contained details of demographics, symptoms, diagnoses, and outpatient and hospital records, including tests, and drug prescriptions. All patients aged 18 years or older, except those with cancer or those with death by suicide, formed the source population.

The study sought deaths occurring over 6 years (1995–2001), and experts blinded to patient exposure to antipsychotic drugs reviewed those that could possibly be regarded as sudden cardiac death. Sudden cardiac death was defined as death occurring within 1 hour after onset of acute symptoms, and if the death was recorded as sudden or acute cardiac death, or similar. If death was not witnessed, unexpected death of anyone seen in a stable medical condition less than 24 hours previously and with no evidence of a non-cardiac cause was used. For each case of sudden death up to 10 controls matched for age, sex, and practice were chosen.

Exposure was defined as current use, past use (longer than 30 days since end of last prescription), or non-use of antipsychotics. Type of antipsychotic, dose (DDD defined as recommended daily dose for an adult for schizophrenia), and duration of use were also noted. Known risk factors for sudden cardiac death were also collected from databases, and used in adjusting results.

There were 582 cases of sudden cardiac death in a population of 250,000 adults over the period, an incidence of 1 per 1000 per year. Controls (4463) were available for 554 cases, of which 334 deaths were witnessed. The

**Table 5.4.5** Numbers of cases of sudden cardiac death and controls, and use of antipsychotic medicines

| Use of antipsychotic medicine | Cases | Controls |
|---|---|---|
| Total patients | 554 | 4463 |
| Non-use | 520 | 4352 |
| Past use | 15 | 74 |
| Current use | 19 | 37 |
| **Of which** | | |
| Butyrophones | 12 | 13 |
| Thioxanthenes | 1 | 3 |
| Lithium | 3 | 9 |
| Phenothiazines | 3 | 12 |
| Others (atypical) | 2 | 7 |
| **At doses of** | | |
| ≤ 0.5 DDD | 14 | 33 |
| > 0.5 DDD | 5 | 4 |

mean age was about 72 years and 60% were men. Known conditions and behaviours (heart failure, diabetes, smoking) and cardiovascular drugs were all associated with increased sudden cardiac death.

Most of the cases and controls did not use antipsychotics, or had done so only in the past (Table 5.4.5). Only 19 (3.4%) cases and 34 (0.8%) controls were current users of antipsychotics, and in these the adjusted odds ratio for increased sudden cardiac death was 3.3 (95% CI, 1.8 to 6.2; Figure 5.4.2). There was a somewhat higher association between use of antipsychotics and sudden cardiac death in witnessed deaths than unwitnessed deaths.

The numbers of users of different types of antipsychotics was small for each group (Table 5.4.5), but for users of older antipsychotics (haloperidol, for instance) the odds ratio was 7.3 (2.8 to 19) based on 12 cases and 13 controls using this group. No other group reached statistical significance but, based on small numbers of cases and controls using them, higher doses were also associated with more frequent cardiac death (Figure 5.4.2), but only five cases and four controls were using doses above 0.5 DDD (Table 1). There was no difference between longer or shorter periods of use.

This is a detailed study, looking at a large population with excellent recording of patient details, and with a large number of sudden

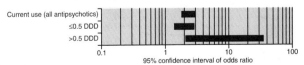

**Figure 5.4.2** 95% confidence interval of the odds ratio associating antipsychotic use or dose with sudden cardiac death.

cardiac death events. Only 19 of these events occurred in people using antipsychotics, on which the whole thesis rests. For any further analysis, by type of drug, by dose of drug, or by duration of use of drug, the numbers of cases mainly fall to single figures. Most of these analyses contain so few cases or controls that there must be a risk that they will be wrong just by the random play of chance.

So the best evidence we have is still limited, despite the quality and validity and size of the population. We can be reasonably sure that anti-psychotics are associated with something like a threefold increase in sudden cardiac death, and perhaps that older antipsychotics may be worse. We cannot be sure that newer antipsychotics, or lithium, or phenothiazines are without effect.

## Commentary

These examples are all recent, and are all good-quality studies based on excellent databases and first-class case finding. They exemplify several of the problems that exist for observational studies used to look at adverse events. Most importantly, although there may be many, often very many, people in the databases, the number of events is often small. Once subdivision begins based on type of drug, or dose, or duration of use, or some other variable, the number of cases associated with that subdivision often becomes very small very quickly.

And there is a need for trying to understand subdivisions. With anti-psychotics, dose was clearly likely to be an important characteristic. For rhabdomyolysis with statins, it was particular lipid-lowering drugs, especially combinations of drugs. For polyneuropathy, what was important was the definition of a case, of the adverse event itself.

For every good study like these, there will be many studies that do not make the grade. It is not uncommon to see far-reaching conclusions drawn from a handful of cases in studies with many faults. The message for readers is to use common sense, and for observational studies to check on issues like numbers of events, case finding and definition, dose, and other criteria that might make a particular study valid or invalid.

## References

1. Bradford-Hill, A. (1966). The environment and disease: association or causation? *Proceedings of the Royal Society of Medicine* **58**, 295.
2. Gaist, D. et al. (2001). Lipid-lowering drugs and risk of myopathy: a population-based follow-up study. *Epidemiology* **12**, 565–9.
3. Gaist, D. et al. (2002). Statins and risk of polyneuropathy. A case-control study. *Neurology* **58**, 1333–7.
4. Thompson, P.D. et al. (2003). Statin-associated myopathy. *Journal of the American Medical Association* **289**, 1681–90.
5. Graham, D.J. et al. (2004). Incidence of hospitalized rhabdomyolysis in patients treated with lipid-lowering drugs. *Journal of the American Medical Association* **292**, 2582–90.
6. Straus, S.M. et al. (2004). Antipsychotics and the risk of sudden cardiac death. *Archives of Internal Medicine* **164**, 1293–7.

# 5.5   Systematic reviews of adverse events

Systematic reviews of adverse events can be of various types. Adverse events may be identified through randomized trials, or through observational studies, or through a combination of these plus case reports, when they are called teleoanalyses [1, 2]. There is no prior reasoning to tell us that any one is better than any other, because it depends on the type and frequency of the adverse event of interest.

Common adverse events are more likely to be best observed in clinical trials and, despite poor reporting, meta-analysis of randomized trials should be the best source for evidence, especially if performed using clinical trial reports (of which more later). Rare, serious adverse events are likely to be best examined through observational studies, and systematic reviews demonstrate why they are superior to single studies in estimating frequency. Teleoanalyses are really interesting, but there are few of them. They are harder intellectually, both to produce and to read, but they can provide a considerable insight into adverse event importance, especially where there is a biological progression from lesser to greater harm.

This section will provide examples of all three approaches. There are no simple rules that can tell you when a study is good or poor, but rules developed for efficacy analyses will generally be applicable here also.

## Systematic reviews of randomized trials

Two systematic reviews epitomize the benefits of good systematic reviews of adverse events: first from published data looking at a relatively rare adverse event, and second from a systematic review of more and less common adverse events from a different data source.

### Aspirin and gastrointestinal bleeding

Aspirin is now well known as a cause of gastrointestinal bleeding. A systematic review [3] assessed the incidence of gastrointestinal haemorrhage associated with long-term aspirin therapy. It found and used 24 randomized trials with 66,000 patients, where aspirin was compared with placebo or no treatment. Treatment duration was 12–60 months, and various aspirin formulations were used including standard, modified release, and in many cases unspecified. Patient numbers varied from a few hundred in a trial, to many thousands. The dose of aspirin varied between 50 and 1500 mg daily.

The main analysis was by dose, split between those taking less than 163 mg daily, and those taking more. The results can be seen in Figures 5.5.1 and 5.5.2. In each case there was great variation in bleeding rates, both for aspirin and for placebo, probably reflecting difference in trial duration, size, and baseline risk. Small and short studies would be expected to have fewer events than large and long studies. Table 5.5.1 summarizes the evidence.

But we can do more. For instance, from data provided in the paper we can calculate that, at the lower dose of aspirin (50–163 mg daily), the weighted average duration of studies was 51 months. So the absolute annual rate of bleeding with and without aspirin can be calculated, the

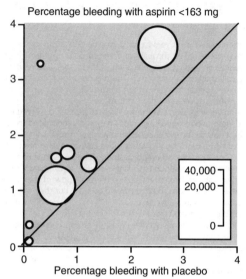

**Figure 5.5.1** Gastrointestinal bleeding with aspirin 50–163 mg daily.

difference found, and the increased risk because of low dose aspirin calculated on an annual basis. In this case (Table 5.5.2) the increased risk is 1 in 530 per year. For higher dose aspirin, where the studies were of shorter duration, the annual risk increase was 1 in 160.

This analysis assumes that the rate of gastrointestinal bleeding is constant with time (largely borne out by large coxib studies), and does not take into account any potential differences in baseline risk between different groups of people (for instance, age is a major determinant of baseline risk of gastrointestinal bleeding, and the absolute annual placebo risks are different for lower and higher doses of aspirin in Table 5.5.2).

The real strength of the analysis is that it provides absolute values for risk in several ways, one or more of which is likely to be understandable and usable by patients and professionals.

### Adverse events of opioids

Putting results into absolute terms can be particularly helpful, and is a technique that can be used even with multiple comparators in clinical trials. For instance, a systematic review of published trials of opioid drugs and combinations of opioids and paracetamol used in chronic non-malignant pain (mainly arthritis and musculoskeletal disorders) used the method of giving a simple prevalence [4].

The prevalence of a variety of adverse events in several conditions is shown in Figure 5.5.3. Knowing what is likely to happen with a drug, despite

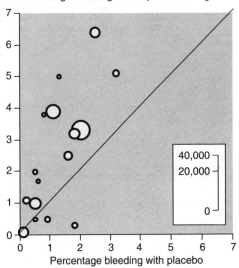

**Figure 5.5.2** Gastrointestinal bleeding with aspirin 163–1500 mg daily.

having some caveats about the validity of the studies, at least provides some information. For instance, the prevalence of constipation found with opioids in Figure 5.5.3 is about that seen in the US adult population (Section 5.1).

### Adverse events of celecoxib

A systematic review and meta-analysis of adverse events and tolerability of celecoxib in osteoarthritis and rheumatoid arthritis had information from 31 trials lasting between 2 weeks and 1 year, with 39,600 patients [5]. The main methodological feature of this review was that it used information not from published papers, but from clinical trial reports.

**Table 5.5.1** Summary results by dose of aspirin

| Daily dose of aspirin (mg) | Number of | | % bleeding with | | Relative risk (95% CI) | NNH (95% CI) |
|---|---|---|---|---|---|---|
| | Trials | Patients | Aspirin | Placebo | | |
| 50–163 | 8 | 49,927 | 2.3 | 1.5 | 1.6 (1.4–1.8) | 118 (92–164) |
| 163–1500 | 16 | 16,060 | 3.0 | 1.4 | 2.0 (1.6–2.6) | 62 (48–85) |

**Table 5.5.2** Absolute risks with placebo and aspirin

| | Absolute risk (%) | Weighted mean duration (months) | Absolute risk per year (%) | Absolute risk frequency per year (1 in) |
|---|---|---|---|---|
| **Aspirin dose 50–163 mg daily** | | | | |
| Placebo | 1.5 | 51 | 0.35 | 283 |
| Aspirin | 2.3 | 51 | 0.54 | 185 |
| Absolute difference | | | 0.19 | 531 |
| **Aspirin dose 163–1500 mg daily** | | | | |
| Placebo | 1.4 | 30 | 0.6 | 179 |
| Aspirin | 3.0 | 30 | 1.2 | 83 |
| Absolute difference | | | 0.6 | 156 |

Clinical trial reports are the main report of a trial produced by a pharmaceutical company or an independent clinical trial organization. They are usually very detailed, and with that detail comes length. Typically they will run into hundreds, perhaps thousands, of pages, with much detail, especially about adverse events. In this review, for instance, there were 180,000 pages of information for 23 trials, with slightly shorter but exten-

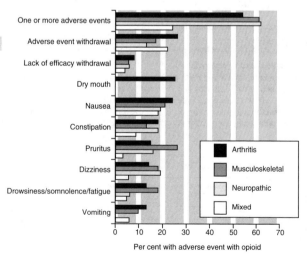

**Figure 5.5.3** Adverse events with opioids in chronic non-malignant pain.

sive clinical trial summaries for the remaining eight. In all there were over 200,000 pages of information, about five pages per patient. Most published studies have perhaps 3000 words to cover a trial, with a few tables and figures. Information then becomes compressed, and much essential information is omitted [6].

It is also the case that even good published clinical trials truncate reporting of adverse events, mainly though space limitation. This may mean that adverse events occurring at rates below 10%, or 5%, or 3%, are not reported, however important that adverse event may be. Clinical trial reports do not have such restrictions, and provide a comprehensive report of every adverse event.

It is not appropriate here to reprise an enormously complex and detailed review, but rather to demonstrate what can be achieved by these methods. Table 5.5.3 shows just some of the comparisons that were made, between licensed doses of celecoxib (200–400 mg daily) and placebo, paracetamol 4000 mg daily, rofecoxib 25 mg daily, and with NSAIDs at their maximum daily dose. A comparison of all doses of celecoxib with NSAIDs was also made, and various sensitivity analyses were presented.

### Systematic reviews of observational studies

These are less common than systematic reviews of randomized trials, and suffer from the fact that many older observational studies were of poor quality, or rather small, with few events. One example [7] concerning gastrointestinal bleeding with NSAIDs epitomizes the best from systematic review and meta-analysis of observational studies.

The review chose to use only epidemiological studies associating NSAID use and upper GI problems published in the 1990s, because the authors considered these to be of higher quality and bigger size than previous studies. To be included studies had to:

- be case control or cohort studies on non-aspirin NSAIDs;
- include data on bleeding, perforation, or other serious upper gastro-intestinal tract event resulting in hospital admission or referral to a specialist;
- have data to calculate relative risk.

Eighteen such studies were found. All had specific definitions of exposure and outcome and similar ascertainment for comparison groups. All but two attempted to control for potential confounding factors, like age, sex, history of ulcer, or concomitant medicines.

The main results are summarized in Figures 5.5.4 and 5.5.5. Compared with non-users, NSAID users had a higher risk of upper GI bleed (UGIB) when they were current NSAID users and used a higher dose. The duration of use was unimportant, but different NSAIDs had different risks, with ibuprofen (especially doses below 2400 mg a day) being least harmful.

The effect of ulcer history and age is shown in Figures 5.5.6 and 5.5.7. People with a history of ulcer or with a previous bleed who took NSAIDs were at much greater risk than those with no history of ulcer who took NSAIDs. Older folk who took NSAIDs were at greater risk than under 50s who took NSAIDs.

In this set of high-quality studies, there was a clear effect of size (in terms of the number of cases of upper gastrointestinal bleeding in each study) on the estimate of relative risk of upper gastrointestinal bleed with NSAID.

**Table 5.5.3** Some adverse event (AE) comparisons available for celecoxib in a review

| Event | Celecoxib dose | | | | |
|---|---|---|---|---|---|
| | 200–400 mg daily | | | All doses | |
| | Placebo | Paracetamol 4000 mg | Rofecoxib 25 mg | NSAID top daily dose | NSAID top daily dose |
| All-cause discontinuation | − | − | = | = | − |
| LoE discontinuation | − | − | = | + | = |
| AE discontinuation | = | = | = | − | − |
| GI AE discontinuation | = | = | = | − | − |
| Any AE | + | = | = | = | = |
| Treatment–related | + | = | = | = | = |
| Serious AE | = | = | = | = | = |
| GI tolerability | = | = | = | − | − |
| Nausea | = | = | = | − | − |
| Vomiting | = | = | = | − | − |
| Abdominal pain | = | = | = | − | − |
| Dyspepsia | + | = | = | − | − |
| Diarrhoea | + | − | = | − | − |
| Clinical ulcers and bleeds | ND | ND | ND | − | − |
| Cardiac failure | ND | ND | ND | = | = |
| Raised creatinine | = | ND | ND | = | ND |
| Hypertension | = | ND | = | = | = |
| Oedema | + | = | − | = | = |
| Haemoglobin fall | = | ND | ND | − | − |
| Haematocrit fall | = | ND | = | − | − |
| Endoscopic ulcers | = | ND | ND | − | − |

+, Increased with celecoxib; =, no difference; −, decreased with celecoxib; ND, no data.

The pooled estimate was 3.8 (3.6–4.1). With fewer than 1000 cases, the result of individual studies was highly variable (Figure 5.5.8), and with 200 or less the relative risk ranged from below 1 to almost 8—between no effect and a massive effect. Clearly, size of study and number of events are major determinants of the weight we give to any result. Yet many individual studies of adverse events extrapolate to whole populations, sometimes from only a few tens of events.

### Teleoanalysis

In all of what is termed evidence-based medicine, the concept of teleoanalysis, bringing together evidence from different forms of evidence, is the

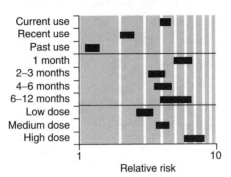

**Figure 5.5.4** Risk of UGIB for NSAID for users compared with non-users.

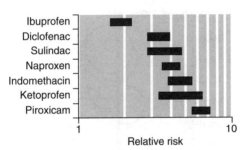

**Figure 5.5.5** Risk of UGIB for particular NSAIDs for users compared with non-users.

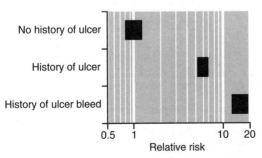

**Figure 5.5.6** Effect of history of ulcer in users of NSAIDs.

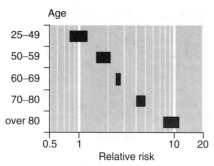

**Figure 5.5.7** Effect of age in users of NSAIDs.

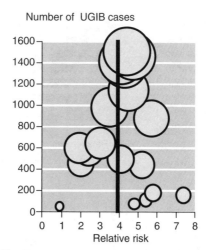

**Figure 5.5.8** Effect of size of study in determining overall relative risk of GI bleeding for NSAID users compared with non-users.

newest, and perhaps the least researched as yet. For adverse events, though, it is one of the most interesting areas. There are some splendid and thought-provoking examples, so this part of this section will use a number of examples, most of which come from a research group based in Geneva, with links to Oxford. All are from the pain and anaesthesia literature.

These reviews were predicated on the idea that, to some extent, many adverse events have a biological progression. That is, a mild form of the event is relatively common, a more severe form is less common, whilst the most severe form is very rare indeed (Figure 5.5.9). In the figure, adverse

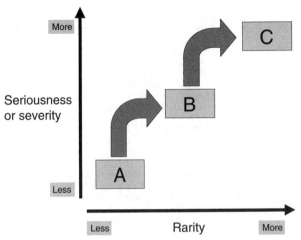

**Figure 5.5.9** Biological progression for adverse event.

event B is more severe and rarer than A, and adverse event C is more severe and rarer than B. There may be circumstances where adverse events progress through one level of harm to another, or where different manifestations of the same harm are more severe but rarer than others.

Whichever relationship one event has to another, the point is that the incidence of mild adverse events is relatively easy to establish compared with that of rare adverse events. If we know the incidence of a common adverse event and the relative incidence of progression from that level of harm to the next, more serious, level, then we can establish the incidence of that more severe level of harm, and so on. In order to have all this knowledge, we need information from many different study architectures.

The benefits of teleoanalysis include being able to provide absolute estimates of risk of adverse events, rather than relative risks or some other statistical output that few could understand and even fewer could use. Three examples will help understand how the process works, and what it can deliver.

### Propofol and bradycardia

The first of these studies examined the incidence of bradycardia with a drug called propofol, used for the induction of anaesthesia [8]. The review used a systematic search for any type of report of bradycardiac events during propofol anaesthesia, and also requested information from 38 national reporting centres, as well as from the manufacturer. Events other than bradycardia that were likely to be related (like asystole and death) were also sought.

The authors found 65 published reports (randomized trials, case series, and case reports), with additional information from drug monitoring centres. There were 1444 cases of bradycardia, 86 asystoles, and 24 deaths. For bradycardia, propofol, compared with other anaesthetics, had an NNH of 11 overall, but as low as 4 in paediatric strabismus surgery. One patient in every 660 had an asystole with propofol. So, in absolute terms, in adults undergoing surgery studied in controlled trials, the risks were that 1 in 8 would have bradycardia and 1 in 660 would have an asystole. The risk of bradycardia-related death was 1.4 in 100,000. Controlled trials and observational studies tended to produce somewhat different estimates.

### NSAIDs and gastrointestinal bleeding

A similar situation of a biological progression pertains with gastrointestinal problems associated with NSAIDs [9]. Many patients suffer gastrointestinal symptoms, some have frank bleeding, and some of those with frank bleeding can die because of it. A systematic review attempted to quantify the risks, beginning with a systematic literature search for any use of NSAID or aspirin lasting at least 2 months. The search sought data on gastrointestinal ulcer, bleed, or perforation, or death, and, in particular, information about progression from one level of harm to the next, more serious, level. It used:

- 15 RCTs (> 15,000 cases);
- 3 cohort studies (215,000 cases, 800,000 controls);
- 6 case-control studies (3000 cases);
- 20 case series or reports (11,800 cases).

There was a consistent finding that events were found with NSAID or aspirin more frequently than without them, whether the event was an endoscopic ulcer, symptoms, bleeding, or death. Bleeding or perforation with NSAID in RCTs occurred in 0.7% of patients, while bleeding or perforation with or without NSAIDs led to death in 6% to 16% (average 12%). With 2 months of treatment with NSAID or aspirin:

- 1 in 5 will have an endoscopic ulcer;
- 1 in 70 will have a symptomatic ulcer;
- 1 in 150 will have a bleeding ulcer;
- 1 in 1200 will die of a bleeding ulcer.

### Subarachnoid haemorrhage and cardiopulmonary dysfunction

Teleoanalysis is a technique that can be applied not just to adverse events of interventions, but also adverse events of medical conditions, and has been applied to the neurological deficit and cardiopulmonary dysfunction of patients with spontaneous subarachnoid haemorrhage [10]. The systematic review looked for studies of any architecture with more than 10 patients with subarachnoid haemorrhage. It reported on randomized trials, case control studies, and uncontrolled case series.

There were a surprising number of results, relating to electrocardiographic abnormalities, creatine phosphokinase and troponin levels, as well as pulmonary oedema and death. It concluded that cardiopulmonary dysfunction is more likely to occur with increasing neurological deficit. While not a surprising result in itself, the important thing again was the use of information from diverse sources to provide absolute risk figures for unwanted outcomes.

## Commentary

Systematic review and meta-analysis of adverse events is a useful advance over non-systematic methods, or using inadequate amounts of data. Once the statistics have been dealt with, tremendously useful information can be obtained, of real value to patients and to professionals. The message is that some very good people are doing some very bright things in this area, and it will have growing importance as increasing attention is paid to the unintended consequences of treatment.

## References

1. Wald, N.J. and Morris, J.K. (2003). Teleoanalysis: combining data from different types of study. *British Medical Journal* **327**, 616–18.
2. Aronsen, J.K. (2005). Unity from diversity: the evidential use of anecdotal reports of adverse drug reactions and interactions. *Journal of Evaluation in Clinical Practice* **11**, 195–208.
3. Derry, S. and Loke, Y.K. (2000). Risk of gastrointestinal haemorrhage with long term use of aspirin: meta-analysis. *British Medical Journal* **321**, 1183–7.
4. Moore, R.A. and McQuay, H.J. (2005). Prevalence of opioid adverse events in chronic non-malignant pain: systematic review of randomised trials of oral opioids. *Arthritis Research and Therapy* **7**, R1046–R1051.
5. Moore, R.A. *et al.* (2005). Tolerability and adverse events in clinical trials of celecoxib in osteoarthritis and rheumatoid arthritis: systematic review and meta-analysis of information from clinical trial reports. *Arthritis Research and Therapy* **7**, R644–R665.
6. Gøtzsche, P.C. (2001). Reporting of outcomes in arthritis trials measured on ordinal and interval scales is inadequate in relation to meta-analysis. *Annals of the Rheumatic Diseases* **59**, 407–8.
7. Hernández-Diaz, S. and García Rodriguez, L.A. (2000). Association between nonsteroidal anti-inflammatory drugs and upper gastrointestinal tract bleeding and perforation: an overview of epidemiological studies published in the 1990s. *Archives of Internal Medicine* **160**, 2093–9.
8. Tramèr, M.R. *et al.* (1997). Propofool and bradycardia: causation, frequency and severity. *British Journal of Anaesthesia* **78**, 642–51.
9. Tramèr, M.R. *et al.* (2000). Quantitative estimation of rare adverse effects which follow a biological progression—a new model applied to chronic NSAID use. *Pain* **85**, 169–82.
10. Macrea, L.M. *et al.* (2005). Spontaneous subarachnoid hemorrhage and serious cardiopulmonary dysfunction—a systematic review. *Resuscitation* **65**, 139–48.

# 5.6 Adverse drug reactions

This section may not contribute a huge amount to understanding evidence about adverse events in clinical trials, or rare or particular adverse events. Rather it is presented to explain just how big the problems are with adverse events in the real world, and how different forms of evidence sometimes come into play. There is also a terminology problem, whether this is about adverse drug effects or adverse drug reactions. We have chosen to use the terms adverse drug reactions or events as used by the authors of the papers we quote.

Adverse drug reactions (ADRs) comprise an important part of evidence about adverse events, which by some accounts are responsible for many deaths, though this is disputed. However much people argue about the precise numbers of ADRs that occur, there is clear evidence that, whatever the number is, it is not small. It might be prudent, then, to examine some key papers about ADRs, about how many there are, and about how they may be reduced.

An adverse drug event (ADE) is defined as an injury resulting from medical intervention relating to a drug. This definition is different from that of an adverse drug reaction (ADR), defined by WHO as 'noxious and unintended, and which occurs at doses used in man for prophylaxis, diagnosis, or therapy'. The ADR definition is likely to be idiosyncratic and rare, and would, for instance, not include an unintended misprescription of a larger than therapeutic dose of a drug which caused harm because it was an overdose. Such an event would be an ADE. It should not occur, and is likely to be preventable. Not everyone favours the term adverse drug event [1].

## Early evidence

An investigation from Boston set out to assess the incidence and preventability of ADEs and potential ADEs, and to analyse these events in order to develop prevention strategies [2]. According to the introduction to the paper, which summarizes some of the information about ADEs, there were many more deaths from adverse drug problems than from road traffic accidents.

All adults at the Brigham and Women's Hospital (726 beds) and Massachusetts General Hospital (846 beds) admitted to any of 11 units over 6 months were included in the study. Obstetric units were not included. The 61 non-obstetric adult units were stratified between hospitals, whether medical or surgical and whether intensive or general care. Study units were then selected randomly using a random number generator. Three methods were used to identify incidents.

1. Nurses and pharmacists were asked to report incidents to nurse investigators.
2. A nurse investigator visited each unit twice daily on weekdays to solicit information.
3. The nurse investigator reviewed all charts at least daily.

The primary outcome was an ADE, and a secondary outcome a potential ADE (an example would be a patient with known sensitivity to penicillin who was given penicillin, but did not react). To discover the cause of preventable ADEs, persons involved were interviewed and the results investigated by a multidisciplinary team.

All incidents were evaluated independently by two physicians who classified them according to the following criteria: whether or not an ADE or potential ADE had occurred; severity; preventability; and, if an error had occurred, the type of error and the stage in the process at which it occurred. Reviewers were asked to consider ADEs as preventable if they were due to an error or were preventable by any means currently available.

In the study period, there were 4031 admissions to the study units, comprising 21, 412 patient-days (about 10% of the 214,000 patient-days in adult, non-obstetric units at the two hospitals). The study found 247 ADEs and 194 potential ADEs. Extrapolated, this amounted to 1900 ADEs per hospital per year with, for every 100 admissions, 6.5 ADEs and 5.5 potential ADEs. Of all ADEs, 1% were fatal, 12% life-threatening, 30% serious, and 57% significant. The rate of ADEs was highest in medical intensive care units (19 per 1000 patient-days) and relatively similar among surgical intensive care and medical and surgical general care units (9–11 per 1000 patient-days).

Over 50% of all ADEs were associated with the use of analgesics (30%) or antibiotics (24%). No single drug accounted for more than 9% of ADEs. Analgesics were the leading drug class associated with preventable ADEs, and half of these involved misuse or malfunction of infusion pumps or devices (epidural catheters or patient-controlled analgesia). Table 5.6.1 shows the data by actual numbers in the study, by the rate per 100 admissions, and by extrapolation to events per hospital per year. It is instructive that even the lowest of these event rates adds up to a significant number of patients.

### Preventable ADEs

Seventy (28%) of 247 ADEs were preventable and 83 (43%) of 194 potential ADEs were intercepted before the drug was given. Errors resulting in preventable ADEs occurred most often at the stages of ordering (56%) and administration (34%); transcription and dispensing errors were uncommon. Errors were more likely to be intercepted if they occurred early in the process—48% at the ordering stage but none at administration of the drug.

### Cost

ADEs generate costs to the patient, costs to the hospital through treating the effects of the ADE, and costs (at least potentially) of medical negligence claims. The hospital cost alone was estimated to be $2000 per event—

**Table 5.6.1**   ADEs reported

| Event | Number | Rate per 100 admissions | Number per hospital per year |
|---|---|---|---|
| All ADEs | 247 | 6.5 | 1923 |
| Due to analgesics | 73 | 1.9 | 568 |
| Due to opiates | 57 | 1.5 | 444 |
| Preventable ADEs due to pump or device malfunction | 9 | 0.2 | 70 |

making about $3.8 million per hospital per year. $1 million of this was preventable, notwithstanding the human cost.

*Lesson*
How might a hospital improve the quality of its drug delivery process? To get the full flavour of the lessons from this study, read the paper and some of the many useful references. In précis the lessons are:
1. Have an effective mechanism for systematically collecting and feeding back data about ADEs.
2. The organization must look for preventable ADEs, not just ADRs.
3. System change must be directed at specific parts of the process where error can occur, or where errors can be minimized.
The total quality improvement perspective assumes that most providers are doing their best in the current system. Major improvements in system performance require redesign of systems rather than pushing people harder with the current system. Better systems should promote fewer errors and include effective mechanisms for catching those that do occur. They also cost less.

This study compares with an Oxford study [3] in which adverse drug reaction data on 20,695 consecutive acute general medical admissions to seven general medical wards at the John Radcliffe Hospital were collected between April 1990 and March 1993. This was a spontaneous reporting scheme in which nurses, pharmacists, doctors, and medical students were invited to report adverse drug reactions occurring in patients during hospital admission. Deliberate or accidental overdoses were not included, nor were patients who were not admitted overnight to hospital. There were 1420 reports to the Oxford scheme, a rate of 6.9%.

## A meta-analysis of all evidence

A meticulous meta-analysis examined ADRs both in US hospital inpatients and those patients admitted with an adverse drug reaction [4]. The searching strategy was heroic, and included examination of a number of electronic databases together with postal questionnaires to researchers. Studies were restricted to US hospitals, since the bulk of information was from that country. The methods and definitions are meticulously laid out, allowing those who are interested in the figures to follow all the manipulations.

The outcome the researchers used was the WHO definition: any noxious, unintended, and undesired effect of a drug that occurs at doses used in humans for prophylaxis, diagnosis, or therapy. This excludes therapeutic failures, intentional or accidental poisoning or drug abuse, and adverse effects due to errors in administration or compliance. A serious ADR was defined as one that requires hospital admission, prolongs hospital stay, is permanently disabling, or results in death. Serious ADRs therefore include fatal ADRs, which were also analysed separately.

The main results (based on 33 million US hospital admissions in 1994) are shown in the Table 5.6.2. They show that 2.1% of inpatients experienced a serious ADR, and that 4.7% of hospital admissions were due to a serious ADR. Fatal ADRs occurred in 0.19% of inpatients and 0.13% of admissions.

Overall, it was estimated that some 2.2 million serious ADRs would have occurred in 1994, with 106,000 of them fatal. Although the reports covered some four decades, there was no evidence of any systematic change in the

**Table 5.6.2** Incidence of adverse drug reactions in the USA in 1994

| | Number of Studies | Patients studied | Incidence of ADR (95% CI) | Estimated number (thousands, with 95% CI) |
|---|---|---|---|---|
| **ADRs in patients while in hospital** | | | | |
| Serious | 12 | 22,500 | 2.1 (1.9–2.3) | 702 (635–770) |
| Fatal | 10 | 28,900 | 0.19 (0.13–0.26) | 63 (41–85) |
| **ADRs in patients admitted to hospital** | | | | |
| Serious | 21 | 28,000 | 4.7 (3.1–6.2) | 1547 (1033–2060) |
| Fatal | 6 | 17,800 | 0.13 (0.04–0.21) | 43 (15–71) |
| **Overall ADR incidence** | | | | |
| Serious | 33 | 50,500 | 6.7 (5.2–8.2) | 2216 (1721–2711) |
| Fatal | 16 | 46,600 | 0.32 (0.23–0.41) | 106 (76–137) |

rate of serious ADRs, and the population studied was similar to that in the US hospitals. Medical wards were overrepresented, though the authors did considerable work to investigate how this might have affected results using the most conservative estimates (not much effect was found). Issues like hospital setting (teaching versus non-teaching), and possible errors in compiling data in the original reports are dealt with thoroughly.

This report suggested that fatal ADRs rank from the fourth to the sixth leading cause of death in the USA after heart disease, cancer, and stroke, and similar to pulmonary disease and accidents. Costs associated with ADRs were estimated at up to $4 billion a year. This is an important clinical issue. Those who want to think about it, and how it might be tackled, should read, digest, and understand this careful and thoughtful piece of work. It should be noted that there have been major disagreements with the work as well [5], mainly because of interpretations of clinical homogeneity and heterogeneity, and whether that is important.

### More meta-analyses

Two later systematic reviews of the world literature [6, 7] confirm the size of the problem and provide some insights about what to look for.

#### Beijer and de Blaey [6]

This Dutch study looked for studies relating hospital admission to adverse drug reaction. Excluding papers about drug and alcohol abuse, and drug-related problems during hospital stay, they were left with 68 studies. They used a WHO definition of ADR that excluded therapeutic failure, intentional and accidental poisoning, and drug abuse.

There were 6000 ADR-related admissions in a total of 124, 000, giving an overall rate of 4.9%, but with large interstudy variation. Almost all of the variation was found in small studies (especially those with just a few hundred patients), with more consistent results in larger studies. The variation could be related just to size or to special circumstances examined in particular studies. Subgroup analysis looked at elderly versus non-elderly (over 65 was the usual criterion). Here the ADR admission rate was 16.6%, compared with 4.1% in younger people. Analysis by condition or medicine was not possible, but year of publication and type of hospital made no difference.

The authors attempted to calculate what the cost was to the Dutch health-care system in 1998, and came up with the range of 186 million to 430 million euros a year. This is based on estimates that a significant proportion of ADR-related admissions in the elderly are preventable.

### Wiffen et al. [7]

The Oxford study used a similar if wider search strategy looking for:

- hospital medical record review whilst patient was in hospital or later review;
- follow-up survey after release from hospital;
- case-control, cohort;
- sample of patients versus all patients with ADRs.

Primarily the ADR rate was the key outcome, rather than admissions from ADR, though the ADR rate could be the proportion of patients or admissions. Admission because of an ADR and ADR whilst in hospital were also examined separately. Several pre-specified sensitivity analyses were defined.

The Oxford study used 69 unique studies with evaluable data on 412,000 patients, with an overall ADR rate of 6.7%. Of the 69 studies, 54 were prospective with an ADR rate of 5.5% (193,000 subjects) and 15 were retrospective with an ADR rate of 7.7% (220,000 subjects). Larger studies tended to have lower ADR rates than small studies (Figure 5.6.1).

Neither geographical setting nor publication before or after 1985 made much difference, except when clinical setting was added (Table 5.6.3). Studies in general medicine after 1985 had a lower ADR rate than those before (3% versus 9%), and those in older people had a higher rate in post-1985 studies (20% versus 4%). Adverse drug reactions were also examined by specialist clinical setting (cancer, emergency departments, for instance) and with specific classes of medicines, and by gender and culture. ADR rates in inpatients and admissions with ADRs were similar. Several studies examined the interaction between age and number of medicines taken. Older age, and increasing numbers of medicines, especially in women, were associated with ADR rates of between 20% and 50%.

Calculating from the number of accident and emergency visits and inpatient days, the rates of ADR likely from UK, European, and US studies, and average stays, the estimate for the burden on the UK NHS was equivalent to about 15–20 400-bed hospitals. This would consume about 4% of available bed-days and cost about £380 million annually.

## Errors can be avoided and ADRs reduced

Is there evidence that giving health-care professionals better tools makes them perform the complicated tasks they do better? A systematic review [8] of computer-based clinical decision support systems (CDSS) shows two things. It demonstrates that there are many studies in a wide variety of different clinical areas. Studies using CDSS in a clinical setting by a health-care practitioner and assessing the effects prospectively with a concurrent control were sought. Five databases, reference lists, and conference proceedings were searched.

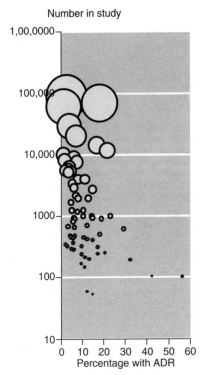

**Figure 5.6.1** ADR rate in studies of different sizes.

Sixty-five studies were found (Table 5.6.4). Of 15 studies of drug dosing systems, 60% found benefit. Of 19 studies on preventive care systems, 74% found benefit. Of 26 studies in other clinical areas, 73% found benefit. Only

**Table 5.6.3** ADR rates with specialty and age of study

| Speciality | Pre/post-1985 | Number of subjects | ADR rate % (95% CI) |
|---|---|---|---|
| General medicine | Pre | 60, 401 | 8.5 (8.2–8.7) |
| General medicine | Post | 243, 803 | 2.9 (2.8–3.0) |
| Geriatric | Pre | 11, 212 | 4.3 (3.9–4.7) |
| Geriatric | Post | 3488 | 20 (19–21) |
| Paediatric | Pre | 469 | 4.2 (2.4–6.0) |
| Paediatric | Post | 837 | 3.1 (1.9–4.3) |

**Table 5.6.4** Health-care professional performance in studies of CDSS

| Study area | Studies showing benefit/total |
|---|:---:|
| Drug dosing systems | 9/15 |
| Diagnostic aids | 1/5 |
| Preventive care systems | 14/19 |
| Other medical care | 19/26 |
| All CDSS studies | 43/65 |

one of five diagnostic decision support systems found benefit; that one used a system to identify postoperative patients at risk of respiratory complications for physiotherapy.

The systematic review is a terrific bit of work. But the question left incompletely answered is whether computer systems can contribute significantly to reduce adverse drug events in hospitals. Two US examples show exactly what can be achieved [9, 10].

### Boston [9]

In the Brigham and Women's Hospital, which is a 726-bed tertiary referral centre, the use of a physician computer order-entry (POE) system was evaluated, in which doctors wrote all drug orders online. The study had a baseline period during which an audit of medication errors was examined, followed by implementation of the POE system and re-audit. Incidents were identified by three mechanisms: nurses and pharmacists reported incidents; an investigator visited the wards twice daily to solicit information; and patient charts were examined daily by an investigator.

The main outcome was the number of non-intercepted serious medication errors. These were either errors preventable by systems currently in use, or had the potential for harm but did not result in injury.

Use of the POE system prevented more than half of the serious medication errors. There were just under 11 of these per 1000 patient-days at baseline, and under 5 per 1000 patient-days during use of the POE system. Potential errors that had not been intercepted fell most, by 84%. Preventable errors fell by 17%.

The authors concluded that their system could be extended to different drug types, such as sedatives (where errors actually rose, but which had not been included in their original system), and by extending the system in other ways. They also show that the cost of running a POE system for their large, complicated hospital would be of the same order as money saved directly. When other costs, like extra work caused by serious drug errors, or malpractice litigation, were included, it could save $5–10 million a year. The system could both save money and improve quality of care.

### Phoenix [10]

The Good Samaritan Regional Medical Centre in Phoenix is a 650-bed referral centre. It has an integrated hospital information system. A multidisciplinary team of professionals met and identified 37 drug- or class-specific areas where adverse drug events might be expected. The system was modified so that, if circumstances arose where an adverse drug event might occur (digoxin toxicity was one example), then a pharmacist or

**Table 5.6.5**  Adverse drug event alerts

| Event | Number | Per 1000 admissions | Per cent |
|---|---|---|---|
| Non-obstetric admissions | 9306 | | |
| ADE alerts | 1116 | 120 | 100 |
| Evaluator needed to alert physician | 794 | 85 | 71 |
| True potential adverse drug events | 596 | 64 | 53 |
| Physicians unaware of potential for harm | 265 | 28 | 24 |
| Changes in treatment | 265 | 28 | 24 |

radiologist was alerted. If necessary, the physician attending the patient was contacted.

Over 6 months there were 9306 non-obstetric admissions. There were 1116 alerts (Table 5.6.5). Physicians needed to be contacted 794 times, and 596 times the event had not been recognized. The average time taken for each contact was 15 minutes.

The rates of clinically unrecognized events varied in different clinical circumstances. For instance, more than half of the potential problems for renal toxicity with the use of radiocontrast media had been recognized previously, but it was felt that potential benefit outweighed potential harm. Using some literature data on costs, the authors calculated that the potential saving to their 650-bed hospital was some $3 million a year, and could be more if the system were extended to other areas.

## Commentary

These are two different types of interventions. One depends on putting systems in place to stop mistakes happening. The other depends on real-time interventions to stop mistakes when they happen. Both had a major effect in stopping medication errors in large, complex institutions. Both would improve patient care. Both would reduce costs.

Concentrating on stopping bad things happening is what quality control is all about. These are two excellent examples of how to do it. Moreover, all three papers have extensive referencing of a wealth of literature in this area, and are worth reading for that alone.

The bottom line, though, is that in the real world adverse drug events or reactions are major drivers of health-care. They have large negative consequences in their own right, and are a major reason why people do not take medicines they are properly prescribed, leading to much additional loss of quality health-care. Insufficient time has been devoted to evidence around adverse events.

## References

1. Aronson, J.K. and Reynolds, D.J.M. Correspondence: adverse drug reactions. (www.jr2.ox.ac.uk/bandolier/band30/b30–9.html).
2. Bates, D.W. et al. (1995). Incidence of adverse drug events and potential adverse drug events. Implications for prevention. *Journal of the American Medical Association* **274**, 29–34.

3. Smith, C.C. *et al.* (1996). Adverse drug reactions in a hospital general medical unit meriting notification to the Committee on Safety of Medicines. *British Journal of Clinical Pharmacology* **42**, 423–9.
4. Lazarou, J. *et al.* (1998). Incidence of adverse drug reactions in hospitalized patients: a meta-analysis of prospective studies. *Journal of the American Medical Association* **279**, 1200–5.
5. Kvasv, M. *et al.* (2000). Adverse drug reactions in hospitalized patients: a critique of a meta-analysis. *MedGenMed* **2** (2), E3.
6. Beijer, H.J. and de Blaey, C.J. (2002). Hospitalisations caused by adverse drug reactions (ADR): a meta-analysis of observational studies. *Pharmacy World and Science* **24**, 46–54.
7. Wiffen, P.J. *et al.* (2002). Adverse drug reactions in hospital patients: a systematic review of the prospective and retrospective studies. *Bandolier Extra*, June 2002, (*www.ljr2.ox.ac.uk/bandolier/extra.html*).
8. Hunt, D.L. *et al.* (1998). Effects of computer-based clinical decision support systems on physician performance and patient outcomes. *Journal of the American Medical Association* **280**, 1339–46.
9. Bates, D.W. *et al.* (1998). Effect of computerized physician order entry and a team intervention on prevention of serious medical errors. *Journal of the American Medical Association* **280**, 1311–16.
10. Raschke, R.A. *et al.* (1998). A computer alert system to prevent injury from adverse drug events. Development and evaluation in a community teaching hospital. *Journal of the American Medical Association* **280**, 1317–20.

# 5.7 Adverse events: final thoughts

When writing about adverse events, and the evidence of adverse events, two things are certain. Firstly, it always leaves the writer with a sense of being unsatisfied, because there is so much to say, because much will have been omitted, and because we just do not know all the rules about evidence. Secondly, some clever person somewhere will disagree with something you say, and have a good reason for doing so.

Perhaps these reasons have prevented people from trying to do more. Whatever you do, you will be criticized.

But that is perhaps the past rather than the reality now. We have increasing examples where a more evidential line is taken, even in case reports. For instance, a case report of two cases of a knotted intravascular device or catheter were presented together with a systematic review of the literature with a further 113 reported cases [1].

What we learn is that the mortality associated with the event was 8%, that open cardiotomy was required in five cases, but that in 62% of cases withdrawal of the catheter was achieved successfully without surgery. That we can have systematic reviews on case studies or series like this is a reflection of the ease with which we can now search the medical (and other) literature, often from the comfort of our desks. Electronic searching for adverse events may be less reliable than searching for studies of efficacy [2], and personal experience indicates that heroic measures may be needed to do find all studies on adverse events. But a consequence of more information being available electronically is that systematic reviews accompanying case reports are becoming more common, and the case reports more interesting, and often better reported.

On the other hand, though we have lots of systematic reviews of various types of evidence around adverse events, they do not always agree, and we do not usually know which is correct. The main example to date relates to amiodarone [3]. Here adverse event rates for different outcomes were approached in three ways: by a meta-analysis of clinical trials; spontaneous reports in journals; and spontaneous reports sent to the WHO.

The rank order of ADRs differed in the three data sets. This was not expected and, while different numerical results might have been expected, with different ADR rates in the different reporting methods, the rank order of one adverse event to another should have been reasonably consistent. The fact that it was not should make us think. It may be that amiodarone, for one reason or another, is just different from other drugs or interventions. It may be that different adverse reactions arouse more interest and therefore more spontaneous reporting than others. It may be something else entirely.

Whichever of these, or any other, explanation is finally shown to be the most likely, we have in the meantime to treat adverse drug reactions, or adverse events due to interventions, very carefully. They are important in their own right, not just afterthoughts. Working out better ways of examining the evidence about adverse events, and which way is best, will be a major challenge.

Recent events with the withdrawal of some cox-2 specific inhibitors show how important an increase in cardiovascular events from 1% to 2%

in patients not normally treated with these drugs may be, and how such effects can be hard to detect without specific long-term trials, or without particularly strong signals emanating from higher-than-licensed doses. When there are other treatment options, then withdrawing the drug is an inevitable political sequel, even when other treatment options have other severe adverse events. What is important for the future is having ways in drug development of identifying the potential risk and, after drug launch, better ways of picking up these problems.

## References

1. Karanikas, I.D. *et al.* (2002). Removal of knotted intravascular devices. Case report and review of the literature. *European Journal of Vascular and Endovascular Surgery* **23**, 189–94.
2. Lemeshow, A.R. *et al.* (2005). Searching one or two databases was insufficient for meta-analysis of observational studies. *Journal of Clinical Epidemiology* **58**, 867–73.
3. Loke, Y.K. *et al.* (2004). A comparison of three different sources of data in assessing the frequencies of adverse reactions to amiodarone. *British Journal of Clinical Pharmacology* **57**, 616–21.

# 6.1 Health economics and management

This section is not intended to be a primer on health economics, and certainly not to define in detail how it is done. It is intended rather as an aid to understanding for those of us who find the topic intimidating. It is also intended as a way of looking at the evidence around health economics. There are two ways of doing this.

One is to claim that 98% of health economics is bunk, and so is management, and move on to something more interesting.

The alternative is to claim that 98% of health economics is bunk. But isn't that interesting, and why is it bunk, and surely management is really important otherwise the last few hundred years of capitalist growth and expansion wouldn't have occurred, and we would all be subsistence farmers working for some guy with chain mail and a very large sword?

This book aims to be close to the second of these, but in a 'lite' fashion. The simple fact is that health economics drives most health-care decision-making, but often in a rather poor way. Throwing up one's hands is not an option, and all of us have to at least try to get our brains around it. And it really isn't that difficult to get to grips with what may be unfamiliar jargon, but what amounts to rather simple concepts. Of course, there is much controversy about detail, quite rightly, but that is an area we really don't need to get into, because broad brush is better.

Some health economists might be scandalized at the statement that 98% of health economics is bunk, while others would agree. How is it possible to make a statement like that? Mainly because much of health economics is involved with cost-effectiveness (explanation of terms comes in the next section, so for now just accept the words).

Cost-effectiveness is to do with two things, cost, and effectiveness. Now health economists know lots about costs, and spend much time arguing about it. But by and large, and certainly in the past, they knew little about effectiveness. Effectiveness was often taken from tiny individual trials (usually the ones that particularly supported a proposition) rather than from systematic reviews and meta-analyses of studies fulfilling criteria of quality, validity, and size. While costs might have been right, effectiveness almost never was. So it is possible to claim that most health economics is bunk, but that is a retrospective view of a dynamic and increasingly important part of an evidence-based world.

At least three things are needed to run health-care effectively. These are evidence on effectiveness, evidence on cost, and evidence on how to make a change (Figure 6.1.1). Only if we have all three will our overall effort be effective and efficient. On all three our knowledge is inadequate, but on some it is more inadequate than on others.

## Perspective

One concept we have to grasp early on is that of perspective. If we want a health economic answer on a topic, we have to ask from whose perspective do we do the calculations? Take an example like TNF-alpha treatment in early rheumatoid arthritis. This is an expensive treatment, with a current cost of about £8000 (about $14,000; 12,000 euros) a year in drugs alone,

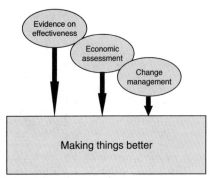

**Figure 6.1.1** Essential evidence for effective and efficient health-care.

but it is a treatment that in the right patient can be highly effective. If it isn't working or has adverse events, treatment is stopped. Patients with early rheumatoid arthritis are relatively young, with the prospect of many years of employment before them, paying taxes. We know that most patients with rheumatoid arthritis leave paid employment within a few years of diagnosis.

From the point of view of a patient in the UK, the treatment would be highly desirable. It keeps them well, and they don't have to pay for the treatment in a socialized health service. For the patient this is a 'good buy'.

From the point of view of the health service, the prospective outlay is over £8000 a year for perhaps many years. There may be good evidence of cost-effectiveness, and some offsets in lower costs of other treatments, but this will put a strain on prescribing budgets, and it will involve questions over affordability. For a health service with limited budgets, this may not be such a 'good buy'.

From the point of view of society, this is a treatment that could, arguably, keep a person gainfully employed and paying taxes instead of being dependent in whole or in part on state benefits. Society benefits greatly from this, offsetting any cost society pays for keeping a person well. For society this is a 'good buy'.

This is a simple example, and many are nothing like as simple as this. But it serves to point out the problem of health-care delivery. In almost all circumstances, there is a fixed resource from which to supply an almost unlimited demand. Increasing expectations by consumers of what health-care can deliver, technological advances that fuel that increased expectation, and demographic changes resulting in more older people, when older people have more chronic health problems, all feed the increasing demand.

The role of health economics is to provide information about costs, calculated in standard ways, to inform decision-making. Health economics does not make the decisions. Once treatments or procedures have a health economic 'tick' that they meet some limit of cost-effectiveness, then decisions over affordability and equitable distribution of that which is cost-effective are for others.

## Value

One concept that is rarely considered is that of value. Value has several different dictionary meanings. One is the worth of something, an amount expressed in money or another medium of exchange that is thought to be a fair exchange for something. In this sense it is pretty similar to cost-effectiveness, as traditionally expressed in health economics. But another meaning is one we probably need to capture as well, that of the worth, importance, or usefulness of something to somebody. Take the example of TNF-alpha in rheumatoid arthritis: it is clearly valuable to keep people healthy and contributing, rather than sick. However much health economics tries to ascribe monetary units to health, there are aspects of value that cannot be captured.

In health economics value is usually measured with cost as the numerator and health outcome as the denominator. Health outcome is usually provided as a quality-adjusted life year (QALY), roughly a year of perfect health (see later). What we get is cost per QALY, and long lists of cost per QALY have been produced, for various interventions [1]. A number of examples are shown in Table 6.1.1.

Decision-making is then based upon what is affordable. Attempts have been made to link evidence and cost in decision-making, perhaps one of the best being shown in Figure 6.1.2 [2]. Evidence here is graded, so that (roughly) level I evidence would be from systematic reviews of properly conducted randomized trials, level II from at least one well conducted randomized trial of appropriate size, level III from observational studies, and level IV from opinion. Low cost per QALY and good evidence is

**Table 6.1.1** Cost per QALY for health-care interventions

| Intervention | £/QALY (1990 prices) |
| --- | --- |
| Neurosurgical intervention for head injury | 240 |
| GP advice to stop smoking | 270 |
| Neurosurgical intervention for subarachnoid haemorrhage | 490 |
| Antihypertensive treatment to prevent stroke (45–69 years) | 940 |
| Pacemaker implant | 1100 |
| Hip replacement | 1180 |
| CABG (left main vessel disease, severe angina) | 2090 |
| Kidney transplant | 4710 |
| Heart transplant | 7840 |
| Home dialysis | 17,260 |
| Hospital dialysis | 21,970 |

Cost per QALY (£,000)

| Evidence | <3 | 3–20 | >20 | >30 |
|---|---|---|---|---|
| I | Strongly support | Strongly support | Limited support | Not supported |
| II | Strongly support | Supported | Limited support | Not supported |
| III | Supported | Limited support | Limited support | Not supported |
| IV | Not proven | Not proven | Not proven | Not proven |

**Figure 6.1.2**   Decision-making on evidence and cost.

supported, while high cost per QALY and lower levels of evidence are not supported.

This looks like a rough and ready way of looking at things, but it has an appeal, because it at least incorporates evidence. Not all systems do that. Even sensible and useful criticisms of current thinking about health economic evaluations seeking to include issues of value [3] fail to examine the evidence on which value assessments are made.

## Commentary

Health economics is a valuable additional aid to decision-making. Just like NNTs, and EBM, it is a tool, not a rule. Health economics is absorbing the lessons of evidence from clinical trials and, while it may not always be correct in what it does, it is a vigorous and flourishing discipline that we should be encouraging. We also need to learn how it works and how we can use it to our benefit.

## References

1. Tengs, T.O. *et al.* (1995). Five-hundred life-saving interventions and their cost effectiveness. *Risk Analysis* **3**, 369–90.
2. Stevens, A. *et al.* (1995). Quick and clean: authoritative health technology assessment for local health care contracting. *Health Trends* **27**, 37–42.
3. Coast, J. (2004). Is economic evaluation in touch with society's health values? *British Medical Journal* **329**, 1233–6.

## 6.2 Health economic terms and meanings

Health economics has its own jargon, and one of the difficulties with understanding the subject is understanding the jargon. A few pages, then, on the meanings of various terms.

### Quality-adjusted life year (QALY)

Outcomes from treatments and other health-influencing activities have two basic components—the quantity and quality of life. Life expectancy is a traditional measure with few problems of comparison—people are either alive or not.

Attempts to measure and value quality of life are a more recent innovation, with a number of approaches. Particular effort has gone into researching ways in which an overall health index might be constructed to locate a specific health state on a continuum between, for example, 0 (= death) and 1 (= perfect health). Obviously, the portrayal of health like this is far from ideal, since, for example, the definition of perfect health is highly subjective and it has been argued that some health states are worse than death. These measures have a number of uses, from identifying public health trends to develop strategies, to assess the effectiveness and efficiency of health-care interventions, or to determine the state of health in communities.

The quality-adjusted life year (QALY) has been created to combine the quantity and quality of life. The basic idea of a QALY is straightforward. It takes 1 year of perfect health-life expectancy to be worth 1, but regards one year of less than perfectly healthy life expectancy as less than 1. Thus an intervention that results in a patient with previously perfect quality of life living for an additional 4 years, but where quality of life fell from 1 to 0.6, produces 2.4 QALYs over the 4 years. The same patient may have had perfect quality of life for 1 year without the intervention, so for that year he lost 0.4 QALY with the intervention. The number of QALYs gained was therefore 2.4 − 0.4 = 2.0.

QALYs can therefore provide an indication of the benefits gained from a variety of medical procedures in terms of quality and life and survival for the patient. Another example is shown in Figure 6.2.1, where treatment provides a bigger area under the QALY/time curve than does no treatment.

It is no use pretending that QALYs are anything but a crude measurement. It is necessary to be aware of their limitations—with the possibility of more research making the process more sophisticated and useful.

The use of QALYs in resource allocation decisions does mean that choices between patient groups competing for medical care are made explicit. QALYs have been criticized because there is an implication that some patients will be refused or not offered treatment for the sake of other patients and, yet such choices have been made and are being made all the time. However big the pot, choices still have to be made.

International comparisons of QALYs and chronic diseases that show quite large differences between different conditions in different countries [1] have been made. Despite this, conditions like arthritis, chronic lung

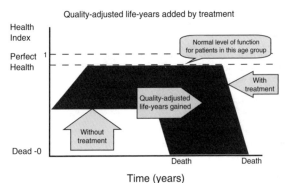

**Figure 6.2.1**    QALY calculation.

disease, and congestive heart failure tend always to have higher negative impacts on quality of life.

### Cost-effectiveness

Cost-effectiveness studies measure the net cost of providing a service, as well as the outcomes obtained. Cost-effectiveness analysis (CEA) is one of the techniques of economic evaluation designed to compare the costs and benefits of a health-care intervention to assess whether it is worth doing.

The choice of technique depends on the nature of the benefits specified. In CEA the benefits are expressed in non-monetary terms related to health effects, such as life-years gained or symptom-free days, whereas in cost–utility analysis they are expressed as quality-adjusted life-years (QALYs) and in cost–benefit analysis in monetary terms. As with all economic evaluation techniques, the aim of CEA is to maximize the level of benefits in terms of health effects relative to the resources available.

Costs are seen differently from different points of view. In economics the notion of cost is based on the value that would be gained from using the same resources elsewhere, known as the opportunity cost. Those resources used for one purpose are not available for another, so benefits that would have been derived in alternate purposes have been sacrificed. In simple terms, you can't have your cake and eat it. It is usual to assume that the price paid reflects the opportunity cost and to adopt a pragmatic approach to costing and use market prices wherever possible.

In CEA it is conventional to distinguish between the direct costs and the indirect costs associated with the intervention, together with what are termed intangibles, which may be difficult to quantify, but are often consequences of the intervention and should be included in the cost profile. Some definitions help.

- Direct costs. Medical: drugs; staff time; equipment. Patient: transport; out-of-pocket expenses.

- Indirect costs. Production losses; other uses of time.
- Intangibles. Pain; suffering; adverse effects.

It is essential to specify which costs are included in a CEA and which are not, to ensure that the findings are not subject to misinterpretation.

Using CEA with different treatments or programmes requires that cost-effectiveness ratios (CERs; note that this is a different CER to the control event rate we met earlier) are calculated for each programme and placed in rank order:

CER = Costs of intervention/health effects produced (e.g. life-years gained).

If we have three interventions with different costs and benefits, then a simple calculation can help decide which makes sense (Table 6.2.1). In example 1, cost-effectiveness analysis would dictate that C should be given priority over A since it has a lower CER, but, in order to decide which to implement, the extent of resources available must be considered. Here it is reasonably simple, because both the total cost and CER are in favour of C. B is discarded because it has a higher cost per life-year gained, and is more expensive overall.

Example 2 is a bit more difficult. Here D, E, and F are closely matched. Yet they have increasing cost overall balanced with increased effectiveness. When resources are unconstrained, F is an obvious choice because it produces most benefit. Where resources are constrained, however, the most beneficial option may not be the one that is chosen. Here the argument is finely balanced, and any constraints favour D or E over F.

### Incremental cost-effectiveness ratio

Where the arguments are finely balanced, incremental cost-effectiveness ratios (ICERs) can help. The different interventions are ranked by increasing effectiveness, on the basis of securing maximum effect rather than considering cost, and ICERs are calculated as shown in Table 6.2.2. The ICER is the difference in costs between interventions divided by the difference in benefits between interventions. The least effective intervention has the same average CER as its ICER, because it is compared with the alternative of doing nothing.

**Table 6.2.1** Cost-effectiveness calculation

| Intervention | Cost (£) | Benefit (unit) | Cost-effectiveness ratio (£/unit of benefit) |
|---|---|---|---|
| **Example 1** | | | |
| A | 100,000 | 1010 | 99 |
| B | 120,000 | 800 | 150 |
| C | 80,000 | 1000 | 80 |
| **Example 2** | | | |
| D | 100,000 | 1000 | 100 |
| E | 120,000 | 1250 | 96 |
| F | 150,000 | 1350 | 111 |

**Table 6.2.2**   Incremental cost-effectiveness ratios

| Intervention | Cost (£) | Difference in costs | Benefit (unit) | Difference in benefit | Incremental cost-effectiveness ratio (£/unit of additional benefit) |
|---|---|---|---|---|---|
| **Example 1** | | | | | |
| B | 120,000 | 120,000 | 800 | 800 | 150 |
| C | 80,000 | −40,000 | 1000 | 200 | −200 |
| A | 100,000 | 20,000 | 1010 | 10 | 2000 |
| **Example 2** | | | | | |
| D | 100,000 | 100,000 | 1000 | 1000 | 100 |
| E | 120,000 | 20,000 | 1250 | 250 | 80 |
| F | 150,000 | 30,000 | 1350 | 100 | 300 |

With this sort of table, negative ICER values are preferred, because they demonstrate an improvement both in units of benefit and in cost. Where the value is positive, it tells us the cost of each additional unit of benefit for that choice, which is not the same as the average benefit.

In example 1, intervention C is preferred over intervention B, but A would probably be excluded because of the high cost per additional unit of benefit for A over C. Each of the 10 additional units of benefit would cost £2000, compared with the £80 each for C, the lowest cost per unit of benefit. If the resources are available, that may be the choice, but where resources are constrained, we know the cost of each **additional** unit of benefit for equitable decisions to be made.

In example 2, we can buy 250 more units of benefit for only £80 each with intervention E, at lower cost than in the base case of intervention D. But intervention F is much more expensive at £300 per additional unit of benefit.

Cost-effectiveness analysis, with incremental cost-effectiveness ratios, can indicate which of a number of alternative interventions represents the best value for money. The quality of the analysis is highly dependent on the quality of effectiveness evidence. Sensitivity analyses can always be employed to test the robustness of any conclusions.

Figure 6.2.2 is a visual guide as to how to use cost-effectiveness, which might be a lot simpler for some of us. In general, if the costs are lower and the effects are greater, this will dominate all other choices. Higher costs but more effects can be cost-effective. Lower costs but lower effects may be useful where resources are severely restricted, but paying more for less effect is dumb and should be excluded.

### Cost utility

Cost utility refers to a cost analysis where the unit of benefit is according to some utility, like QALY. Here we have cost information in terms of £/QALY. The advantage of cost utility is that it should allow us to compare different interventions doing different things with different outcomes, in

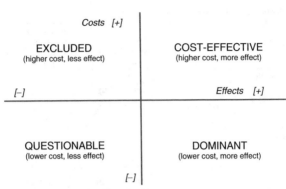

**Figure 6.2.2**  Using cost-effectiveness.

different heath states. We can do this because our inputs are in the same unit, monetary value, and our outputs are also in the same unit, quality-adjusted life years.

Utilities are values that represent the strength of an individual's prefer-ence for specific outcomes under conditions of uncertainty. Health utilities are preferences for specific health states or treatments. They provide an approach to the comprehensive measurement of health-related quality of life. Measuring health utilities involves three steps: defining a set of health states of interest; identifying individuals to provide judgements of the desirability of each health state; and aggregating across the individuals to determine scale values for each health state.

The issues that need to be addressed in any utility study include ensuring that the relevant attributes and levels of health are incorporated into the measurement instrument, determining the appropriate preference-scaling method to elicit utilities, deciding the appropriate subjects whose prefer-ences should be evaluated, and minimizing the impact of context effects on the results.

The methods that have been used to collect data on utilities include the standard gamble approach, the time trade-off approach, rating scales, and the willingness-to-pay approach. Collecting information on health utilities, and which is best, is beyond the scope of this little book.

## Cost minimization

If health effects are known to be equal, only costs are analysed and the least costly alternative is chosen. For instance, if we have two drugs for migraine, which are equally effective, but A costs £4 a tablet and B costs £8 a tablet, the obvious thing is to use A.

Not every patient might be able to manage with A, because A doesn't work for them, or because they have adverse events with A. In that case B might be better, even though it is more expensive. But this simple analysis suggests that a strategy of starting patients with A, and using B if A fails, will minimize costs for the maximum benefit.

Not all cost minimization analyses are that simple, but a surprising number are, and yet this technique is still often not used.

### Discounting

£1000 in your hand today is more valuable than £1000 in 10 years time. It will have less value because of inflation and because you have foregone the use of the £1000 in the intervening 10 years, either to use or to invest. If you had the £1000 now you may have put it into an interest-bearing account at 5%, say. If so, in 10 years time the £1000 would have grown to about £1600. In other words, had you waited 10 years for £1000, it would be worth only about £610 when you received it.

In health economics, if benefits are delayed or deferred to some future date, then you have to discount their future value. The effects of discounting are obviously related to a discounting rate. To halve the value of a future benefit takes about 70 years at a 1% discounting rate, 24 years at 3%, 14 years at 5%, and 8 years at 10%. The discounting rate chosen is therefore rather important. There is ongoing debate as to whether health outcomes as well as costs should be discounted, and whether rates should be constant or variable [2].

### References

1. Alonso, J. et al. (2004). Health-related quality of life associated with chronic conditions in eight countries: results from the International Quality of Life Assessment (IQOLA) Project. *Quality of Life Research* **13**, 283–98.
2. Severens, J.L. and Milne, R.J. (2004). Discounting health outcomes in economic evaluation: the ongoing debate. *Value in Health* **7**, 397–401.

# 6.3 Reflections on quality of health economic studies

There are difficulties for any of us in both understanding a health economic study and knowing how good it is. Quality criteria and scoring systems are being developed and tested, but it is first worth looking at a study from Australia [1] detailing problems with economic evaluations.

The study was based on 326 major applications to the Australian Pharmaceutical Benefits Scheme between 1994 and 1997. Pharmaceutical companies submit information used to determine reimbursement issues. The applications are reviewed in detail, including checking literature, and rerunning searches, validating key assumptions then, and checking computer or other models. A technical subcommittee then reviews the submission and makes a final recommendation to the federal health minister. Problems with submissions were regarded as significant if both the evaluators and the technical subcommittee considered that the problem could have a serious bearing on the decisions made.

Most applications involved new drugs, or major changes to indication, conditions of use, or price. Of the 326 submissions, 279 (86%) were economic analyses based on randomized trials, with 238 (73%) containing direct comparisons of a new agent and a chosen comparator. Indirect comparisons with a common comparator were used in 41 (13%). Twenty-six (8%) were based on quasi-experimental designs and 21 (6%) were based on uncontrolled data (Table 6.3.1). Meta-analyses were used in 64 of the submissions.

Serious problems of interpretation were found in 218 (67%) submissions, and 31 had more than one problem, giving 249 serious problems in total. The main problems in these 218 submissions are shown in Table 6.3.2.

Examples of problems encountered included:
- no randomized trials;
- identification of additional trials contradicting claims;
- trials of poor quality;
- trials too small;
- trials too short;
- trials not appropriate for indication;
- inappropriate subgroup analysis;
- surrogate rather than actual outcomes;

**Table 6.3.1**  Types of studies used in economic evaluations

| Design | Number | % |
|---|---|---|
| RCT direct comparison | 238 | 73 |
| RCT indirect comparison | 41 | 13 |
| Quasi-experimental | 26 | 8 |
| Uncontrolled | 21 | 6 |
| Total | 326 | 100 |

**Table 6.3.2** Types of problem found in the 218 submissions that had problems

| Problem | Submissions | Details | Per cent |
|---------|-------------|---------|----------|
| Trial efficacy issues | 154 | Availability of trials | 5 |
| | | Poor quality trials | 12 |
| | | Interpretation of results | 13 |
| | | Use of surrogate outcomes | 6 |
| | | Determining therapeutic equivalence | 26 |
| Comparator issues | 15 | Uncertainty about choice of comparator or inappropriate comparator | 6 |
| Modelling issues | 71 | Technical aspects of the model | 10 |
| | | Unsubstantiated assumptions | 6 |
| | | Uncertainty about costs | 13 |
| Calculation errors | 9 | Errors introducing serious inaccuracies in estimation of cost-effectiveness ratios | 4 |

- choice of comparator;
- economic models based on inadequate information;
- calculation errors.

None of these problems should be any surprise to readers of *Bandolier*, because they have featured regularly in its pages as problems in assessing evidence. That pharmaceutical companies in Australia failed to recognize these issues in 1994–97 should concern us for two reasons. The first is that most companies are now multinational and the second is that there was no improvement observed over the period of the study.

The authors are really quite gentle with the sponsors of the submissions, rightly identifying that pharmacoeconomic analysis is often a difficult and complex process. They do not believe the problems arose from any deliberate intent to deceive, but rather from a failure to take on board the requirements of quality evidence, process, and transparency.

## Judging quality in economic studies 1

We now have at least two similar but slightly different scoring systems. The most developed and tested is the Quality of Health Economic Studies (QHES) instrument [2]. This collected information from a large number of international health economists to estimate weights for a number of different criteria. Validation was achieved by having 60 individuals with health economics expertise who graded three cost-effectiveness studies. The exercise resulted in 16 criteria, scored individually with weights of 1 to 9 (Table 6.3.3). A study could have a maximum score of 100/100, and a minimum of 0/100.

The QHES scoring system has been applied to a number of studies in gastroenterology. It was first applied to 30 economic analyses in

**Table 6.3.3** QHES grading system for cost-effectiveness studies

| | Criterion | Points | Yes | No |
|---|---|---|---|---|
| 1 | Was the study objective presented in a clear, specific, and measurable manner? | 7 | | |
| 2 | Were the perspectives of the analysis (societal, third-party payer, etc.) and reasons for its selection stated? | 4 | | |
| 3 | Were variable estimates used in the analysis from the best available source (randomized controlled trial best, expert opinion worst)? | 8 | | |
| 4 | If estimates came from a subgroup analysis, were the groups pre-specified at the beginning of the study? | 1 | | |
| 5 | Was uncertainty handled by statistical analysis to address random events, or sensitivity analysis to cover a range of assumptions? | 9 | | |
| 6 | Was incremental analysis performed between alternates for resources and costs? | 6 | | |
| 7 | Was the methodology for data abstraction (including the value of health states and other benefits) stated? | 5 | | |
| 8 | Did the analytic horizon allow time for all relevant and important outcomes? Were benefits and costs that went beyond 1 year discounted (3% to 5%) and justification given for the discount rate? | 7 | | |
| 9 | Was the measurement of costs appropriate and the methodology for the estimation of quantities and unit costs clearly described? | 8 | | |
| 10 | Were the primary outcome measures for the economic evaluation clearly stated and did they include the major short-term, long-term, and negative outcomes? | 6 | | |
| 11 | Were the health outcomes measures/scales valid and reliable? If previously tested and valid and reliable measures were not available, was justification given for the measures/scales used? | 7 | | |
| 12 | Were the economic model (including structure), study methods and analysis, and the components of the numerator and denominator displayed in a clear transparent manner? | 8 | | |
| 13 | Were the choice of economic model, main assumptions, and limitations of the study stated and justified? | 7 | | |
| 14 | Did the authors explicitly discuss direction and magnitude of potential biases? | 6 | | |

**Table 6.3.3**    (contd.)

|  | Criterion | Points | Yes | No |
|---|---|---|---|---|
| 15 | Were the conclusions/recommendations of the study justified and based on study results? | 8 | | |
| 16 | Was there a statement disclosing the source of funding for the study? | 3 | | |
| **Total points** | | 100 | | |

gastro-oesophageal reflux disease [3]. Most studies scored between 50 and 74 points (Figure 6.3.1). Most studies used appropriate cost and health outcome measures according to the authors of the analysis, though this could be questioned because the scoring system lacks rigour in its approach to health outcomes evidence. Very few studies stated their perspective, or reasons for the selection of any particular perspective. Most did not perform an incremental analysis.

A second analysis in gastroenterology was much wider and more ambitious in its approach [4]. English-language health economic studies published between January 1980 and January 2004 were sought in the area of digestive diseases. Studies were identified from journals with an impact factor above 1, using an electronic search strategy. The aim was to assess the studies for quality, and to assess factors predicting high quality. Quality was assessed using the QHES instrument.

Of the 186 health economic studies found, 29% were scored as high quality and 52% as fair quality (Figure 6.3.2). Quality scores were higher in more recently published papers (Figure 6.3.3). The following questions had positive scores only infrequently.

• Question 2. Were the perspectives of the analysis (societal, third-party payer) and reasons for its selection stated? This was mentioned in only 17% of studies.

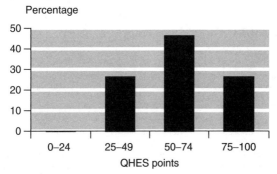

**Figure 6.3.1**    QHES scores of 30 economic analyses in reflux disease.

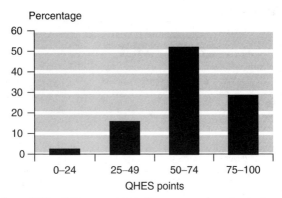

**Figure 6.3.2**  QHES scoring of 186 health economic studies in digestive diseases.

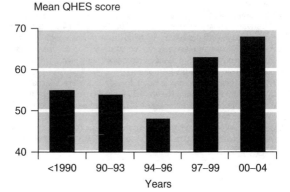

**Figure 6.3.3**  Mean QHES scores over years 1990 to 2004.

- Question 7. Was the methodology for data abstraction (including the value of health states and other benefits) stated? This was mentioned in only 26% of studies.
- Question 14. Did the authors explicitly discuss direction and magnitude of potential biases? This was mentioned in only 29% of studies.

The review also sought factors predicting high quality, and concluded that these were authors having advanced training in health services, studies using decision-analysis software package (against not using one), studies receiving federal funding, and studies citing guidelines for health economic studies in the reference list.

### Judging quality in economic studies 2

More recently a second scoring system, the Consensus on Health Economic Criteria (CHEC), was developed by talking to expert health economists [5]. This one has 19 criteria, and is similar to QHES although it does not yet have points, but rather a yes/no response for each of the criteria. At the time of writing, no evaluations of health economic analyses using this have been found, but it is included (Table 6.3.4) because it is a useful guide to health economic study quality, for readers of studies, and writers of them (as for CONSORT, QUOROM, etc.).

**Table 6.3.4**    CHEC-list scoring system

|   | CHEC-list | Yes | No |
|---|---|---|---|
| 1 | Is the study population clearly described? | | |
| 2 | Are competing alternatives clearly described? | | |
| 3 | Is a well-defined research question posed in answerable form? | | |
| 4 | Is the economic study design appropriate to the stated objective? | | |
| 5 | Is the chosen time horizon appropriate in order to include relevant costs and consequences? | | |
| 6 | Is the actual perspective chosen appropriate? | | |
| 7 | Are all appropriate and relevant costs for each alternative identified? | | |
| 8 | Are all costs measured appropriately in physical units? | | |
| 9 | Are costs valued appropriately? | | |
| 10 | Are all important and relevant outcomes for each alternative identified? | | |
| 11 | Are all outcomes measured appropriately? | | |
| 12 | Are outcomes valued appropriately? | | |
| 13 | Is an incremental analysis of costs and outcomes of alternatives performed? | | |
| 14 | Are all future costs and outcomes discounted appropriately? | | |
| 15 | Are all important variables, whose values are uncertain, appropriately subjected to sensitivity analysis? | | |
| 16 | Do the conclusions follow from the data reported? | | |
| 17 | Does the study discuss the generalizability of the results to other settings and patient groups? | | |
| 18 | Does the article indicate that there is no potential conflict of interest of study researchers and funders? | | |
| 19 | Are ethical and distributional issues discussed appropriately? | | |

## Commentary

Having quality scoring systems is clearly good stuff, and it is good to know that health economic analyses are getting better with time (Figure 6.3.3). Not everything is as rosy as it could be, though.

Health economics is essentially a product both of health outcomes, and of costs. Whatever the structure of the study, these are the two critical components. The two scoring systems, and many health economic evaluations, are strong on costs, if a little weaker on other aspects, like perspective. They are not strong on health outcomes evidence. There may be comments about using information from randomized trials, but awareness about evidence and knowledge about pitfalls of evidence are just not strong enough to give us confidence. Consumers of health economics studies, and that means decision-makers and policy-makers, have to wake up to the fact that they have to be critical, and know that any health economic study, however technically competent, is only as good as the health outcome evidence it uses. If that is flawed, the study is useless, however many points it scores.

## References

1. Hill, S.R. *et al.* (2000). Problems with the interpretation of pharmacoeconomic analyses. A review of submissions to the Australian Pharmaceutical Benefits Scheme. *Journal of the American Medical Association* **283**, 2116–21.
2. Chiou, C.F. *et al.* (2003). Development and validation of a grading system for the quality of cost-effectiveness studies. *Medical Care* **41**, 32–44.
3. Offman, J.F. *et al.* (2003). Examining the value and quality of health economic analyses: implications of utilizing the QHES. *Journal of Managed Care Pharmacy* **9**, 53–61.
4. Spiegel, B.R. *et al.* (2004). The quality of published health economic analyses in digestive diseases: a systematic review and quantitative appraisal. *Gastroenterology* **127**, 403–11.
5. Evers, S. *et al.* (2005). Criteria list for assessment of methodological quality of economic evaluations: Consensus on Health Economic Criteria. *International Journal of Technology Assessment in Health Care* **21**, 240–5.

# 6.4 Guidelines

Guidelines are important, and are proliferating. They can be individual, local, regional, or national, and often many variants of the same guidelines exist at the same time. Guidelines should be updated regularly. Most importantly, they should be based on the best available evidence. The evidence is that many, perhaps most, are not.

On the face of it guidelines seem like a good idea because they should condense all the best knowledge and experience to give individual practitioners the confidence that, within limits, they can aspire to the same level of practice as the best in their field.

### Variability of guidelines

Not all guidelines are created equal and there are examples of great variability between the advice of guidelines. One revelation from Newcastle concerned guidelines for anticoagulation for atrial fibrillation in the UK [1]. In 1996 various people and organizations in England, Wales, and Scotland were contacted about the existence of guidelines for anticoagulant treatment of atrial fibrillation. These included regional and national NHS bodies, professional and charitable institutions, and members of mailing lists of audit organizations. They represented purchasers and providers of health-care and relevant national organizations.

Guidelines were defined as documents produced to help clinicians decide which patients should be given anticoagulant drugs. Drafts, or documents designed for single specialized units, or to provide guidance once warfarin treatment had begun were not included. Where possible, guideline developers were interviewed using a semistructured method about how guidelines had been developed. All included guidelines were applied to the same 100 consecutive patients with atrial fibrillation aged 65 years or older identified in a community survey. Details of risk factors for stroke or contraindications for treatment were obtained.

The overall response rate was 66% (350/534), yielding 48 documents of which 20 fulfilled the requirements for definition of a guideline. They varied from a single page to 28 pages, were primarily for use by general practitioners, and affected populations from 12,000 to 500,000.

Guidelines were not systematically developed. A group of people developed about half of them, and the other half were developed by a single individual. About half had some outside consultation, but about a quarter had no external review. Distribution was haphazard and few had educational meetings to introduce the guideline. Only one was explicitly claimed to be evidence-based, and had outside consultations from a health economist and clinician, with external review and local consultation, with wide distribution, and an educational meeting to introduce the guideline.

When applied to 100 consecutive patients, the number recommended for anticoagulation by the guidelines ranged from 13 to 100 (Figure 6.4.1). Only one patient would have had anticoagulant treatment recommended by all of the guidelines, but every patient would have been recommended for anticoagulation by at least two guidelines (but not the same two). Target INR values varied between 1.2 to 1.5 and 2.5 to 3.0.

Number of patients with AF recommended for anticoagulant

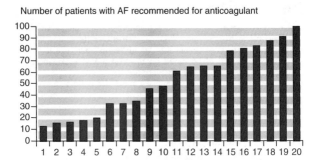

Individual guideline

**Figure 6.4.1** 20 evidence-based anticoagulation guidelines in the UK applied to the same 100 consecutive patients.

### Evidence base of guidelines

Another examination of the evidence base of guidelines comes from Greece [2]. Researchers looked for guidelines published in 1979, 1984, 1989, 1994, and 1999 in six prestigious English language journals (*Annals of Internal Medicine, British Medical Journal, Journal of the American Medical Association, New England Journal of Medicine, Lancet,* and *Pediatrics*). The definition of what constituted a guideline was specific and included all articles containing the words guideline or recommendation or other characteristic words in the title or abstract, and which had a main focus on prevention or therapeutic interventions.

For each guideline, the reference lists were scrutinized and articles were characterized as a randomized trial, systematic review, meta-analysis, or none of these. All cited articles were found in MEDLINE and full records and abstracts were scrutinized. The full paper was retrieved and read in the case of any uncertainty about whether it was a randomized trial. This also applied to articles published before 1966.

Where guidelines had references, contained fewer than two citations of randomized trials, and cited no systematic reviews, a full MEDLINE search was performed up to the year of publication of the guideline.

There were 191 guidelines identified in these six journals for the years searched, predominantly from the USA (86%). Group authorship was most common (84%). Of the 191 guidelines only 12 (6%) had performed a systematic review, but 130 (68%) made no mention about a lack of evidence. Thirty-six guidelines (19%) had no references.

Randomized trials made up a minority of the citations (Table 6.4.1). Only 8% of the citations were randomized trials, and fewer than 1% were systematic reviews or meta-analyses of randomized trials or epidemiological studies. The proportion of guidelines not citing any randomized trials fell from 95% in 1979 to 53% in 1999 (Figure 6.4.2). Only about one guideline in 10 cited a systematic review or meta-analysis.

**Table 6.4.1** Citations in 191 guidelines in six prestigious medical journals

| Type of publication cited | Number | Per cent of total citations | Mean citations per guideline |
|---|---|---|---|
| Total from 191 guidelines | 4853 | 100 | 25.4 |
| Randomized trial | 393 | 8.1 | 2.1 |
| Systematic review | 19 | 0.4 | 0.1 |
| Meta-analysis of randomized trials | 23 | 0.5 | 0.1 |
| Meta-analysis of epidemiological studies | 11 | 0.2 | 0.1 |
| Books/pamphlet/brochure | 719 | 14.8 | 3.8 |
| Abstract | 122 | 2.5 | 0.6 |

Thirty-nine guidelines had fewer than two randomized citations with no systematic review. Because 30 were in paediatrics, 10 of these were chosen at random, and 19 in all were the subject of specific searches. In 12 of the 19, additional relevant randomized trials were found. The number of additional randomized trials was 1 to 194 per topic.

#### How to make guidelines work

There is increasing awareness that guidelines have to be produced in relation to both the evidence available and what patients think. We have a good example of this [3]. Briefly, a number of extensive literature searches were performed to generate information on:

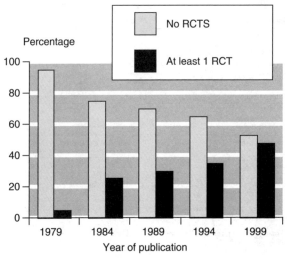

**Figure 6.4.2** Evidence from RCTs in guidelines.

- effectiveness of anticoagulation and antiplatelet therapy;
- absolute risk of stroke and stroke outcomes in atrial fibrillation;
- risk of adverse effects in patients treated with anticoagulants;
- utility values of health states associated with anticoagulation;
- costs of outcomes.

A decision model used a hypothetical cohort of patients, with patients able to move from one state to another—as, for instance, if a patient had a major stroke, or bled, or died. Information on this was obtained from the systematic reviews. The model was run for 1512 combinations of age, sex, blood pressure, and risk factors, and assessed in terms of quality-adjusted life-years (QALYs) and costs. A guideline development group that included various medical specialties met to define the scope and to develop specific questions for review and modelling and advise on the guideline produced.

Because of the lack of published information, health utilities were determined by interviews with 57 patients representative of those in clinical practice, if a little younger than average. Low health utility was given to major stroke, and moderate utilities to minor strokes and bleeds (Table 6.4.2). Table 6.4.2 shows the mean, median, and modes on scales of 0 (immediate death) to 1 (normal health).

There were four distinct outcomes from the decision model, and these are shown in Table 6.4.3, together with the decision made on the basis of each outcome.

In most cases treatment led to lower costs. In only 12 of the 1512 cases modelled was there a reduced cost per QALY. Results for 12 age and sex

**Table 6.4.2** Health utility values associated with anticoagulation

| Health state | Utility value | | |
|---|---|---|---|
| | Mean | Median | Mode |
| On warfarin with GP | 0.95 | 0.99 | 1.00 |
| On warfarin with outpatients | 0.94 | 0.98 | 1.00 |
| Major bleed | 0.84 | 0.88 | 1.00 |
| Mild stroke | 0.64 | 0.68 | 0.63 |
| Major stroke | 0.19 | 0.00 | 0.00 |

**Table 6.4.3** Model outcomes and clinical decisions

| Model outcome | Clinical decision |
|---|---|
| Treatment produces QALY gains and cost savings | Definitely treat |
| Treatment produces QALY losses and higher costs | Definitely do not treat |
| Treatment produces higher QALYs but with higher costs | Treat if cost per QALY is acceptable |
| Treatment produces QALY losses at lower costs | Definitely do not treat |

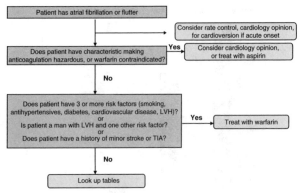

**Figure 6.4.3** Treatment algorithm.

groups were tabulated using the classification in Table 6.4.3, and these are available in the original paper as simple look-up figures.

A treatment algorithm was produced for certain clear-cut cases, and with treatment decisions for patients not fulfilling these clear-cut definitions based on the look-up tables. The algorithm is shown in Figure 6.4.3.

In a consecutive community sample of 207 patients with atrial fibrillation, 116 (56%) had no contraindications to treatment. There were 46 women, 13 aged between 65 and 74 years and 33 aged 75 years or older. There were 70 men, 19 aged between 65 and 74 years and 51 aged 75 years or older.

The proportion of patients above predefined risk threshold and recommended for treatment with warfarin was almost 100% in each group when the utility of warfarin was 1.0. When it fell to 0.92, the proportion dropped dramatically (Figures 6.4.4 and 6.4.5).

## Commentary

The Greek review [2] interestingly looked at parameters associated with citing randomized evidence in guidelines. Guidelines funded by government and professional bodies were worse (cited fewer RCTs and systematic reviews) than those with university and private (usually pharmaceutical) sources of funds. The lesson is that we should not take any guideline on trust, without a sceptical examination of how it has been arrived at, and whether it has followed good practice for guideline development. Because this is a fast-moving area, with acceptance of the use of evidence now much greater than in the period of the study, it is highly likely that guideline development is getting better, though not all may be so. Guidelines still need to be looked at with a degree of scepticism, and bearing in mind that not all patients are the same.

We have an important piece of work about how guidelines can and should be developed [3], especially when contrasted with the way in which anticoagulation guidelines were developed previously. What this shows is

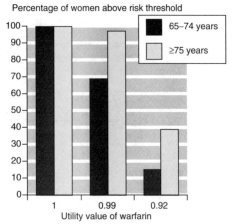

**Figure 6.4.4** Proportion of women above the risk threshold for warfarin treatment for different utility values.

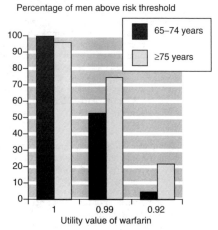

**Figure 6.4.5** Proportion of men above the risk threshold for warfarin treatment for different utility values.

that anticoagulation treatment may be applied successfully to almost all patients, but that that conclusion is exquisitely sensitive to how individual patients see the impact of warfarin therapy on their lives. It re-emphasizes, if that were necessary, that the choices of individuals are extremely important in making decisions about prophylaxis.

We do know that guideline implementation strategy is an associated difficult area [4]. A systematic review of implementation strategies concluded that there was an imperfect evidence base [4]. There is little evidence that the strategies make much difference in and of themselves.

## References

1. Thomson, R. *et al.* (1998). Guidelines on anticoagulant treatment for atrial fibrillation in Great Britain: variation in content and implications for treatment. *British Medical Journal* **316**, 509–13.
2. Giannakakis, I.A. *et al.* (2002). Citation of randomised evidence in support of guidelines of therapeutic and preventive interventions. *Journal of Clinical Epidemiology* **55**, 545–55.
3. Thomson, R. *et al.* (2000). Decision analysis and guidelines for anticoagulation therapy to prevent stroke in patients with atrial fibrillation. *Lancet* **355**, 956–62.
4. Grimshaw, J.M. *et al.* (2004). Effectiveness and efficiency of guideline dissemination and implementation strategies. *Health Technology Assessment* **8**, 6.

# 6.5   Care pathways

We hear a lot about guidelines, which are supposed to ensure that the right patient gets the right treatment. This is a rather glib statement, but is underpinned by some interesting ideas, including:

- diagnosis: treating the right patient;
- treatment: treating the right patient right;
- organization: treating the right patient right at the right time;
- pathway: treating the right patient right at the right time and in the right way.

Guidelines are supposed to cover this, but they mostly cover just the first two steps. There is more to delivering good care than that. It requires good organization—what one might call management, except that many of us now see that word as meaning anything but organization. And it requires that we perform actions in ways that are known to deliver good quality care.

A care pathway is analogous to a manufacturing guide in industry. There may be many different ways of assembling a television or car, but each one is assembled in the same way on a production line, because that is the best and cheapest way of doing so, for a product that works and that the customer wants.

Care pathways, or treatment protocols, should be the quality-assessed and evidence-based way of consistently delivering high-quality care for a particular circumstance. This section will examine the evidence that they do, and see if there are any lessons to be learned about how to prepare a care pathway.

### Care pathways/treatment protocols

The unique biology of individual patients, with their special circumstances, drives diagnosis and treatment. Yet individuals are often sufficiently similar one to another to make a treatment protocol based on evidence seem worthwhile. Even if it simply ensures that nothing important is missed, it should reduce error and might improve results. To that end treatment protocols, or clinical pathways, critical pathways, or care paths have been developed and are used.

Do they deliver? This is not just being precious about evidence, but has real importance. Treatment protocols often require more front-end resources. Where the biggest constraint is one of capacity, as is the case in the NHS right now, we need to know that professionals' time is likely to be used to the best advantage.

Treatment protocols are often used in hospital, where the advantage might be reduced length of stay. Where beds are restricted or waiting times long, greater throughput could be a major efficiency benefit.

Looking for evidence from randomized trials that care pathways or treatment protocols deliver the goods is not easy, but we searched PubMed using a variety of free-text terms, and scanned reference lists and reviews. What follows is not an exhaustive systematic review, but the papers we found. There are a number of examples, in different situations with different goals and outcomes, all in secondary care. For each we give a brief outline of the method and results.

### Hip and knee replacement [1]

This study in Australia randomized patients admitted for standard hip or knee replacement to:

- standard reactive treatment, where the treating team responded to the will and condition of the patient in providing postoperative care;
- proactive treatment in a care pathway, where specific goals were set each day for the patient and treating team, using a special written protocol listing milestones to be achieved, tests ordered, and daily tasks for patient and team members.

The main outcome was length of stay, but others collected included complications (wound infection, chest infection, deep vein thrombosis, for instance) and readmission rates.

The 92 patients randomized to the pathway and 71 to control were similar in age, weight, and co-morbid conditions. Those treated in the pathway sat out of bed and were ambulant earlier, and were discharged after 7.1 rather than 8.6 days (Figure 6.5.1). There were fewer complications, and the proportion readmitted within 3 months was 4% for the pathway, against 13% for controls.

Reduced length of stay did not increase the complication rate. There might have been a concern, perhaps, about whether the patients were having too little time in hospital resulting in more complications and higher readmissions later on. Readmissions did not increase, but fell. No costs or resource allocation are given in the paper, but there is no indication that this care pathway would cost more to provide better quality of care.

### Fractured neck of femur [2]

Another Australian study randomized (by date of birth) patients with uncomplicated fractured neck of femur to usual care or to a clinical pathway. The main components of this pathway included an admission information checklist, specific pathway documentation specifying responsibilities and timing, with a discharge package, and with discharge planning begun on admission.

The 55 patients randomized to the pathway and the 56 randomized to control were similar in age and weight. Those treated in the pathway had earlier mobilization, and were discharged after 6.6 rather than 8.0 days. There were no more in-hospital complications (24% versus 26%), and the proportion readmitted within 1 month was 4% for the pathway, against 11% for controls, though these last two were not statistically different.

This was a small study in a unit already operating with an on-site rehabilitation unit and quite short background length of stay. Patients included those who, on admission, were confused (40%), had a co-morbid condition (33%), or who did not speak English (26%), so that the population studied was not overselected. Their mean age was 83 years.

### Inpatient asthma management [3]

In this study from Johns Hopkins, a paediatric multidisciplinary team combined to create the care pathway plus a weaning protocol, designed for asthma patients between 2 and 18 years of age. Patients being admitted with a primary diagnosis of asthma exacerbation were randomized to a bed on the intervention unit (in which staff had been trained in the pathway) or a control unit in which they received standard care.

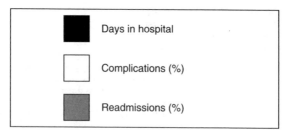

Days, or per cent

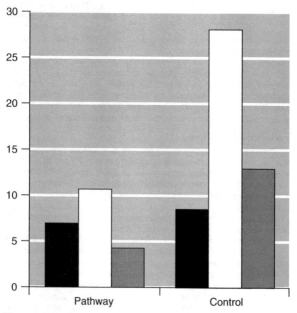

**Figure 6.5.1** Outcomes in knee and hip replacement.

There were 55 patients treated using the clinical pathway, and 55 usual care controls. Patients were similar apart from clinical path children being slightly older. The duration of hospital stay was significantly shorter using the clinical pathway (40 versus 54 hours, Figure 6.5.2) with a larger percentage discharged in the first day (38% versus 15%). The pathway also resulted in less use of beta-agonists. The average cost was almost US $1000 per patient lower for patients in the clinical pathway.

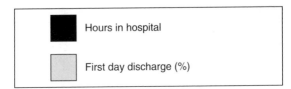

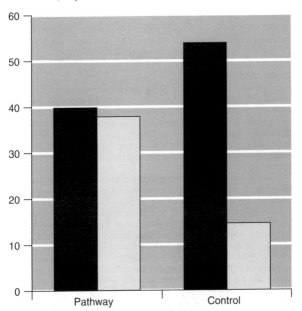

**Figure 6.5.2** Outcomes in asthma management in children.

A particularly detailed and interesting paper, this. It shows shorter stay, better outcomes, and lower cost. One problem was that only a quarter of eligible patients could be enrolled in the study because of bed shortages.

### Community-acquired pneumonia [4]

A critical pathway for treating patients with community-acquired pneumonia had three main components: use of a clinical prediction rule to assist admission decisions, treatment with levofloxacin (a fluoroquinolone antibiotic with good oral bioavailability and broad antimicrobial activity), and practice guidelines for care of inpatients. Nineteen hospitals were randomized to continue conventional management or implement the critical pathway.

Over 6 months 1743 patients were evaluated. Hospitals using the critical pathway had an 18% reduction in the admission of low-risk patients (only 31% of patients in the pathway were low risk compared with 49% of admissions in the comparison period). Those treated in hospitals using the pathway spent 1.7 fewer days in hospital (5.0 versus 6.7 days), despite having more patients with moderate or severe disease at admission. Patients at hospitals implementing the pathway were also much more likely to be treated with a single antibiotic (64% versus 27%). There was no difference in the rate of adverse clinical outcomes (intensive care admission, mortality, readmission, complication) or quality of life indicators.

Combining the lower admission rate and reduced hospital stay, this care pathway resulted in a reduced cost of treating each case of US $1700. This was with no reduction in quality of care or clinical outcomes.

## Stroke rehabilitation [5]

An integrated care pathway for stroke patients based on evidence of best practice and professional standards was developed and coordinated by an experienced nurse in London. Eligible patients were those with persistent impairment within 2 weeks of the event. Exclusions were those with severe premorbid conditions or cognitive disability, or who had only mild deficits not needing rehabilitation. The stroke rehabilitation unit had two independent teams of carers, and the care pathway was introduced in one of them.

There were 76 patients in each group, with a mean age of 75 years and no difference at baseline. There was no difference between the groups in outcomes, length of stay, institutional admission, or mortality.

This negative result could, of course, be due to the fact that care was already so good that it could not be bettered. The average length of stay was about 50 days, but the standard deviation was a huge 20 days, indicating the large variations between patients. Issues other than those in the study may have influenced this, and there could have been cross-over between the two teams. Whatever the reason, the additional cost of a coordinating nurse made the pathway more expensive at no benefit.

## Use of laboratory tests [6]

Prospective randomized studies of patients undergoing elective surgery or acute medical admissions using clinical pathways were examined for use of laboratory tests in this Australian study.

In the elective surgery study of 224 patients, use of laboratory tests was reduced by about 70% using the care pathway (1 versus 3 tests per patient for hernias; 3 versus 7 tests per patient for cholecystectomy). For acute medical admissions, there were 12 versus 16 tests per patient using the care pathway. These were mainly haematology and clinical chemistry tests. Estimated cost reductions were of the order of A$68 (£26) per patient.

There was no suggestion that patient care was in any way impaired by this reduction in laboratory testing. As laboratory tests have often been shown to be over-used, this outcome is a beneficial effect from using a care pathway.

### Heart failure [7]

This randomized study from Johns Hopkins concerned patients at high risk of coronary heart failure readmission. This was defined by the presence of one or more of a rather long list that included age over 70 years, low left ventricular ejection fraction, and at least one admission for heart failure in the previous year. An intervention team involved a telephone nurse coordinator, a heart failure nurse, a heart failure cardiologist, and the patient's primary physician.

The cardiologist designed and documented a treatment plan for all study patients before randomization and saw patients at baseline and after 6 months. The primary care physician delivered the interventions and looked after all non-heart failure problems. The heart failure nurse visited patients on a monthly basis, and the telephone coordinator also kept in contact. In the usual care control group the cardiologist's plan was documented without further intervention.

Two hundred patients were enrolled, and the two groups were similar at baseline. There were fewer heart failure hospital admissions or deaths over 6 months using the care pathway (49% versus 73%; Figure 6.5.3). Patients in the care pathway group were more likely to hit targets of treatment (weight, diet, vasodilators), and have stable or improved symptoms. Inpatient and outpatient resource use had similar costs, though the care pathway group tended to have lower costs and shorter lengths of stay. For every 10 patients treated in the care pathway, one fewer would have died or had a hospital admission for heart failure compared with usual care. Better quality was delivered at the same cost.

### Community-acquired lower respiratory tract infection (LRTI) [8]

The study was conducted in the medical wards of a single hospital in Antrim. All adult patients admitted with a primary diagnosis of LRTI during December 1994 to February 1995 formed the control group. Diagnoses were made on clinical grounds supplemented with X-rays in most cases. Patients received empirical treatment before development of a treatment protocol.

After development and institution of a treatment protocol in November 1995, all patients admitted with a primary diagnosis of LRTI from December 1995 to February 1996 formed the intervention group. The treatment protocol consisted of measuring the severity of the condition according to age more than 60 years, respiratory rate above 30 breaths/minute, diastolic blood pressure below 60 mmHg, white cell count below 4 or above 20 billion cells/L, new confusion, new atrial fibrillation, and multiple lobe involvement on X-ray. One point was given for the presence of each of these, and treatment instituted depending on severity:

- moderate (score 2 or less): oral amoxycillin/clavulanic acid every 8 hours;
- severe (score 3 or more): intravenous cefuroxime every 8 hours;
- very severe (score 3 or more and $pO_2$ less than 8 kPa on 28% oxygen): intravenous cefuroxime every 8 hours and intravenous erythromycin every 6 hours.

Protocol development was with the involvement and support of all consultant physicians. Introduction involved presentations, seminars, and ward

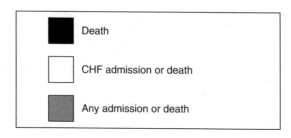

Per cent

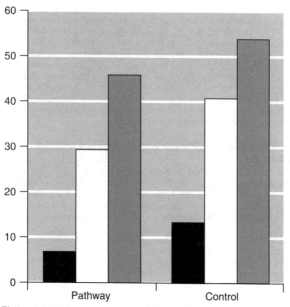

**Figure 6.5.3**  Outcomes in heart failure management in the community.

discussions; involvement of new junior medical staff; distribution of written summaries of the protocol; posting the algorithm in all wards; and encouragement of implementation by clinical pharmacists. Details of patients and outcomes were collected on a customized data collection form. Treatment success was a major improvement or complete resolution of all signs and symptoms. Treatment failure was persistence or progression of signs and symptoms, or development of new clinical findings, or death from the

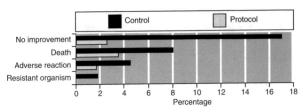

**Figure 6.5.4** Results in Antrim before and after protocol for LRTI.

primary diagnosis, or discontinuation of medicines because of adverse reaction.

There were 112 patients in the control group, and 115 in the treatment protocol group. Their mean age was about 68 years, with a mean onset of about 5 days at admission. Two-thirds were moderate and one-third severe on admission. There were no differences between the groups, and no patient was very severe on admission. Most patients (99%) had an X-ray. The only significant difference in laboratory testing was that 98% of patients on the protocol had a sputum cultured, while only 55% of controls had this test.

There were 35/112 treatment failures (31%) on control and 9 (8%) on the protocol. The outcomes and reasons for the failures are shown in Figure 6.5.4. Protocol was better than control for every outcome or reason for failure. For every four patients on the protocol there was one fewer treatment failure than if the protocol had not been used (NNT 4.3; 95% CI, 3.0–7.4).

Control patients had a mean length of stay of 9.2 days. Those on the protocol had a mean length of stay of only 4.5 days. The overall average cost per patient was £2024 for controls but only £1020 for those on the protocol, a saving of £1000 per patient. Most savings came from lower bed costs and lower antimicrobial costs (£11 protocol versus £54 control).

Adopting a treatment protocol delivered better care at lower cost. Protocol construction and implementation was exemplary. This is a study worth reading, although individual hospitals may want to institute different regimens because of local differences.

### Emergency admission with pneumonia [9]

A similar study to that in Antrim had been conducted before in Pennsylvania. This retrospective time series study looked at three cohorts of patients admitted to an emergency department with community-acquired pneumonia, before and after the introduction of a critical pathway.

A multidisciplinary group established a pneumonia pathway detailing the recommended sequence of clinical actions and decisions from the time of arrival in the emergency department, and through hospital admission to discharge. It recognized the need for a standardized set of antibiotic regimens, depending on where the patient came from, and based on national US guidelines. A key feature of the pathway was early recognition, diagnosis, and prompt antibiotic treatment of pneumonia.

All patients admitted with pneumonia during a 3-month period immediately before the introduction of the pathway, over the period 10–12 months afterwards, and over the period 34–36 months afterwards formed the subjects in the survey. Each period was for 3 months, and the same inclusion criteria were applied. These were age 18 years or more, admission to emergency department with primary diagnosis of pneumonia and radiological evidence at time of admission, and a discharge diagnosis of pneumonia. Not included were patients with antibiotics administered before admission, with HIV infection, extensive stay in hospital because of another diagnosis, or repeat admission with the 3 month assessment period.

In the three periods 63, 96, and 122 patients, respectively, were admitted. The mean age of patients was in the mid-70s, about equally distributed between the sexes. Vital signs were similar between the three cohorts, as was the frequency with which symptoms were reported.

One of the process-of-care goals was to reduce the time to antibiotic administration in the emergency department. In the cohort admitted before pathway initiation, the mean time was 315 minutes and 58% of patients had antibiotic administered in the emergency department. The proportion administered antibiotics in the emergency department increased to over 90% in both post-initiation cohorts, with mean time to antibiotics down to 170 minutes.

The main gains were in mortality in hospital, which fell from 10 to 5% (Figure 6.5.5), and in length of stay, which fell from 10 to 6 days. The decline in mortality was not statistically significant, given the small number of deaths that actually occurred.

There are several interesting things about this paper. Unusually, it has assessed the effect of the care pathway not just in the period immediately after introduction, when effects might be expected to be greatest, but 1 and 3 years later. The findings were that, if anything, results continued to improve, showing that initial benefits can be maintained.

It sought rapid diagnosis and treatment using standardized antimicrobial therapy, treating the right patient right in the right way and at the right time. This not only improved the quality of care (fewer deaths), but must have reduced costs. Four fewer days in hospital is between £800 and £1000 less cost per patient, just as was seen in Antrim. There is more to it than that,

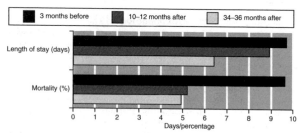

**Figure 6.5.5**  Effect of a clinical pathway for pneumonia on length of hospital stay and mortality.

though. Fewer days in hospital means less stress on a capacity constrained system. In reality, we should increase the cost savings to take account of this very important finding.

### Clinical pathway for bronchiolitis [10]

A multidisciplinary team generated this guideline for infants of 1 year or younger admitted with a first-time episode of typical bronchiolitis. The method of guideline development was described in detail, and included exact information from hospital data systems about children admitted with the condition and a systematic review of literature relating to the condition. A series of order sheets and scoring instruments were developed and subjected to peer and institutional review before being implemented.

The guideline was not formally made into a clinical pathway and, specifically, clinicians did not have to document when guideline goals were met or recommendations not followed.

Evaluation of the guideline was by a retrospective comparison of children admitted in the first 8 or 9 weeks after it had been implemented and children admitted in the same 8-week period over the 4 years before the guideline was introduced.

There were 1300 records for children admitted before implementation, and 229 admitted after implementation, of whom 181 had a guideline admission order. There were no differences between the two groups for a number of characteristics.

The main results of implementing the pathway were reduced length of stay (by an average of half a day) and reduction in overall cost (by US $400 or 37%). Use of beta-agonists was reduced, but not antibiotics, where use was high at 56%. A later report [11] extended the observations for 2 additional years, and confirmed the reduction in costs, especially bed occupancy and respiratory care. This guideline was so very close to being a clinical pathway that it is included in this section. It has been used as the basis of other pathways.

### Another clinical pathway for bronchiolitis [12]

Many children are admitted to hospital with bronchiolitis, and it is known that bacterial infection requiring antibiotics is a factor in only a very small proportion. Despite this, many children receive unnecessary antibiotics. This adds to costs, has the possibility of adverse reactions, and could serve to increase microbial resistance to antibiotics. Reducing this unnecessary antibiotic prescribing is thus a goal for a quality service.

The development of the clinical pathway is not well described, but its intent was to reduce inappropriate antibiotic use. It consisted of a detailed order set, inclusion and exclusion criteria, criteria for admission and discharge, and educational material on bronchiolitis and the specific goals of the pathway. Parent and family material was included, explicitly emphasizing the evidence that antibiotics are rarely indicated in this condition.

All patients admitted through one complete winter season after the introduction of the pathway formed the patient cohort. The review was by an involved investigator, and children on the pathway were matched to a group of children who met the inclusion criteria for pathway use but who were not managed on the pathway. Inclusion was viral respiratory infection with wheezing and respiratory distress in children over 4 weeks of age.

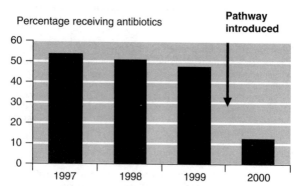

**Figure 6.5.6** Antibiotic prescribing for 3 years before and 1 year after pathway introduction.

Matching was done on the basis of age, disease severity, and socioeconomic status.

There were 96 children treated on the pathway and 85 not treated on the pathway. The two groups were indistinguishable in terms of severity indices. Antibiotics were used in just 9% of children on the pathway, compared with 27% off the pathway. Length of stay was half a day shorter on average on the pathway, and average cost was reduced by US $1000 (from $3200 to $2200). There was no increase in unplanned admission after discharge on the pathway.

For the 3 years before the implementation of the clinical pathway, antibiotic use occurred in about half of children with the condition. In the year after implementation this fell to 13% (Figure 6.5.6).

This may not be the very best of study architectures, and we do not know why some children were treated on the pathway and others off it. Though the two groups of children appeared to have very similar characteristics, the non-random approach may have led to the introduction of some biases.

### Clinical care pathway for colon resection [13]

Here we have a straightforward before and after study. The intervention was a care pathway for patients undergoing colon resection. It involved at-home bowel preparation before admission, preoperative patient education about length of stay and return of bowel function, standardized anaesthetic, and, to some extent, surgery, and standardized postoperative care, discharge, and post-discharge education for patients.

One strength of this study was that it involved all patients undergoing this surgery with a single surgeon at one hospital, from start of practice. It was therefore comprehensive, and the comparison was between patients operated on before the new pathway and those operated on after the care pathway was initiated.

Length of stay (days)

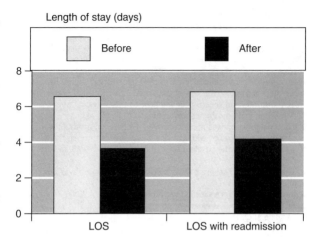

**Figure 6.5.7** Length of stay (LOS) for colon resection before and after care pathway introduction.

There were 138 patients, 52 before and 86 after pathway initiation. The two groups were broadly similar, though the after group patients were somewhat younger, at 62 years, than the before pathway group, with an average age of 69 years.

The length of hospital stay was reduced from an average of 7 days before the pathway to 3.7 days after the pathway. There were somewhat more readmissions after the pathway (10% versus 2% before), but including this additional time in hospital made no difference to the average length of stay saved (Figure 6.5.7). There were fewer complications in patients treated on the pathway (12% versus 25% before).

Hospital costs fell with the new pathway. Before, these averaged US $8800, and afterwards $6500, an average saving for each patient of $2300. When the costs of readmissions were added, the before and after costs rose to $9300 and $7100, and the average saving was still $2200.

The implementation of a comprehensive care pathway resulted in no loss of quality of care. It was cheaper because patients spent less time in hospital. Of course, elective surgery lends itself to the use of care pathways, given that the environment in which it occurs is well managed, and not constantly assailed by the vagaries of bed crisis, blocking, or emergency surgery.

### Improving pain control after Caesarean section [14]

In Warwick, a baseline audit involving case note review and interviews with 30 mothers suggested that pain control after Caesarean section was not always satisfactory. Pain was not being routinely assessed and it limited function, stopping some mothers from feeding and bathing their babies.

This prompted the formulation of a local protocol for the management of post-Caesarean pain, with input from different professions. Key features of the protocol were the introduction of formal pain assessments, the use of pre-printed prescription labels to apply to drug charts, and the introduction of self-medication by mothers. The introduction of self-medication was supported by intensive one-on-one education and discussion for professionals, and a patient information leaflet. Reflecting a three-step approach, the leaflet explained how mothers should handle mild, moderate, and severe pain and how to seek advice if needed.

A re-audit in 31 mothers showed that:

- Maternal function was much improved. Only seven mothers were not caring for their babies with just one giving pain as the reason (the other six in SCBU). In the baseline audit, the numbers were 13 and 10, respectively.
- The incidence of severe pain at rest and on movement was down by about 30%.
- Mothers were more satisfied with their pain control. Over 40% (13/31) rated pain control as excellent compared with about 20% (7/30) in the baseline audit (Figure 6.5.8).

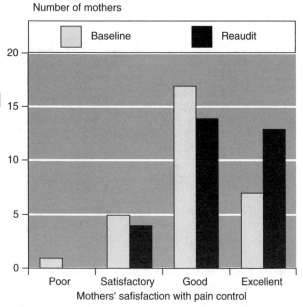

**Figure 6.5.8** Satisfaction of mothers with pain treatment in initial and subsequent audit.

The length of stay of mothers was not recorded in the baseline audit but subsequent examination of hospital records revealed an encouraging reduction of 1 day between the baseline and reaudit. Based on the hospital's average number of Caesarean sections (438 a year), the average reduction of 1 postoperative day suggests a saving of about £95, 000 per annum, or 438 bed-days. It could be argued that these savings are a direct consequence of the new protocol because there have been no other policy or operational changes in the care of mothers after Caesarean section.

What is interesting about the Warwick experience is that, although small, it demonstrates what can be achieved in even relatively small institutions by simple management techniques. Again, the result is better quality of care delivered at a lower cost.

### Treating the right patient right

All of the examples we have looked at so far have in common that patients entering the care pathways had well defined conditions. It was clear which were the right patients, and it was mainly the right treatments and their right organization being examined. Finding the right patients to treat is a somewhat different matter, and there are examples of where finding the right patient to give the right treatment is the key.

Two examples follow, both randomized trials, demonstrating the importance of giving the right treatment to the right patient, a defining issue for care pathways. One examines rehabilitation for back pain and the other treatments for acute migraine.

### Acute migraine attacks [15]

A number of strategies can be used to treat acute migraine attacks, each utilizing some part of the evidence base.

- For instance, the initial attack could be treated with aspirin or simple analgesic and, if or when that fails, a triptan could be used. That is a step strategy within an attack.
- A different approach may be to try aspirin or simple analgesic for a few attacks. It will work for some but, for those for whom it does not work, a triptan may be an alternative treatment. That is a step strategy across attacks, and is probably the strategy most likely to be used in the UK as it is probably seen as the cheapest.
- A third way would be to assess the individual patient for the severity of the disorder, and then to treat appropriately: mild disease might be treated with aspirin or simple analgesics, while more severe disease might be treated with a triptan. This would be stratified care.

It just so happens that a randomized controlled trial indicates that stratified care produces the best results.

The trial was randomized, but open-label, and examined multiple migraine attacks for patients with an established diagnosis of migraine according to International Headache Society criteria. Patients completed the MIDAS questionnaire [16], which measures lost time in three domains of activity. Patients were assigned a grade of disability from I (little or infrequent disability), grade II (mild or infrequent disability), grade III (moderate disability), to grade IV (severe disability). Patients with grade II–IV disability were included. Randomization was to:

1. stratified care. Grade II patients received aspirin 800 to 1000 mg plus metoclopramide 10 mg for all six attacks. Those with grade III or IV received zolmitriptan 2.5 mg.
2. step care across attacks. Patients treated the first three attacks with aspirin 800 to 1000 mg plus metoclopramide 10 mg. Those without adequate relief took zolmitriptan 2.5 mg for the next three attacks.
3. step care within attacks. Patients treated all attacks with aspirin 800 to 1000 mg plus metoclopramide 10 mg first. If adequate relief was not obtained by 2 hours, they then took zolmitriptan 2.5 mg.

In the three treatment groups, 1062 patients were randomized. Twenty per cent of patients withdrew or were lost for various reasons, mostly innocuous. Only 3% withdrew because of an adverse event, and 0.2% because of deteriorating condition. Groups were well balanced.

More patients had a 2-hour headache response with the stratified care strategy than with either step care strategy (Figure 6.5.9). More patients were pain-free at 2 hours with the stratified care strategy than with either step care strategy (Figure 6.5.10).

Adverse events were equally common in all three groups, and were predominantly mild and transient. Adverse event study withdrawals were evenly distributed across the groups.

Most guidelines would probably use a step up approach, similar to that of step up across attacks, but with many more steps. Because of the time involved and because of repeated failure of treatment, some patients simply become disenchanted and seek other forms of treatment. Treating the appropriate patient appropriately from the beginning is a better bet.

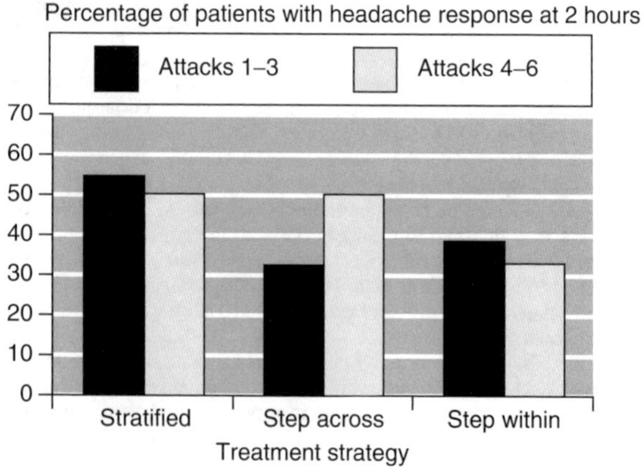

Percentage of patients with headache response at 2 hours

**Figure 6.5.9** Two-hour headache response for up to six migraine attacks with different treatment strategies.

Percentage of patients pain free at 2 hours

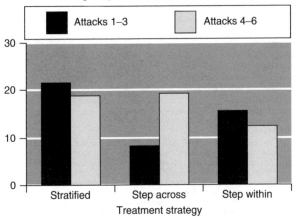

**Figure 6.5.10** Two-hour pain-free response for up to six migraine attacks with different treatment strategies.

It takes less time, is more effective, and is without the 'hassle factor' for patient and doctor. This is exactly what evidence-based medicine was supposed to be about, and reading the definition of EBM in the context of this trial is rewarding.

### Pulling it all together

Care pathways do not start from nowhere and nothing. It is not as if what we do usually is badly awry, and our experience in modern health-care systems is the opposite. These large, complex, organizations looking after millions of individual people do a simply marvellous job for most people most of the time.

While recognizing that, none of us could or would claim that everything is perfect. There is always room for improvement as our technology, experience, and support services improve. The issue is often not one of no change, but often one of too much change, but of the wrong sort.

In industry, care pathways would be called something else; it is a mix, perhaps, of good practice and quality control, plus a large helping of ongoing quality improvement. After all, care pathways involve not one action, but many, often in a complex package of care. In these complex packages, it is the combining of individual interventions in a management framework suited to local needs and abilities that is the critical factor.

Many of the examples cited here have things in common. They frequently:

- examine the external evidence for individual technologies;
- combine this with local knowledge and experience and conditions;

- involve a number of different disciplines of people in a team decision, and create ownership of the product;
- measure the results of the actions;
- have information systems feeding back to the team on a timely basis;
- amend the pathway in the light of results.

They also have in common that they usually deliver a better quality of care, and almost always manage to do this at lower cost. That is perhaps the single most important result—better quality at lower cost. This goal is exactly the one most sought after by commissioners and the folk who hold the purse strings. Of course, care pathways cannot and will not work in an environment of chaos, and they demand a certain basic structure that is reasonably constant. That may be obvious, but is still worth saying.

## References

1. Dowsey, M.M. *et al.* (1999). Clinical pathways in hip and knee arthroplasty: a prospective randomised controlled study. *Medical Journal of Australia* **170**, 59–62.
2. Choong, P.F. *et al.* (2000). Clinical pathway for fractured neck of femur: a prospective, controlled study. *Medical Journal of Australia* **172**, 423–7.
3. Johnson, K.B. *et al.* (2000). Effectiveness of a clinical pathway for inpatient asthma management. *Pediatrics* **106**, 1006–12.
4. Marrie, T.J. *et al.* (2000). A controlled trial of a critical pathway for treatment of community-acquired pneumonia. *Journal of the American Medical Association* **283**, 749–55.
5. Sulch, D. *et al.* (2000). Randomized controlled trial of integrated (managed) care pathway for stroke rehabilitation. *Stroke* **31**, 1929–34.
6. Board, N. *et al.* (2000). Use of pathology services in re-engineered clinical pathways. *Journal of Quality in Clinical Practice* **20**, 24–9.
7. Kasper, E.K. (2002). A randomized trial of the efficacy of multidisciplinary care in heart failure outpatients at high risk of hospital readmission. *Journal of the American College of Cardiology* **39**, 471–80.
8. Al-Eidan, F.A. *et al.* (2000). Use of a treatment protocol in the management of community-acquired lower respiratory tract infection. *Journal of Antimicrobial Chemotherapy* **45**, 387–94.
9. Benenson, S. *et al.* (1999). Effects of a pneumonia clinical pathway on time to antibiotic treatment, length of stay, and mortality. *Academic Emergency Medicine* **6**, 1243–8.
10. Perlstein, P.H. *et al.* (1999). Evaluation of an evidence-based guideline for bronchiolitis. *Pediatrics* **104**, 1334–41.
11. Perlstein, P.H. *et al.* (2000). Sustaining the implementation of an evidence-based guideline for bronchiolitis. *Archives of Pediatric and Adolescent Medicine* **154**, 1001–7.
12. Wilson, S.D. *et al.* (2002). An evidence-based clinical pathway for bronchiolitis safely reduces antibiotic overuse. *American Journal of Medical Quality* **17**, 195–9.
13. Stephen, A.E. and Berger, D.L. (2003). Shortened length of stay and hospital cost reduction with implementation of an accelerated clinical care pathway after colon resection. *Surgery* **133**, 277–82.
14. Bandolier (1999). Do-it-yourself pain control. *ImpAct* **1**(4), 6–7.
15. Lipton, R.B. *et al.* (2000). Stratified care vs step care strategies for migraine: the disability in strategies of care (DISC) study: a randomized trial. *Journal of the American Medical Association* **284**, 2599–605.
16. Stewart, W.F. *et al.* (2000). Validity of the migraine disability assessment (MIDAS) score in comparison to a diary-based measure in a population sample of migraine sufferers. *Pain* **88**, 41–52.

# 6.6   Evidence-based management

Is there an evidence base for management? There certainly is, but not necessarily as we who work in health-care understand it. Two personal Bandolier stories to make the point, both from a while ago, but echoed more recently as well, contrasted with another story about health-care improvement.

### Story 1

In the Radcliffe Infirmary in the 1980s, personal computers were banned, except for research. Out of my research fund I bought a £3500 Superbrain (two 64k drives for the techies, and a lot of money for the 1980s). The problem was that, when it rained in a certain way and the wind blew at a certain strength from a certain direction, water flowed through a light fitting in the ceiling and all over my desk. So this enormously expensive computer (1980s don't forget) was sat next to a red plastic bucket.

By chance Frank, the hospital engineer, happened to walk through just at the right time and promised to get the problem fixed. A plumber duly arrived, went off to the roof space, and returned about 20 minutes later. He explained that there was a vent in the roof and, when it rained in a certain way and the wind blew at a certain strength from a certain direction, water collected and came through the light fitting on to my desk.

'But could you fix it?' I asked. 'What did you do?'

'No problem, sir.' was the reply. 'I took the bucket upstairs.'

### Story 2

Clinical budgets were first introduced in Oxford at the same time as an early screening programme for neonatal hypothyroidism funded by the Regional Health Authority (RHA). The accountants running the budget exercise set an unrealistically low non-staff budget for the biochemistry labs, and we told them the actual figure, but they said not to worry, it was only an exercise.

A year later the third set of accountants wanted to know how we were going to deal with our 'overspend' of £8000. Conveniently, the RHA grant for neonatal hypothyroid screening was also £8000.

'Take the money, but don't do the tests', was their suggestion. But what about the five or six children affected by neonatal hypothyroidism whom we would not detect in the next year? We explained that they would, at best, be intellectually impaired.

'Ah', they replied, 'that's the mental health budget!'

### Story 3 The Esther project

'Esther' is not a real patient, but her persona as a grey-haired, ailing, but competent elderly Swedish woman with a chronic condition and occasional acute needs has inspired impressive improvements in how patients flow through a complex network of providers and care settings in Höglandet, Sweden.

Esther was invented by the team of physicians, nurses, and other providers who joined together to improve patient flow and coordination of care for elderly patients of a six-municipality region in Sweden. The productive work done on Esther's behalf led the Jönköping County Council, responsible for the health care of 330,000 residents living around

Höglandet, to become one of two international teams participating in the 'pursuing perfection' initiative. This programme, launched by the Robert Wood Johnson Foundation, was designed to help physician organizations and hospitals dramatically improve patient outcomes by pursuing perfection in all their major care processes. (The Institute of Healthcare Improvement (www.ihi.org/idealized/idpf/index.asp:IHI) serves as the national programme office for this initiative.)

The Esther Project had six overall objectives:
1. security for Esther;
2. better working relations in the entire care chain;
3. higher competence through the care chain;
4. shared medical documentation;
5. quality through the entire care chain;
6. documentation and communication of improvements.

The Esther project team consisted of physicians, nurses, social workers, and other providers representing the Höglandet Hospital and physician practices in each of the six municipalities. They were divided into two subgroups: the strategy group, and the project management group.

To establish a clear picture of where the problems existed, team members conducted more than 60 interviews with patients and providers from throughout the system. Together they analysed the results, which included such statements as 'patients in a nursing home rarely see their doctor' and 'a patient getting palliative care at home was in contact with 30 different people during one week'.

During the 3-year project, they were able to achieve the following improvements.

- Hospital admissions for heart failure fell from approximately 580 in 1998 to 460 in 2000.
- Hospital-days for heart failure patients decreased from approximately 3500 in 1998 to 2500 in 2000.
- Waiting times for referral appointments with neurologists decreased from 85 days in 2000 to 14 days in 2001.
- Waiting times for referral appointments with gastroenterologists fell from 48 days in 2000 to 14 days in 2001.

## Operational research

The Esther project might be regarded as a type of operational research project, which is a key technique for management, though almost unknown in health-care management in some parts of the world. Operational research (operations research in the USA) is the application of scientific method to the management of organized systems. It attempts to provide those who manage organized systems with an objective and quantitative basis for decision. It is normally carried out by teams of scientists or engineers from a variety of disciplines, and often working with people involved in the organization and with detailed knowledge of it. Operational research is concerned with the decisions that control the organization, and how managerial decisions could and should be made.

It is easier to understand what operational research is all about with an example, and there is none better than the example that led to the creation of the discipline.

The origins of operational research are inextricably linked with the development of radar in the late 1930s. Radar was not 'invented' in Britain, and the first patent for a radar-like detection apparatus was granted in Germany in 1904. But in the mid-1930s the British developments under the leadership of Robert Watson-Watt meant that a practical radio detection and location (hence radar) system was developed.

But there was a problem. Though aircraft could be detected, fighter interceptors could not be brought into play in time for them to be effective. The RAF thought the answer was 'better' radar. But as a result of an initiative of A.P. Rowe, the superintendent of the research station involved with radar, a team of scientists showed military leaders how to use the system effectively. The answer was simple—better communications between radar station, RAF high command, and the fighter stations. It was the telephones, stupid!

Operational research was used by British and American teams throughout the Second World War for all sorts of purposes. After the war it became a central principle of much US industry. The British forgot about it, although there is a UK operational research society (www.orsoc.org.uk).

Operational research comes down to a few simple actions: formulating the problem; constructing a model; deriving a solution; testing the model and solution; and implementing and controlling the solution.

### Operational research in health-care

Where can we find examples of operational research in health-care? Actually, that's not easy. There doesn't seem to be a readily accessible literature, or a place where operational research is used systematically in health-care.

A sister publication of *Bandolier*, a journal called *ImpAct*, aimed to find folk in the NHS who had found ways of making inspirational and lasting change for the good of patients, staff, and the organization as a whole. It ran from 1999 to 2001, when the meagre funding it received from government was withdrawn. As an aside, the idea behind *ImpAct* has resurfaced on several occasions, all with much more lavish funding, but yet to make any impression.

In retrospect, many of the examples featured in *ImpAct* were *de facto* examples of operational research, and involved describing the problem, modelling different possible solutions, deriving one that seemed most likely to work, testing the solution, and implementing it.

Searching the literature using PubMed and the words operational and research in the title gives little to look at. But there are a some good examples from rural South Africa.

Rabies is an important disease in rural South Africa. The state provides vaccine and immunoglobulin to people after suspected exposure to rabies virus by bite, scratch, or mucosal splash. A simple standardized telephone survey was used as a rapid tool for operational research into the reliability and effectiveness of the programme. Startling deficiencies in the availability of treatment led to decisive corrective action [1].

Another paper from the same team examines a series of operational research initiatives for malaria treatment, again in rural South Africa [2]. Part of the reason for developing a programme was the recognition that diagnostic services were a shambles. Methods were poor, agreement between centres was non-existent, and some clinics never received any results from the samples they sent in.

This led to the introduction of a new diagnostic test for use in the field with excellent accuracy, field-testing of different and better tests, and a confidential inquiry into malaria deaths, all as part of continuously improving the service and the treatment of malaria.

All this is referenced, but the interesting thing about this paper is that the subject was used for teaching a module for a master's degree in public health, with participants from South Africa and Australia. While there were some concerns from participants, the comments about using operational research were enthusiastic.

## A worked example: gastro-oesophageal reflux

Back in the 1990s, advice from the Department of Health in the UK on the treatment of reflux disease was that the most cost-effective way of treating it was to begin with lifestyle advice (avoid spicy food and alcohol, and raise the head of the bed), and when that didn't work move on to treatments like alginates, and when that didn't work use histamine antagonists (H2A), and when that didn't work try proton pump inhibitors (PPI; though usually after endoscopy, which also has a high cost and a finite morbidity and mortality associated with it). This advice failed to take account of the fact that most people in clinical trials and practice were older women.

A piece of operational research [3] sought to examine the hypothesis, testing various treatment options based on evidence. There was a three-fold comparison:

1. Stepped treatment 16 weeks:
   (a) lifestyle advice 4 weeks; then
   (b) gaviscon 4 weeks; then
   (c) H2A 4 weeks; then
   (d) PPI 4 weeks.
2. Histamine antagonist 8 weeks immediately.
3. Proton pump inhibitor 8 weeks immediately

Using information from systematic reviews, the research was able to show that using a proton pump inhibitor immediately cost less per cure than either of the alternative strategies (Table 6.6.1). It was the high cure rate that made the difference, and made it more cost-effective than the guideline strategy even when costly and possibly dangerous endoscopy was omitted.

Just look at healing rates from a later systematic review [4] comparing different treatments, given as percentage of people healed at 8 weeks, using endoscopic healing as the end point (Figure 6.6.1).

**Table 6.6.1**  Cost of three alternative strategies for reflux oesophagitis

| Strategy | Total cost (£) | Months taken | Cure in primary care (%) | Cost per cure (£) |
|---|---|---|---|---|
| Stepped treatment | 224,000 | 4 | 75 | 298 |
| Histamine antagonist | 318,000 | 2 | 44 | 722 |
| Proton pump inhibitor | 185,000 | 2 | 78 | 237 |

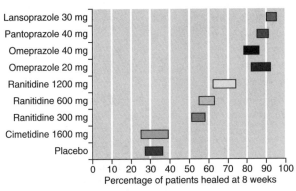

**Figure 6.6.1** Endoscopic healing at 8 weeks.

This sort of representation shows not only the expected proportion of patients cured, but also those not cured. Patients who are not cured presumably have other things happen to them—more visits to the GP or outpatients, more drugs, more diagnostics, more endoscopy. That also consumes resources. Perhaps we should think about the balance between the simple costs of treatment, usually the acquisition costs of the medicines, and the consequences of not being cured.

So let us assume that the consequences of not being cured for moderate or severe gastro-oesophageal reflux disease is about £100. It could easily be this, given the cost of a GP visit as about £16, an outpatient visit at £65, an endoscopy at £200 and a course of drugs from about £20 to £70 per month. Doing a few sums, it is clear that proton pump inhibitors are cheaper than histamine antagonists and doing nothing, both in cost per patient healed at 8 weeks (Figure 6.6.2) and in total cost (Figure 6.6.3).

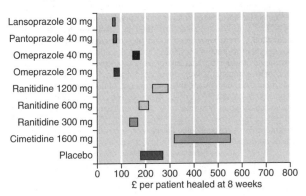

**Figure 6.6.2** Cost for each patient healed at 8 weeks.

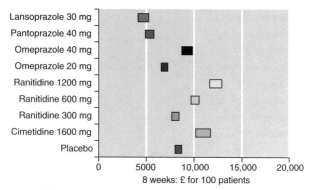

**Figure 6.6.3**    Total cost of treatment.

A study from Stanford confirms this view of the world [5] demonstrated for the UK previously [3], and concludes that step down treatments are likely to be the most cost-effective when success rates with proton pump inhibitors are above 59%, which they clearly are at 4 or 8 weeks. This is now part of guidance in the UK, at least as an option.

It is also useful to know what happens in practice. A simple but important example from the pages of *ImpAct* (issue 2) helps. The example comes from a primary care practice in Manchester.

Repeat prescriptions account for about 75% of items and 80% of the costs of all prescribing. Within this overall picture reflux is a common relapsing condition and a common cause of consultations in general practice. Although the majority of patients suffering from this condition self-medicate with over the counter preparations, those visiting their GP still represent a significant workload for primary care. Expenditure by practices on H2-antagonists for these patients is likely to be significant. The Beswick surgery in Manchester decided to look for ways to reduce repeat prescribing.

The first step was to collect together information to help the practice understand current knowledge about the condition and treatments. This allowed them to become confident about the effectiveness of alternative treatments. It was clear that omeprazole was the most effective maintenance therapy in patients with reflux oesophagitis.

To help them understand the consequence of their initiative the practice identified 32 patients with reflux who were being prescribed histamine-antagonists or other treatments (11 different treatments). They developed a protocol for a review of treatment, including the patient's view of their treatment. The protocol guided discussion about the incidence of pain, the use of medicines (what is used and how frequently), and related lifestyle issues. A key feature of the consultation was the objective of 'negotiating' with the patient a change to a daily dose of omeprazole 20 mg with related emphasis on the need to take the full prescribed course. A notional 'agreement' between the GP and the patient was the intended outcome

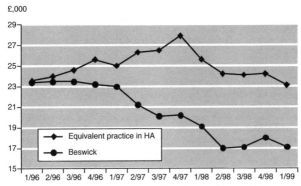

£,000

**Figure 6.6.4** Spending on acid-suppressing medicines in Beswick and a typical practice for the area.

of this review. Patients' progress was reviewed after an 8-week treatment programme.

The 8-week review showed that 17 of the 32 patients required continuing repeat prescriptions. These were changed to omeprazole 20 mg or 10 mg daily because the evidence is that this is better than histamine-antagonists for maintenance therapy. The other 15 patients required no repeat prescriptions, were given omeprazole 20 mg as pulsed therapy to tailor their needs, and were invited to attend surgery if the problems returned. Patients welcomed the process of review. The initiative produced cost savings of £2900 over 6 months in the prescribing budget. The result was happier patients, at lower cost (Figure 6.6.4).

Small initiatives can lead to big savings. £2900 per 6 months for a practice size of 7600 would mean £76, 316 a year for a population of 100, 000, tens of millions across the UK, just by doing the opposite of what was then received wisdom. Moreover, this was entirely predictable, and the process of operational research would have demonstrated it, and had done several years earlier. Better care, less cost. That is the goal, and yet only trivial amounts are spent on the discipline in health-care, at least in the UK, but probably in most places around the world. Most importantly, operational research grows out of evidence.

### Lessons from *ImpAct*

*ImpAct* asked questions of people instituting change in the NHS: 'What was learned by those involved?' *and* 'What are your "tips for success" for others wanting to tackle a similar initiative?' People were expected to be honest about what went right and what went wrong.

Project teams usually do not systematically discuss these questions. They should form part of an essential discussion for all project teams: we all have things to learn. Experience suggests that setting aside time in the middle of a team meeting for 'reflection and learning' is the best solution.

On completion of each case study bottom lines were identified that seemed to have been the key actions to assure success. *ImpAct* bottom lines fit into three groups: those about the impact of patients on the work; those about the people involved; and those about the supporting systems and process.

### Working with patients

It has surprised us that there are only three *ImpAct* bottom lines about *patient* involvement. Perhaps 'working with patients can be a learning process' says it all.

- Working with patients can be a learning process—for both clinical staff and patients.
- Work with volunteers from the community to keep developments going, but be sure that the community supports the endeavour.
- Collaboration between primary and secondary care can impact significantly on little things that make a difference—like the number of patients who don't turn up for appointments.

### The people involved

Ways to encourage innovation and build on the enthusiasm of people working in the NHS are common features of the case studies. There are four main themes. First, ensure that people have time to get involved in development work, though in ways that do not prejudice their clinical responsibilities. Space and time are essential to allow people to adopt new ideas and approaches. Second, find ways to ensure that the existing skills are used to the best effect. Third, initiatives to improve team working are time well spent. Fourth, leadership to harness the skills and release the energy of staff is essential.

### Time

- Time spent telling staff affected by initiatives what is going on is never wasted.
- Make sure that people can get involved—change rosters so that they can attend training sessions.
- Make adopting change easy for clinicians: find ways to facilitate change that do not unduly add pressure to clinical commitments.

### Skills

- Practical training makes things happen.
- Just because people use the language of IT don't assume that they understand it.
- Find ways to value and make the most of the skills and experiences of staff locally—before you bring in 'outsiders.'
- Exploring ways to use therapy assistants offers practical and economic opportunities to improve the quality of care to patients.
- Don't rest on the status quo—encourage innovative ideas and the potential of new roles as ways to improve service quality.

### Teams

- Devote effort and time to training and team building.
- Achieving change can be hard work—share out the tasks—but make sure people know what is expected of them—and when.

- Do not underestimate the positive impact development work can have on staff morale.
- Effective interdisciplinary work requires understanding and communications between team members—it must be worked at—it will not happen by magic.

*Leadership*
- Active—senior—leadership is important when tasks require coordination across large (and small) organizations.
- Avoid the careless use of meaningless (job) titles.

### Systems and processes

The case studies remind us that effective local development work needs good people and good systems. There are four themes about systems and processes. First, value simplicity and don't believe that complex solutions are always needed. Second, build on proven management techniques as a framework for the work. Third, recognize the importance of information and IT systems. These ensure a focus on what needs to change and allow progress to be measured. Fourth, make sure that local channels of communications are open and used to keep people in touch with progress: ignorance breeds doubt.

*Simplicity*
- Efficiency and effectiveness thrive on doing simple things well.
- Small initiatives can lead to big savings.
- Take time out to learn about developments elsewhere when developing new services: don't re-invent the wheel!
- Use pilot studies to verify potential benefits from change and remember —success breeds success.
- Don't believe that complex solutions are bound to be the best—simple approaches can be effective.
- Look for simple practical ways to use IT—don't be tempted by overly elaborate solutions.

*Techniques*
- Using a recognized development model can ensure that effort and resources are used to the best effect.
- Tackling those parts of a process that dictate the pace overall may be the best way to achieve rapid change.
- Don't be afraid to try new ideas—but have the courage to stop if they don't work.
- Look for practical ways to improve and build on existing systems—don't believe that you have to start afresh on everything.
- Be patient and persistent—creating effective services for small groups takes time.
- There are no quick answers.
- Persistence is required if you want to overcome long-standing problems.

*Information*
- Find novel ways of tackling problems: set standards but allow practices to find their own ways to deliver those standards.

- Make sure that you know what needs to change before making detailed plans—don't rely on anecdotes. Make sensible use of questionnaires.
- Investment in time may be worthwhile if it produces a uniform and efficient way of doing things—rather than major change.
- Solutions have to be tailored to the particular problem. Solutions may be different but the process of solving them is the same.

*Communication*

- Time devoted to communications and ensuring that staff affected by initiatives 'know what is going on' is never wasted.
- Services that are outward looking and that care about how others perceive them are more likely to succeed. Influence is born of good relationships, not internal structures and systems.
- Make new services work and be successful—so good that ways have to be found to resolve any funding issues.

### To sum up

Taken together the *ImpAct* bottom lines suggest that good practice thrives where five key activities are integrated, namely:

1. *information*: identifying the need for change, to develop new standards and monitor progress;
2. *communications*: keeping people in touch;
3. *training*: ensuring people and teams have space and time to develop and learn new skills, ideas, and approaches;
4. *involving patients*: ensuring that appropriate arrangements are in place;
5. *management*: ensuring that planned changes happen.

## Commentary

Evidence-based management is not rocket science, nor do we need a new tier of management just to do it. What we need is for ordinary doctors, nurses, scientists, and managers to get to grips with a few simple tools. It needs neither complicated statistics nor any computer assistance other than a simple computer with Excel to do some sums.

There are examples of good evidence-based thinking that have made substantial differences to health-care delivery. Many of these come from laboratory science and quality control. Back in the 1960s and 1970s, quality control in laboratories was in its infancy, at a time when the number of laboratory tests was exploding. New tests, especially, might be done in different ways, and one result was that numerical results from one laboratory would be totally different from those in another. Laboratory people got together, asked questions about the science, put an evidence base in place, implemented good practice, and monitored it. It was also policed, with a result that today a progesterone result on a given sample is much the same the world over. It made a difference. Quality control, the art of knowing just how bad you are at doing something, is a topic for a whole book, but is a crucial part of management. It is why televisions, and cars, and so many consumer goods are better now than they were in the past.

Many decisions are made on the hoof and without proper assessment of the consequences. And, though it is easy to point to prescribing policies, it also applies to many others, including those made in the higher echelons of management. There is no simple answer, certainly not from this source. If this has made you think, then perhaps it has been worthwhile. Operational research may just be one way to begin to stand on the management shoulders of others. We want good, readable books, accessible to all of us (like Muir Gray's book on making health policy and management decisions [6]), that add to the tools we can use to make delivery of health-care better. Another useful source of thinking are the three essays on delivering better health-care by Mike Dunning on the Bandolier Internet site, also available as PDF downloads.

## References

1. Durrheim, D.N. *et al.* (2002). Rabies post-exposure management in South Africa: a telephonic survey used as a rapid tool for operational research. *Tropical Medicine and International Health* **7**, 459–61.

2. Durrheim, D.N. *et al.* (2002). Research that influences policy and practice—characteristics of operational research to improve malaria control in Mpumalanga Province, South Africa. *Malaria Journal* **1**, 9 (*http://www.malariajournal.com/1/1/9*).

3. Phillips, C. and Moore, A. (1997). Trial and error—an expensive luxury: economic analysis of effectiveness of proton pump inhibitors and histamine antagonists in treating reflux disease. *British Journal of Medical Economics* **11**, 55–63.

4. Chiba, N. *et al.* (1997). Speed of healing and symptom relief in grade II to IV gastroesophageal reflux disease: a meta-analysis. *Gastroenterology* **112**, 1798–810.

5. Gerson, L.B. *et al.* (2000). A cost-effectiveness analysis of prescribing strategies in the management of gastroesophageal reflux disease. *American Journal of Gastroenterology* **95**, 395–407.

6. Muir Gray, J.A. (1997). *Evidence-based healthcare*. Churchill Livingstone, Edinburgh.

# 6.7 Trust

Trust: (noun) firm belief that a person or a thing can be relied on; (verb) believe in, rely on. That's the dictionary definition of trust, and it describes perfectly the relationship between the NHS in the UK and the public over 50 years, for most of the time, and will be mirrored by other countries with socialized health-care systems.

That trust is of two sorts. First is trust in the doctors and nurses we see in GP clinics and hospitals, together with an unstated trust in all the unseen support staff in laboratories and offices. Second is trust in the systems of the NHS to deliver the health-care people need, most of the time.

Despite some hard knocks in recent years, there is still an immense amount of trust in the NHS and in health professionals, and within the NHS between health-care professionals. Is there anything the literature can tell us about trust?

### Literature review

Running a PubMed search with trust as a title word pulls up over 300 references, but most of them are about work done in various hospitals (Trusts) or by charities (Trusts). The trouble is that there is a third dictionary definition, that of a 'law arrangement', and the use of trust in that context dominates the literature.

That doesn't mean that there is nothing that the medical (rather than philosophical or theological) literature can tell us about trust. For instance, there is a meta-analysis [1] about trust in leadership. It tells us that direct leaders (supervisors) are a particularly important 'referent' of trust, and, for those who are interested, 'a theoretical framework is offered to provide parsimony to the expansive literature and to clarify the different perspectives on the construct of trust in leadership and its operation'.

### Public trust in health-care systems

The Dutch have taken the issue of public trust in health-care systems to heart, spurred on by finding no reliable way of measuring it. The idea for the research was suggested by economic research into public trust. So they set out to develop a valid and reliable instrument to measure different dimensions of public trust in health-care in the Netherlands [2].

In a first phase, more than 100 people were interviewed to gain insight into the issues they associated with trust. Eight categories of issues that were derived from the interviews were assumed to be possible dimensions of trust. On the basis of these eight categories and the interviews, a questionnaire was developed that was used in the second phase. The questionnaire was sent to 1500 members of a consumer panel; the response was 70%.

Analysis revealed that six of the eight possible dimensions of trust were important. They were trust in:
- patient-focus of health-care providers;
- macro policy level having no consequences for patients;
- expertise of health-care providers;
- quality of care;
- information supply and communication by care providers;
- quality of cooperation.

They concluded, not surprisingly, that public trust is a multidimensional concept, including not only issues that relate to the patient–doctor relationship, but also issues that relate to health-care institutions. Their instrument appeared to be reliable and valid. Similar efforts have been directed at measuring patient trust in primary care physicians [3].

### Does patient trust matter?

One answer from California would suggest that it does matter, to the patients themselves, their doctors, and to health-care systems [4].

This was an observational study of visits by 732 patients to offices of 45 physicians (16 GPs, 18 general physicians, and 11 cardiologists) in the university and HMO systems in and around Sacramento. Patients and physicians were surveyed before, immediately after, and 2 weeks after an outpatient visit. Patient trust was measured using a nine-item scale, with items selected from previous patient focus groups and validated trust scales.

Patients were divided into tertiles of low trust, moderate trust, and high trust, and outcomes examined according to these tertiles.

The results were interesting. Overall patient trust was high—a mean of 87 when the data were transformed into a scale of 0 to 100, with a range of 14 to 100. Nearly three out of 10 patients rated their trust as perfect. But low trust was associated with lower patient satisfaction and had other negative consequences.

For instance, patients in the lowest tertile of pre-visit trust were much less likely to receive medical information, new medication, or a diagnostic test that they requested (Figure 6.7.1) or believed they needed. Two weeks after the consultation, patients in this same low trust tertile were less satisfied with the care provided, fewer of them intended to adhere to the advice given by their physicians, and fewer of them had symptom improvement (Figure 6.7.2).

Patients with low pre-visit trust were more likely to report that they had asked for medical information, though their physicians did not report this association. Both patients and physicians reported higher likelihood of a request for new medication in patients with higher pre-visit trust. There

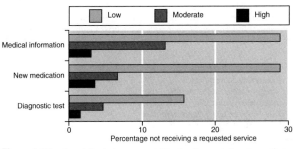

**Figure 6.7.1** Association between pre-visit trust and requested service not being provided (patient report).

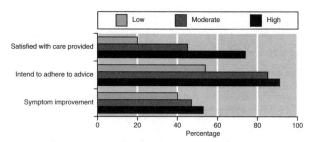

**Figure 6.7.2** Association between pre-visit trust and outcomes at 2 weeks.

was no other significant association between trust and the request for, or provision of, other services.

So, despite there being little difference in service provision between patients, low pre-visit trust meant that patients were less satisfied with their treatment. Their doctors found that the visits were more often more demanding than average in patients with lower pre-visit trust.

### Can doctor–patient trust be improved?

There is at least one small, randomized trial to attempt to improve patient trust [5]. With only 20 physicians enrolled, even though there was a net improvement in 16 of 19 specific patient-reported physician behaviours in physicians receiving the intervention when compared with those receiving a control intervention, there was, not surprisingly, no statistical significance. Similar results have been seen in a non-randomized study [6].

### Trust in general

Perhaps one of the most interesting essays on trust comes from an editorial [7] in the *Journal of the American Medical Association* that examined issues of trust between the American Medical Association and the journal following the departure of George Lundberg as its editor. The editorial discusses many topics, and has some interesting comments on academic freedom. For our purposes, though, it has some pertinent words on trust-damaging and trust-building behaviours.

These are summarized below. Most of us, if pushed, would have come up with similar lists and, while the points in the boxes were directed towards organizations rather than individuals, much the same general principles will apply.

### Trust-damaging behaviours
• Unwarranted interference.
• Excessive criticism (especially in the public arena without right of reply).
• Coercive or threatening behaviour.
• Dishonesty or being disingenuous.
• Wilfulness or recklessness.

### Trust-building behaviours
• Mutual recognition of accountability.
• Shared vision.

- Explicit strategic objectives.
- Tactics left unstated.
- Free and frequent flow of information.

## Commentary

Trust is hard won, but easily lost. The increasingly robust examination of scientific and clinical evidence can hardly help individuals at the coalface rather than in pointy-headed academia. It is not surprising that distrust rather than trust seems to be the pervading tone. But perhaps 'seems' is the operative word. When asked, most health-care professionals trust their colleagues, most patients trust their doctors and nurses, and even most pointy-headed academics are happy to share control if there is a real problem.

Trust is like quality. We get neither by avoiding hard questions, but when the hard questions are asked and answered, building on what we have gets easier. We know where the rock is, and that we have to avoid the sand. It is just strange that trust is so little researched.

## References

1. Dirks, K.T. and Ferrin, D.L. (2002). Trust in leadership: meta-analytic findings and implications for research and practice. *Journal of Applied Psychology* **87**, 611–28.
2. Straten, G.F. *et al.* (2002). Public trust in Dutch health care. *Social Sciences in Medicine* **55**, 227–34.
3. Hall, M.A. *et al.* (2002). Measuring patients' trust in their primary care providers. *Medical Care Research Reviews* **59**, 293–318.
4. Thom, D.H. *et al.* (2002). Patient trust in the physician: relationship to patient requests. *Family Practice* **19**, 476–83.
5. Thom, D.H. (2000). Training physicians to increase patient trust. *Journal of Evaluation in Clinical Practice* **6**, 245–53.
6. Thom, D.H. *et al.* (1999). An intervention to increase patients' trust in their physicians. *Academic Medicine* **74**, 195–8.
7. Davies, H.T.O. and Rennie, D. (1999). Independence, governance, and trust. *Journal of the American Medical Association* **281**, 2344–7.

# 7.1 Introduction

In any book, once you have dealt with all the obvious topics, there is a ragbag of interesting issues left over that just don't fit easily into any other section and are too small for a section to themselves. Looking at evidence is no exception, so what we have decided to do is to put all these interesting leftovers into a section all of its own.

Some of the issues we will cover in this section include good examples for us to draw upon to make a point. For instance, Bandolier is often asked what evidence there is on a topic; often there is none, or appears to be none, but again there is often more than you think. There is also a problem when it appears that evidence is set in granite, but where received wisdom says one thing and the evidence seems to go in the opposite direction.

There are other topics for which there is truly limited, but interesting, evidence. Communicating risk is one example. Questions about fraudulent research or conflicts of interest are others.

What joins all these themes together is the simple fact that we have no clear answer to any of them, but we are pretty sure that applying solid rules of evidence can help us even in difficult situations.

# 7.2 Where there is no evidence

There can often be no research on a topic, or anyway little or none you want to read. One of the greatest achievements of the Cochrane Collaboration is that it creates and publishes systematic reviews where no trials have been found. Imagine trying to get a paper with no data published in a mainstream journal? It would be next to impossible.

Yet negative information of this sort is priceless. If a group of worthy souls has had the energy to search through multiple databases, according to strict Cochrane criteria, and found zilch, then that is a very positive negative. It saves all the rest of us having to do the same when faced with the same question. Such reviews often tell us of other types of evidence that they did not include, like case reports, or tell us of the absence of even that type of information. At least we then know what we don't know, and that an answer cannot be found.

Often, though, the world is not as bereft of information as it may seem, especially with the cornucopia of electronic searching available at the click of a mouse. Bandolier gets a little exasperated with media reporting of medical matters, especially the Friday announcements of yet another breakthrough in cancer in a few mice, or an association between rainbows and heart disease. This week it is pain and red hair. Typically, we have a small study in an experimental situation reaching some level of statistical significance, and a good press release gets it into the media; once it is in one media outlet they all have to use it. When you look for real evidence in clinical situations, there is little or none.

Three examples will, we hope, show how we can deal with at least some of these. All three had an involvement from the media in some way, which is why we chose them.

## Serratiopeptidase

A UK national newspaper carried an article about an attractive young woman (photographed, of course) who had a 6-year history of back pain after falling off a motorcycle. The severe stabbing pains disappeared after treatment with silkworm enzyme, a product known as serratiopeptidase. The young woman was free of her chronic pain within a week or so of starting on this treatment. Trials had reportedly found that it killed pain as effectively as NSAIDs, without the gastrointestinal damage. The article then gave examples of other ailments this product would be wonderful for, including arthritis, asthma, heart disease, stroke, and migraine.

Wonderful and all for about £18 a month! With all these brilliant results there must be a plethora of wonderful data in the literature to support it.

At the time the article was published Bandolier did a quick search on PubMed. It found 34 articles, including letters, animal studies, case reports of adverse events, and some comparative trials. There was nothing about back pain, or migraine, heart attack, stroke, or asthma. There were comparative trials in postoperative or traumatic swelling (three of them), two each in ENT disorders and chronic respiratory disease, and one in breast engorgement.

The problem with these trials was small size, poor design, doses not stated, outcomes not defined, mixed medical conditions, and mixed acute and chronic conditions. Of five trials that were randomized and double blind:

- One was completely uninterpretable (and it's not just us being stupid, as so far we have found no one who could understand it).
- Three were positive, but of such poor quality that bias was highly likely.
- One was of high quality, but was negative:
  - it was the largest study (125 patients per group);
  - it was in chronic respiratory disease;
  - it had a placebo control;
  - it found no significant difference between the groups.

Since that search in about 2002, one more randomized trial has been published in chronic airway disease. It was not blind, it was small (29 patients), and it had statistical significance for a not very important outcome. Yet type serratiopeptidase into Google, and you will find about 750 pages, many of them selling it. Fortunately, the third one is a *Bandolier* article pointing out the lack of evidence.

Here the failure to find evidence should support our critical faculties. We know that there is no evidence that this stuff works. We know that it cannot have been tested properly for safety, especially for the rare but serious adverse events that worry us most. This is a biological agent after all; there must be a finite if small risk of severe allergic reaction.

### Ibuprofen and women

A Bandolier researcher in the process of updating a Cochrane review on the analgesic efficacy of ibuprofen in acute pain was told by a chiropractor that there was little point in taking ibuprofen, as it didn't work in women. The source of the assertion was an article from a popular science journal pinned on the wall of the reception area for patients to see.

The article made some sensible points about the relative exclusion of women from clinical trials in the past. It claimed that only in 1993 did the USA make it a legal requirement for women to be included in clinical trials and that on average 52% of subjects in large-scale trials are women, but that this figure included women-only studies. The article implied that women had not been included in analgesic trials of ibuprofen, which is why we did *not* know that ibuprofen did *not* work for women.

The real clinchers were the following:
1. a report of a study of experimental pain in 10 men and 10 women, in which there was a statistically significant response to ibuprofen in men but not women;
2. a comment from a female pain expert who said that this finding was 'dramatic' and had a direct impact for the clinic.

A systematic review of acute pain studies [1] showed that, in 37 trials of ibuprofen in acute pain with 3577 patients:
- 67% of patients in the trials were women;
- 86% of patients were in trials in which over half the patients were women;
- 8 trials enrolled only women and no trial enrolled only men;
- the proportion of patients with at least 50% pain relief from ibuprofen 400 mg was unaffected by the proportion of women included in the trials;
- NNT for 50% pain relief in women was 3.4 (2.6–4.6), not significantly different than that for men of 2.5 (2.0–3.3);

- the general distribution of pain relief was the same for women and men. This was from an updated Cochrane review, but similar information could have been obtained from the review extant at that time. Moreover, entering 'ibuprofen AND (gender or sex)' into PubMed brought up an FDA meta-analysis of 314 (195 women and 119 men) dental pain patients where no differences were found [2]. If one wanted to really make the point about how much evidence there is that ibuprofen works in women, one could add the following.

- A systematic review shows efficacy of NSAIDs, including ibuprofen, for dysmenorrhoea.
- Reviews showing efficacy of ibuprofen in osteoarthritis (predominantly women in the trials).
- Large clinical trials of coxibs showing efficacy of ibuprofen in women in both osteoarthritis and rheumatoid arthritis.
- Evidence that ibuprofen is effective in migraine and headache, and migraine again predominates in women.

So what we had was a small experimental pain study that flew in the face of a wealth of clinical data. It was used to score points about sex difference, and spun a trivial finding into a real problem. What we know about small studies is that they are unreliable, and to that can be added a fact that most pain professionals know, that experimental pain findings rarely if ever extrapolate to clinical importance, or even reproducibility.

A few moments on the Internet with neurons in gear could have shown that everything about this article was just plain wrong.

## MMR vaccines and autism

Publication of a study of 12 selected children with autism and bowel disorders and the association of these with previous MMR vaccination [3] began the controversy linking use of the triple MMR vaccine to autism. The study itself has proved to be highly contentious, with all but one of the authors and the journal in which it was published subsequently repudiating the article and its conclusions.

Although the article itself seemed to make no direct connection, publicity surrounding it made the connection that, because measles virus was present, and because measles virus might have come from the vaccine, and because the children had autism and bowel disorder, then the vaccine caused the problem. That is about as intelligent as saying that because the lights are on and it is dark outside, putting the lights on made it dark outside.

Without dwelling on the problems of the study itself or the concerns that have been expressed over events that may or may not have surrounded it, it is worthwhile noting the features, at least in the popular and media mind, that associated MMR with autism. They included:

- Autism rates had increased following introduction of MMR.
- MMR vaccination led to regression, meaning that children who were developing normally regressed in their development after MMR vaccination.
- MMR vaccination caused a form of autism associated with bowel disorders.
- MMR, but not single vaccines, overwhelmed the immune system.

A huge amount of research of high quality and validity has been assembled subsequently, none of which supports any of these contentions. Over the next few years a host of large, good, epidemiological studies failed to outweigh this single study, at least in the eyes of the media. Only in 2005, almost 7 years later, has the heat transferred to the important question of what does cause autism and what, if anything, can we do to prevent it.

The benefit of immunization was completely overlooked. In Finland, for example [4], much of the push for immunization resulted from the large number of conscript soldiers who fell ill. Before immunization more than a quarter of them contracted clinical mumps. A third of them had orchitis (inflammation of the testicle), a quarter of those (1 in 12 of the total) had bilateral orchitis, and a quarter of them (1 in 50 of the total) were rendered sterile. Mumps contracted during military service was a major cause of infertility in the general population and mumps was a major cause of hearing impairment in children, as well as later deafness. Rubella was also common, with about 1 case per 1000 people a year. Again there was an association with hearing impairment in children, and congenital rubella syndrome (CRS) was a problem. As a reminder to those of us who forget that infectious diseases are not merely inconvenient, when rubella infection occurs during pregnancy, especially during the first trimester, fetal infection is likely and often causes CRS, resulting in abortions, miscarriages, stillbirths, and severe birth defects. Up to 20% of the infants born to mothers infected during the first half of pregnancy have CRS. The most common congenital defects are cataracts, heart disease, deafness, and mental retardation.

In 1982 a major effort was put into vaccinations using a triple MMR vaccine. The programme involved 1000 child health centres, catch-up programmes, and military recruits. Two million people (40% of the population) received 3.5 million doses, and coverage was over 95%.

The number of cases of measles ran at 5000–15,000 in the decades before the introduction of a vaccination programme. Since 1985 the number of cases was tiny, and in 1996 fell to zero [4]. For mumps and rubella, the number of cases was a few thousands to a few tens of thousands a year, but fell sharply after the introduction of MMR to a few hundreds or tens, and since 1997 there have been no cases except cases imported from outside Finland.

In addition, the Finnish National Board of Health and Public Health started a long-term country-wide surveillance system to detect serious adverse events associated with MMR [5]. A series of seminars was held for public health and other involved professionals before the project started, and materials were made available in both official languages (Finnish and Swedish). There was also public information.

In the event of a possible serious adverse event (defined as any temporal association without limit of time between MMR and a life-threatening disorder, triggering of a chronic disease, or hospital admission), a form was completed and forwarded to a central office with a serum sample. A second form and second sample followed 2 weeks later. Forms, envelopes, and collection tubes were available at child health centres and hospitals. The total number of reported vaccine-associated events in 1.8 million people having 3 million vaccinations was 437. Of these, potentially serious adverse events occurred in 169 people, of whom 79 went to hospital. These 169 people were subject to intense scrutiny. About half the reported adverse events could be ascribed to other factors (like other vaccinations given with MMR) on clinical, serological, and epidemiological analyses. No event had an incidence of more than 1 case per 100, 000 doses of vaccine. There were no cases of autism, and no cases of ulcerative colitis, Crohn's disease, or any chronic disorder affecting the gastrointestinal tract.

This large population-based survey demonstrated very great benefits, and little harm.

### Californian experience

A Californian study [6] showed MMR immunization rates by 2 years of age rising from 72% before 1988 to 82% afterwards, with the same preparation used since 1979. During this time the number of cases of autism, about 200 in 1980, increased inexorably to about 1200 by 1994. The trend for increasing autism in California persisted long after the introduction of MMR vaccination, and was not affected by a modest increase in immunization rates in the mid-1980s.

### Danish experience

A retrospective study of all children born in Denmark between 1991 and 1998 provided another insight into the effects of MMR vaccination in a complete population [7]. In Denmark, a system of unique personal identification numbers, linked to vaccination registers and linked information about the diagnosis of autism, makes almost complete follow-up possible. A record review of 40 children with autism by a consultant in child psychiatry confirmed that 37 of the 40 children met operational criteria for autism.

There were 440,655 children vaccinated, and 96, 648 children who were unvaccinated. The mean age of vaccination was 17 months, and 99% of children vaccinated had their first vaccination before they were 3 years of age. Table 7.2.1 shows the number and percentage of children who developed autism or autistic spectrum disorders. There was no statistically significant difference between vaccinated and unvaccinated children for autism or autistic spectrum disorders. There was no association between development of autism and age at vaccination or the interval between vaccination and development of autism, with no clustering at any particular time. About 1 in 1700 children developed autism and 1 in 1250 autistic spectrum disorder whether they were vaccinated or not.

### British experience

A study [8] based on the UK General Practice Research Database included cases of children with a first recorded pervasive developmental disorder (PDD) in the study period (1987–2001), and for each case planned five controls. Controls were individually matched by year of birth, sex, and

**Table 7.2.1** Autism and MMR vaccination in Denmark

|  | Vaccinated | Unvaccinated |
| --- | --- | --- |
| Total number of children | 44, 0655 | 96, 648 |
| Number with autism | 263 | 53 |
| % with autism | 0.06 | 0.055 |
| Number with autistic spectrum disorder | 345 | 77 |
| % with autistic spectrum disorder | 0.078 | 0.08 |

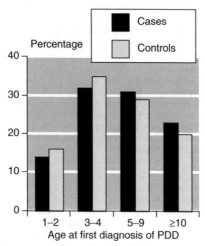

**Figure 7.2.1** Age of first diagnosis of PPD for vaccinated and unvaccinated children.

general practice. Details of vaccination were extracted, together with diagnoses of autism, Asperger's syndrome, or other PDD. The date of provisional diagnosis of PDD was taken as the date of the diagnosis (because final diagnosis could take several months).

There were 1294 cases and 4469 controls. For cases, 78% had MMR vaccination at any age, similar to the 82% for controls. The median age at first MMR vaccination was 1.2 years for cases and controls. The mean age at diagnosis was 5.4 years, with 77% of diagnoses being for autism and 23% for other PDDs. The age at which a PDD was diagnosed was the same in both groups (Figure 7.2.1). Most children were diagnosed after their fifth year.

This paper also sought other studies that assessed the risk of PDD in those who had MMR vaccine and those who did not. Eligible studies were those from which an overall effect measure could be obtained. The results (Figure 7.2.2) showed that risk of a PDD for a child having MMR vaccination was not significantly different from that of a child not having the vaccination. The combined relative risk of 0.87 (0.76–1.001), if anything, pointed to a lower risk with vaccination.

### Japanese experience

In Japan, MMR vaccine was introduced in 1989, but the programme was terminated in 1993 and only single vaccines used thereafter, because of problems with production of MMR in Japan. The experience of Japan therefore constitutes a real-world experiment of replacing triple MMR vaccine with single vaccines. If the proponents of a link between MMR and autism were correct, the result should be that cases of autism fell after withdrawal of MMR.

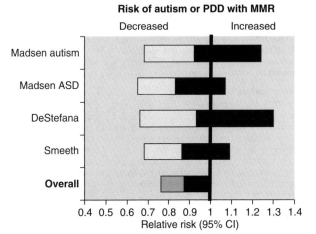

**Figure 7.2.2** Meta-analysis of risk of developing PDD with MMR vaccination (bars show 95% confidence interval of the relative risk, with junction between shades as the point estimate) [8].

The study [9] was conducted in a part of Yokohama with a population of about 300,000, which was stable, or reflected changes typical for Japanese society as a whole, over the period of the study. It had an early detection and intervention system that included specific routine check-ups at 4, 18, and 36 months, working to defined diagnostic criteria. At 18 months, about 90% of children participated in the programme. These services began in 1987, 2 years before introduction of MMR. The study had not only specific diagnostic criteria, but also complete and consistent coverage of a defined population over the time covering the introduction and withdrawal of triple MMR vaccine.

Over the whole period, and with full follow-up to age 7 years, in birth cohorts from 1988 to 1996, 278 children developed autistic spectrum disorder: 158 autism and 120 other autistic spectrum disorders. Of those with autism, 60 had definite regression and another 12 probable regression, according to defined tests. In the 1988 birth cohort, 70% of children had the MMR triple vaccine, falling to 1.8% in the 1992 birth cohort. Thereafter no children had the MMR triple vaccine.

The incidence of all autistic spectrum disorders, and of autism, continued to rise after MMR vaccine was discontinued. The incidence of autism was higher in children born after 1992 who were not vaccinated with MMR than in children born before 1992 who were vaccinated. The incidence of autism associated with regression was the same during the use of MMR and after it was discontinued. The increase of autistic spectrum disorders was evident in children with higher IQ.

The increase in autism and autistic spectrum disorders in this part of Yokohama displays the same increase over time seen in other parts of the world, even when the MMR vaccine was withdrawn. This destroys any possible causative link between use of the vaccine and autism.

Perhaps the most important features of the study were that it comprehensively covered a population, and that the population was served by a special service testing children for developmental disorders, using standard methods over the whole period. The quality and validity of the study is superlative, and the size good.

## Commentary

For MMR the same message about a lack of association between MMR vaccination and autism has been provided by all the epidemiological studies. Despite this, in the media eye this consistent and growing mountain of evidence counted as nothing. Each new piece of information was treated as if it sprang out of nothing. It was the same as for ibuprofen and women.

For both these examples it was as if there were no evidence, when there was masses of good evidence. People involved in the media just couldn't be bothered to find it. Perhaps the evidence that existed just wasn't the evidence they wanted to hear.

The lesson is that there is rarely no evidence, and you can often find out quite a lot in a relatively short time.

## References

1. Barden, J. *et al.* (2002). Ibuprofen 400 mg is effective in women, and women are well represented in trials. *BMC Anesthesiology* **2**, 6. (*http://www.biomedcentral.com/1471-2253/2/6*).
2. Averbuch, M. and Katzper, M. (2000). A search for sex differences in response to analgesia. *Archives of Internal Medicine* **160**, 3424–8.
3. Wakefield, A.J. *et al.* (1998). Ileal-lymphoid-nodular hyperplasia, non-specific colitis, and pervasive developmental disorder in children. *Lancet* **351**, 637–41.
4. Peltola, H. *et al.* (1997). No measles in Finland. *Lancet* **350**, 1364–5.
5. Patja, A. *et al.* (2000). Serious adverse events after measles–mumps–rubella vaccination during a fourteen-year prospective follow up. *Pediatric Infectious Diseases Journal* **19**, 1127–34.
6. Dales, L. *et al.* (2001). Time trends in autism and in MMR immunization coverage in California. *Journal of the American Medical Association* **285**, 1183–5.
7. Madsen, K.M. *et al.* (2002). A population-based study of measles, mumps and rubella vaccination and autism. *New England Journal of Medicine* **347**, 1477–82.
8. Kaye, J.A. *et al.* (2001). Mumps, measles, and rubella vaccine and the incidence of autism recorded by general practitioners: a time trend survey. *British Medical Journal* **322**, 460–3.
9. Honda, H. *et al.* (2005). No effect of MMR withdrawal on the incidence of autism: a total population study. *Journal of Child Psychology and Psychiatry* **46**, 572–9.

# 7.3   Beware received wisdom

Received wisdom is one of those things that can be very helpful when you find it for yourself, but can be really irritating when thrust upon you. If once considers the guidelines and guidance that flow from everywhere these days, it seems as if received wisdom is taking over. Bandolier particularly likes a couple of quotes on wisdom attributed to Mahatma Gandhi and Marcel Proust, respectively, which go something like:

It is unwise to be too sure of one's own wisdom. It is healthy to be reminded that the strongest might weaken and the wisest might err.
We don't receive wisdom; we must discover it for ourselves after a journey that no one can take for us or spare us.

The underlying message is that we need to have our own wits about us, and be alert, because no amount of good work by guideline committees will come up with the right answer for every patient in every circumstance. That means that the neurons have to do a little jig once in a while. To help them, we have chosen two examples, low-dose aspirin and topical NSAIDs.

## Low-dose aspirin

Low-dose aspirin is a good thing for preventing heart attacks and strokes in people who have already had a heart attack, as we showed in Chapter 5.5. For people at high risk, for instance, those who have already had a heart attack, the risk of another over the next 27 months is 17.5% [1], or 8% a year, or 80% over 10 years (more or less). Here the NNT to prevent another event is about 50 in any 1 year, or about 5 over 10 years. Clearly, this is beneficial.

That does not mean that low-dose aspirin is safe for everyone and, at lower levels of risk of cardiovascular disease, the risks of adverse events come much more into play. These are not insignificant, and there is certainly evidence out there that makes one think carefully about the issues when prescribing low-dose aspirin. Two observational studies help, one looking at gastrointestinal harm and one looking at costs of harm with low-dose aspirin.

### Low-dose aspirin harm

One study [2] determined the rate of finished consultant episodes for gastric and peptic ulcer, and for haemorrhage and perforation from 1989/90 to 1998/9, standardized against the European standard population. Information on the number of items dispensed in the community between 1990 and 1999 was also obtained.

Hospital admissions for gastric and peptic ulcer did not change over the period for men and women under 65 years, but rose in older age groups for both men and women, by about 10–30% in 65–74s and 30–40% in over-75s. For duodenal ulcer, finished consultant episodes rose by 25% for men and women aged 65–74 years, and 30–50% for men and women over 75 years.

Prescribing over the period showed major changes. For instance, there was a huge increase in prescribing of proton pump inhibitors (PPI) and selective serotonin reuptake inhibitors, and also in the 75 mg dose of aspirin (Figure 7.3.1). NSAID prescribing did not change over the period.

This observational study cannot link cause and effect between any particular prescribing practice and changes in duodenal ulcer haemorrhage.

Prescribed items ('000)

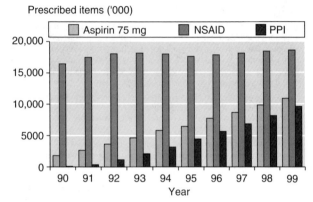

**Figure 7.3.1**  Prescribing of NSAIDs, low-dose aspirin, and PPIs over the 1990s.

Based on the number of prescriptions, assuming each prescription to be for 30 tablets and assuming that one 75 mg tablet was taken a day, then it was calculated that by 1999 there would have been 900,000 more person-years of exposure. Given that low-dose aspirin causes one or two gastrointestinal bleeds per 1000 patients, then low-dose aspirin could account for 1000 to 2000 episodes of gastrointestinal bleeding each year, approximating the 1000 excess admissions actually observed.

*Low-dose aspirin costs*
The costs of low-dose aspirin have been explored in a massive study from Tayside [3]. In this population of about 400,000 people there is a well-established record-linking scheme, so that primary care prescriptions can be linked to medical history, other prescriptions, and hospital admissions and diagnostic interventions.

People who were dispensed one or more prescriptions for low-dose aspirin (defined as not higher than 325 mg per day) at any time over the 6 years of 1990–95 were included if they were new users. For each subject there were 10 age- and sex-matched controls. Study outcomes were:
- hospital admission with a primary diagnosis of renal failure;
- creatinine of 150 μmol/L (the paper says 150 mmol/mL, which is a million times too high);
- hospital admission with a primary diagnosis of upper gastrointestinal event;
- endoscopy;
- histamine antagonist, proton pump inhibitor, or misoprostol prescription.

Of the 17, 244 subjects taking aspirin, 77% were aged 60 or older. There was an average of 2.5 years of observation per patient, during which aspirin was taken for 1.2 years. The implication was that compliance (concordance) was 47%.

Aspirin users had more renal and upper gastrointestinal adverse events (Table 7.3.1). The average annual cost was £18 per person for renal adverse events and £25 for gastrointestinal adverse events, compared with an average £2 for the aspirin and £5.50 for dispensing. These annual average costs were obtained by division of the total cost by the number of years of follow-up, not by years of aspirin exposure. Had the calculations used years of aspirin exposure, then the adverse event costs would be about £100 a year for each person actually taking low-dose aspirin.

A second analysis was limited only to low-risk subjects free of disease at study entry (30% of total) and adjusted for different risk factors between aspirin users and non-users. This produced a lower cost estimate of average annual cost of £2.90 per person for renal adverse events and £2.66 for gastrointestinal adverse events, and a total of £13 per patient per year.

This cost paper produces cogent arguments why the full analysis (called a pragmatic analysis in the paper) is likely to be the most sensible. It makes the point that it did not include costs involved with congestive heart failure nor did it include any costs with any bleeding events not in the upper bowel. It also considers sources of bias, such as use of non-prescribed aspirin or NSAIDs and possible confounding by indication.

The projected annual costs, multiplied pro-rata for Scotland would be £3–11 million, and therefore for the UK would be ten times greater. And, of course, this is for newly treated patients, and with costs at 1996/7 prices.

**Table 7.3.1** Drug costs and costs of renal and upper gastrointestinal adverse events with low dose aspirin

| | Costs (£) over an average follow up of 2.5 years per patient | | | |
|---|---|---|---|---|
| | Aspirin users | Controls | Excess cost | Excess cost (£)/year |
| **Drug costs** | | | | |
| Aspirin | 4.95 | | 4.95 | 1.96 |
| Dispensing cost | 13.89 | | 13.89 | 5.49 |
| Total drug cost | 18.84 | | 18.84 | 7.45 |
| **Renal costs** | | | | |
| Renal admission | 16.02 | 2.20 | 13.84 | 5.47 |
| Dialysis | 44.69 | 13.46 | 31.22 | 12.34 |
| Total renal cost | 60.71 | 15.66 | 45.06 | 17.81 |
| **Gastrointestinal costs** | | | | |
| GI admission | 3.66 | 2.40 | 1.26 | 0.50 |
| Endoscopy | 44.19 | 18.99 | 25.19 | 9.96 |
| Anti-ulcer drugs | 46.72 | 10.95 | 35.80 | 14.15 |
| Total GI cost | 94.57 | 32.34 | 62.25 | 24.60 |
| **Total cost** | 174.12 | 48.00 | 126.15 | **49.86** |

Actual exposure was 1.18 years of the average 2.53 years between the first prescription and end of the study.

It also examined costs per event prevented, using information from the largest meta-analysis. Using the benefit of 16 events prevented per 1000 people treated per year after a heart attack, the cost of one vascular event prevented would be £3330. This used the pragmatic analysis and average costs over 2.5 years, not the 1.2 years of actual exposure, which would double the figure. At lower levels of cardiovascular risk the cost per event prevented rises substantially.

It is interesting to speculate on how many patients, at whatever level of risk, are given the full figures of benefit and harm to help them make up their own minds about treatment. It is also interesting to reflect on the huge increases in prescribing of low-dose aspirin and proton pump inhibitors, and the costs, and wonder whether better targeting of therapy to patients might make even better sense of guidance and received wisdom.

## Topical NSAIDs

How readers react to a section about topical NSAIDs for musculoskeletal pain depends on where they live and what they do. In much of continental Europe topical NSAIDs are accepted as effective, and are much used. In the USA, the FDA has been circumspect, with concerns over efficacy because of limitations in design of older trials. In the UK topical NSAIDs are licensed and are considered effective by many primary care physicians but not by prescribing authorities, so their use is often considered a marker of bad prescribing.

A brief run down of the evidence goes something like this, from two recent systematic reviews [4, 5].

- Topical NSAIDs were well investigated in acute painful conditions (musculoskeletal in nature like strains and sprains) in over 3000 patients in trials using 1-week outcomes.
- Topical NSAID was significantly better than placebo in 19 of the 26 trials, with a pooled relative benefit of 1.6 (1.4–1.7), and NNT of 3.8 (3.4–4.4) compared with placebo for the outcome of half pain relief at 7 days; 65% of patients had at least half pain relief with topical NSAID. Ketoprofen was significantly better than all other topical NSAIDs.
- Topical NSAIDs were well investigated in chronic painful conditions (musculoskeletal in nature) in over 3000 patients in trials using 2-week outcomes.
- Topical NSAIDs were clearly better than placebo in chronic musculoskeletal pain, with an NNT of 4.4 (3.6–5.6) in the best trials; 48% of patients had at least half pain relief with topical NSAID. Studies were generally of short duration, and no single preparation could be shown to be better than another. No study showed oral NSAID to be better than topical NSAID.
- Longer duration trials of topical diclofenac have lasted 12 weeks, and include comparisons with placebo and oral diclofenac 150 mg daily in large, high-quality studies. Topical diclofenac was superior to placebo and as effective as oral diclofenac, but with many fewer serious gastro-intestinal adverse events, and less anaemia [6].
- Local adverse events, systemic adverse events, or withdrawals due to an adverse event were rare, and no different between topical NSAID and placebo.

- Large-scale observational studies fail to associate topical NSAIDs with any increased risk of gastrointestinal bleeding. The mechanism for this safety is very much lower blood NSAID concentrations with topical than oral NSAID, and this should also protect against renal problems of congestive heart failure [7].

What is interesting is that for some patients with limited joint problems, perhaps early in the progression of arthritis, topical NSAID will be an effective and safe option. The weight of evidence is considerable for efficacy and safety. Yet physicians are told that it is 'just the rubbing' and that topical rubefacients are just as effective, when we know that they are not [8].

## Commentary

Just as in the previous section where we were able to castigate the media for their inattention to evidence, and perhaps for choosing evidence they felt fuelled their own agenda, we can see much the same thing happening to medical professionals. We should not adopt a 'holier than thou' attitude. The acceptance and use of evidence within health-care is a long way from fulfilment.

## References

1. Antithrombotic Trialists' Collaboration (2002). Collaborative meta-analysis of randomised trials of antiplatelet therapy for prevention of death, myocardial infarction, and stroke in high risk patients. *British Medical Journal* **324**, 71–86.
2. Higham, J. *et al.* (2002). Recent trends in admissions and mortality due to peptic ulcer in England: increasing frequency of haemorrhage among older subjects. *Gut* **50**, 460–4.
3. Morant, S.V. *et al.* (2003). Cardiovascular prophylaxis with aspirin: costs of supply and management of upper gastrointestinal and renal toxicity. *British Journal of Clinical Pharmacology* **57**, 188–98.
4. Mason, L. *et al.* (2004). Topical NSAIDs for acute pain: a meta-analysis. *BMC Family Practice* **5**, 10 (http://www.biomedcentral.com/1471–2296/5/10).
5. Mason, L. *et al.* (2004). Topical NSAIDs for chronic musculoskeletal pain: systematic review and meta-analysis. *BMC Musculoskeletal Disorders* **5**, 28 (http://www.biomedcentral.com/1471–2474/5/28).
6. Evans, J.M. *et al.* (1995). Topical non-steroidal anti-inflammatory drugs and admission to hospital for upper gastrointestinal bleeding and perforation: a record linkage case-control study. *British Medical Journal* **311**, 22–6.
7. Tugwell, P.S. *et al.* (2004). Equivalence study of a topical diclofenac solution (PENNSAID) compared with oral diclofenac in the symptomatic treatment of osteoarthritis of the knee: a randomized controlled study. *Journal of Rheumatology* **31**, 2002–12.
8. Mason, L. *et al.* (2004). Systematic review of efficacy of topical rubefacients containing salicylates for the treatment of acute and chronic pain. *British Medical Journal* **328**, 995–8.

# 7.4 Wrongdoing

Wrongdoing exists in science and medicine at various levels and is of various types. Mistakes can be made and can be put right [1]. For the purposes of this book, the types of wrongdoing that interest us are where data are manipulated to change a result, frankly fraudulent, or where a conflict of interest develops from potential to actual distortion. None of this has a massive evidence base, and what we have are some cases, often seen and written about from different perspectives. Let's look at them separately.

## Data manipulation, or fraud

### Duplicate publication

We have already met one clear example of data manipulation in Chapter 2.4, when we examined the effects of duplicate publication on expectation of efficacy [2, 3]. The more recent of these investigations examined 56 systematic reviews with 1131 papers and 129,337 subjects. It found 103 duplicates with 12,589 subjects originating from 78 main articles. Sixty articles were published twice, 13 three times, 3 four times, and 2 five times. So almost 10% of the published articles and subjects were in duplicate publications.

The authors identified six duplication patterns:

- (1A) identical samples and identical outcomes (21 pairs);
- (1B) same as 1A but several duplicates assembled ($n = 16$);
- (2) identical samples and different outcomes ($n = 24$);
- (3A) increasing sample and identical outcomes ($n = 11$);
- (3B) decreasing sample and identical outcomes ($n = 11$);
- (4) different samples and different outcomes ($n = 20$).

The prevalence of **covert** duplicate articles, that is, those without a cross-reference to the main article, was 5.3% (65/1234). Of the duplicates, 34 (33%) were sponsored by the pharmaceutical industry, and 66 (64%) had authorship that differed partly or completely from the main article.

Duplication goes beyond simple copying. The importance of covert duplication is that it makes it appear as if there is a larger literature than actually exists. Covert duplication has fooled many clever people doing systematic reviews, people who normally have particular sensitivity to problems in articles. Most of us who are not professional reviewers would be easily fooled.

### Geography and publication bias

We have also met the topic of geography bias [4]. It is an obvious thing to say that many experiments do not work, whether at the bench or in the clinic. Clinical trials are usually designed statistically so that they will come up with a significant result if one is there 80 or 90 times out of 100. So 10 or 20 times out of 100 trials should have a negative result. So, if trials of acupuncture or any clinical intervention from a particular region are positive 99% of time, clearly something is going on. The conclusion drawn is that only positive trials are published, so that this is a form of publication bias. True publication bias, suppressing the publication of negative results, is another form of wrongdoing, as is the selective reporting of trial outcomes [5], though that may be more a reflection of size restrictions on papers.

*Overgood results*

It is difficult to discuss true fraud, the manipulation or manufacture of results, because cases appear so infrequently, and because almost anything one says is liable to be pored over by lawyers looking for an angle. There are clear examples of fraud, for instance, where papers are published from data that are just made up [6]. There are also many suggestions for dealing with fraud that is clear or missed [6], including auditing a proportion of submitted papers down to the original data, much as happens with modern clinical trials. The complexities of getting at research fraud are great, though, and demonstrated by two articles in the *British Medical Journal* in 2005 in which investigations of suspected fraud are outlined [7, 8].

Knowing when to be suspicious is difficult, as there are no rules, though a plethora of trials from a single small organization might make one's antennae twitch. Another concern is when results are very good, in the face of the known power of random chance. An example of this is the effect of policosanol on cholesterol.

Policosanol is a mixture of long-chain primary alcohols isolated from sugar cane wax. The main components are octacosanol (about 65%), triacosanol (about 12%), and hexacosanol (7%). Similar alcohols are found in other plant materials, such as wheat germ and rice bran, and in beeswax. A systematic review [9] found 24 reports of placebo-controlled trials of Cuban sugar cane policosanol, and one of wheat germ policosanol. All studies but one were double-blind. The mean age of patients in the trials was 50–67 years, and there were more women than men. The dose of policosanol used was 2–40 mg/day, with most patients receiving 5–10 mg/day. The duration of the studies ranged from 30 days to 24 months. For the two trials of 24 months, 12-month lipid levels were used in the analysis to make them more comparable with the other studies.

Figure 7.4.1 shows the effects of policosanol on total cholesterol in these studies, most of which had fewer than 100 patients treated with policosanol. There was a consistent effect for the sugar cane product, but no effect for the wheat germ product. There was very much less variability for the policosanol studies than for similar-sized studies of total cholesterol reduction with simvastatin (Figure 7.4.2).

How might we interpret this? This set of trials shows that Cuban sugar cane policosanol reduces total and low density lipoprotein cholesterol by an amount equivalent to that achieved by statins. There are two catches.

The first catch is in the amazing consistency of the results for policosanol from Cuban sugar cane. As Figure 7.4.1 shows, all of the larger trials found exactly the same 15–16% reduction in total cholesterol. This was regardless of patient characteristics, duration of study (though most were longer than 6 weeks), or dose of policosanol. Moreover, almost all studies on Cuban policosanol come from a small number of researchers in a small number of institutions in Cuba. But the very considerable variation in percentage cholesterol reduction for group sizes below 300 patients in simvastatin trials suggests that the consistency in the policosanol studies is rather special.

The second catch is that all these studies used policosanol manufactured by one company. Policosanol manufactured from other sources such as wheat germ has not been effective in lowering cholesterol despite having

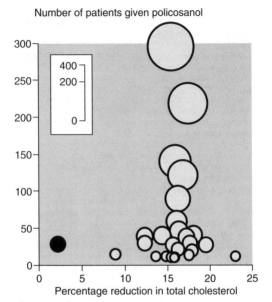

**Figure 7.4.1** Percentage reduction in total cholesterol with sugar cane polico-sanol (light fill) and wheat germ policosanol (dark fill).

very similar chemical composition. The mechanism of action is not under-stood.

To have any confidence we need:
- independent verification from studies outside Cuba on the Cuban poli-cosanol;
- studies of Cuban and other policosanols in non-Hispanic populations;
- these studies should last at least 12 weeks, and compare policosanol with both placebo and statins.

What this graphical way of looking at evidence demonstrates is that over-precision should make us worry about results, especially when trials are small. Variability is the norm. Variability is what we should expect. Lack of variability is a concern.

### Conflicts of interest

Conflicts of interest abound. For instance, a financial conflict of interest (COI) occurs when a person owns shares in a company and writes a paper about a product from that company. It is assumed that natural behaviour is to praise the product in order to increase the company's share price and thus become individually wealthier.

How much of a conflict of interest this actually is might depend on whether the individual held stock personally or through a pension fund

Number of patients given any dose of simvastatin

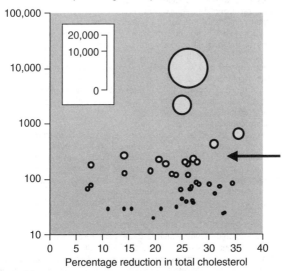

**Figure 7.4.2** Percentage reduction in total cholesterol in randomized studies of simvastatin (any dose) of 12 weeks or longer. The arrow shows the maximum group size in policosanol studies. Note the logarithmic scale for trial size.

divorced from his or her influence, or whether he or she was a major shareholder in a new start-up company, or whether he or she was involved with an intermediate company such as a clinical trials organization or even an academic institution depending on industry grants. It is difficult, and complex, and almost impossible to unravel. To try and address some of the issues, conflict of interest committees have been set up to evaluate faculty financial COI and to develop strategies to eliminate, reduce, or manage such conflicts [10].

This is important. It has also been suggested that the potential threat of funding bias is neither recognized nor taken seriously by clinical investigators [11], over a quarter of whom have industry affiliations [12]. According to some sources, the majority of US and UK consumers now believe that potential gain for scientists could affect research quality and are concerned with the commercialization of research.

Much of the financial intercourse between industry, academia, medical practitioners, journals, and other health organizations is well known, and much discussed. A recent survey of sources of financial support in healthcare organizations in Australia received 29 responses; 17 of these organizations (59%) had received support from one or more pharmaceutical company in the past financial year. Support was predominantly for annual conferences, with some support for continuing medical education, research, travel, and library purchases [13].

When conflicts of interest are unstated things get more difficult. For instance, a review of homeopathy claimed no conflicts of interest. Yet the writers of the original papers were predominantly homeopathic practitioners, as were the authors of the review, receiving a grant from a charity for homeopathy and working in an homeopathic organization. So no conflict of interest there, then.

The absence of industry funding does not imply no conflict of interest. There is no simple answer, but the most sensible thing is to assume that conflicts of interest apply in all cases. Let's take two examples of how prevalent conflict of interest is likely to be.

One study looked at a consecutive series of 332 randomized trials published between January 1999 and June 2001 in 13 leading medical and surgical journals [14]. It found that industry funding was most often associated with drug trials, but that surgical and other interventions often had no reported funding source (Table 7.4.1). Statistically significant results were frequent, occurring in two-thirds or more trials.

A survey in the dermatological literature [15] looked at 179 clinical trials published between October 2000 and October 2003. At least one conflict of interest by at least one author occurred in 43% of these trials. Studies with sponsorship or with conflicts of interest were much more likely to have higher quality scores, adequate blinding, be much larger (median numbers about three times larger in sponsored studies), and be more likely to have a positive result. Sponsored studies were more likely to fulfil criteria of quality, validity, and size.

## Right to publish

A topic not often discussed, but of real importance, is a researcher's right to publish. Research agreements between academia and industry often include a veto on publication if it is in the interest of one or more parties. This will usually be related to early-phase research, where publication might preclude later patents. Industry and academia welcome patents as ways of protecting and benefiting from the results of research, and it might well be considered the proper course of action.

This would not be the proper course of action, though, for clinical research. No veto over clinical research should be allowed, though it can still happen, sometimes at the behest of academic institutions overly reliant

**Table 7.4.1**  Sponsorship in randomized trials

| Funding | Drug | Surgery | Other |
|---|---|---|---|
| Industry (%) | 62 | 18 | 9 |
| Government or foundation (%) | 15 | 11 | 37 |
| None reported (%) | 23 | 70 | 54 |
| Statistically significant outcomes (%) | 64 | 74 | 70 |
| Industry-funded favouring industry product (%) | 34 | 81 | 25 |

on external funding. Insisting on the right to publish is an interesting test of an organization; clinical researchers might wish to work with those who don't have a problem with a right to publish, and be wary or avoid those that insist upon a veto.

### Scientists behaving badly

The thing with quality control is that the more you look, the more problems you find. An electronic survey of over 3600 US scientists asked questions about possible behaviours, using questions built around results of earlier focus groups [16]. Scientists had to answer the questions in a yes or no fashion. The results (Table 7.4.2) show that some behaviours that might be regarded as questionable were not uncommon, although how common and how serious they were varied. For instance, duplicate publication was attested to by about 5% of scientists, about the same order as the number of duplicate publications. Only 0.3% (3 in 1000) falsified data, though 15% ignored data they felt was wrong.

**Table 7.4.2** Percentage of scientists who engaged in various behaviours within previous 3 years. The first 10 questions were the survey 'top ten'

|    | Behaviour | % |
|----|-----------|---|
| 1  | Falsifying or cooking research data | 0.3 |
| 2  | Ignoring major aspects of human–subject requirements | 0.3 |
| 3  | Not properly disclosing involvement in firms whose products are based on one's own research | 0.3 |
| 4  | Relationships with students, research subjects, or clients that may be interpreted as questionable | 1.4 |
| 5  | Using another's ideas without obtaining permission or giving due credit | 1.4 |
| 6  | Unauthorized use of confidential information in connection with one's own research | 1.7 |
| 7  | Failing to present data that contradicts one's own research | 6.0 |
| 8  | Circumventing certain minor aspects of human–subject requirements | 7.6 |
| 9  | Overlooking other's use of flawed data or questionable interpretation | 12.5 |
| 10 | Changing the design, methodology, or results of a study in response to pressure from a funding source | 15.5 |
| 11 | Publishing the same data in two or more publications | 4.7 |
| 12 | Inappropriately assigning authorship credit | 10.0 |
| 13 | Withholding details of methodology or results in papers or proposals | 10.8 |
| 14 | Using inadequate or inappropriate research designs | 13.5 |
| 15 | Dropping observations or data points from analyses based on a gut feel that they were inaccurate | 15.3 |
| 16 | Inadequate record-keeping related to research projects | 27.5 |

## Commentary

This section is not here to frighten, but to inform. Conflict of interest is clearly going to continue to be a major feature in clinical and nonclinical research, and research misconduct clearly requires policing. But to a large extent that policing is already in place with clinical trials research, where good clinical practice guidelines exist, where trials have to pass through extensive ethical considerations, where considerable trial monitoring goes on, and where there are often independent data monitoring committees. There may be conflicts of interest, but these larger trials, often but not always performed by industry, are of high quality and unlikely to be open to abuse.

Proposals by the world's major pharmaceutical industry trade associations, and agreed by major companies, should make complete suppression bias unlikely. Results of all industry-sponsored clinical trials evaluating safety and benefit of a medicine approved for marketing will be publicly available regardless of outcome. Details of all new clinical trials will also be publicly registered in advance, so that patients and clinicians will have information about how to enrol. Both requirements are likely to be adopted by the worldwide pharmaceutical industry during 2005.

Moreover, from July 2005 member journals of the International Committee of Medical Journal Editors will require, as a condition of publication of a trial, that it was registered in a public trials registry before patient enrolment [17]. Such a policy, if extended, should remove much of the disquiet about possible unpublished trials, and should increase transparency in performance and reporting of clinical trials.

It is naïve to assume that, because a paper reaches a particular conclusion, it must be certainly true. Yet many people seem to consider that publication of any piece of research in a peer-reviewed journal provides sufficient credibility for decision-making. It doesn't.

## References

1. Hawthorne, G. *et al.* (2003). Retraction of a paper on maternal diabetes. *British Medical Journal* **327**, 929.
2. Tramèr, M.R. *et al.* (1997). Impact of covert duplicate publication on meta-analysis: a case study. *British Medical Journal* **315**, 635–9.
3. Von Elm, E. *et al.* (2004). Different patterns of duplicate publication. An analysis of articles used in systematic reviews. *Journal of the American Medical Association* **291**, 974–80.
4. Vickers, A. *et al.* (1998). Do certain countries produce only positive results? A systematic review of controlled trials. *Controlled Clinical Trials* **19**, 159–66.
5. Chan, A.W. *et al.* (2004). Empirical evidence for selective reporting of outcomes in randomized trials: comparison of protocols to published articles. *Journal of the American Medical Association* **291**, 2457–65.
6. Lock, S. (1995). Lessons from the Pearce affair: handling scientific fraud. *British Medical Journal* **310**, 1547–8.
7. White, C. (2005). Suspected research fraud: difficulties of getting at the truth. *British Medical Journal* **331**, 281–8.
8. Smith, R. (2005). Investigating the previous studies of a fraudulent author. *British Medical Journal* **331**, 288–91.
9. Bandolier Extra. Policosanol. (*http://www.jr2.ox.ac.uk/bandolier/Ectraforbando/Policosanol.pdf*).
10. Rubin, E.H. (2005). The complexities of individual financial conflicts of interest. *Neuropsychopharmacology* **30**, 1–6.

11. Boyd, E.A. *et al.* (2003). Financial conflict-of-interest policies in clinical research: issues for clinical investigators. *Academic Medicine* **78**, 769–74.
12. Bekelman, J.E. *et al.* (2003). Scope and impact of financial conflicts of interest in biomedical research: a systematic review. *Journal of the American Medical Association* **289**, 454–65.
13. Kerridge, I. *et al.* (2005). Cooperative partnerships or conflict-of-interest? A national survey of interaction between the pharmaceutical industry and medical organizations. *Internal Medicine Journal* **35**, 206–10.
14. Bhandari, M. *et al.* (2004). Association between industry funding and statistically significant pro-industry findings in medical and surgical randomized trials. *Canadian Medical Association Journal* **170**, 477–80.
15. Perlis, C.S. *et al.* (2005). Extent and impact of industry sponsorship conflicts of interest in dermatology research. *Journal of the American Academy of Dermatology* **52**, 967–71.
16. Martinson, B.C. *et al.* (2005). Scientists behaving badly. *Nature* **435**, 737–8.
17. DeAngelis, C.D. *et al.* (2004). Clinical trial registration: a statement from the International Committee of Medical Journal Editors. *Journal of the American Medical Association* **292**, 1363–4.

# Section 8

# Glossary

We use an awful lot of jargon in science and medicine. It is inevitable to keep sentences and paragraphs short, but using a plethora of technical terms can lock newcomers out of the magic circle of initiated cognoscenti. The trouble is that resort to jargon can lead to other difficulties, mainly because people use the same jargon terms to describe different things; the result is confusion, a bit like the order, counterorder, disorder of the battlefield. As far as possible, key technical terms have been explained in the text. Some either have not been used, or perhaps we overlooked defining them. In any event, this glossary is intended as a place of sanctuary if all else fails.

**Absolute risk reduction/increase**. The absolute arithmetic difference in rates of bad outcomes between experimental and control participants in a trial, calculated as the experimental event rate (EER) and the control event rate (CER), and accompanied by a 95% CI. Depending on circumstances it can be reduction in risk (death or cardiovascular outcomes, for instance, in trials of statins) or an increase in benefit (pain relief, for instance, in trials of analgesics).

**Adverse drug reaction**. An appreciably harmful or unpleasant reaction, resulting from an intervention related to the use of a medicinal product, that predicts hazard from future administration and warrants prevention or specific treatment or alteration of the dosage regimen or withdrawal of the product.

**Adverse effect**. As for adverse drug reaction, but applied to all interventions, not just drug interventions.

- The 'safety' of an intervention relates to its potential to cause serious adverse effects. 'Tolerability' relates to medically less important but unpleasant adverse effects of drugs. These include symptoms such as dry mouth, tiredness, etc. that can affect a person's quality of life and willingness to continue the treatment.
- A 'serious' adverse effect is one that has significant medical consequences, such as death, permanent disability, prolonged hospitalization. Indirect adverse effects, such as traffic accidents, violence, and damaging consequences of mood change, can also be serious.
- 'Severe' refers to the intensity of a particular adverse effect. For example, a non-serious adverse effect, such as headache, may be severe in intensity (as opposed to mild or moderate). A 'non-serious' effect, such as impotence, can have major consequences for a person's quality of life.

**Adverse event**. An adverse outcome occurring during or after the use of a drug or other intervention but not necessarily caused by it.

**Average**. A measure for the central tendency of a sample of observations. The term average is most often used for the arithmetic mean, but sometimes also for the median. For instance, suppose the yearly incomes of five people are $50,000, $80,000, $100,000, $120,000, and $650,000, respectively. The arithmetic mean is the sum of these values divided by the number of values, that is, $200,000. The median is obtained by ranking the values (as above) and taking the one in the middle, that is, $100,000. When the distribution is asymmetric, as it often is with income, the mean and the median are not the same, and it can be the case that most people earn less than the mean, with a few people having very high incomes.

Another example is with legs. Most people (99.9%) have two legs. But some have had amputations or accidents, so the average number of legs in the population is less than two. Therefore 99.9% of the population have more legs than average.

**A priori**. *A priori* comparisons are planned in advance of any data analysis. They are more reliable than *post hoc* comparisons.

**Bayes theorem**. Thomas Bayes (1702–61) was a mathematician who first used probability inductively and established a mathematical basis for probability inference (a means of calculating, from the number of times an event has not occured, the probability that it will occur in future trials). He set down his findings on probability in 'Essay towards solving a problem in the doctrine of chances' (1763), published posthumously in the *Philosophical Transactions of the Royal Society of London*. There is a whole school of Bayesian statistics, the subject of many books, though how much is due to Bayes and how much to Richard Price is another matter.

Richard Price was born in Tynton, Llangeinor, in 1723 and was friendly with Bayes before his death, and Bayes's relatives asked Price to examine his unpublished papers. Price realized their importance and submitted 'An essay towards solving a problem in the doctrine of chances' to the Royal Society. In this work Price, using the information provided by Bayes, introduced the idea of estimating the probability of an event from the frequency of its previous occurrences.

In 1765 Price was admitted to the Royal Society for his work on probability. He also began collecting information on life expectation and in May 1770 he wrote to the Royal Society about the proper method of calculating the values of contingent reversions. It is believed that this information drew attention to the inadequate calculations on which many insurance and benefit societies had recently been formed, and Price could be regarded as the father (or at least the midwife) of epidemiology. There have been suggestions that Price contributed more to what we know as Bayes theorem than Bayes himself did.

**Bias**. A dictionary definition of bias is 'a one-sided inclination of the mind'. It defines a systematic disposition of certain trial designs to produce results consistently better or worse than other trial designs. Bias occurs in many different ways in all types of study, and avoiding or checking for known sources of bias is one of the most important elements in assessing the quality and validity of evidence. Unless it is done, it renders any evidence worthless.

**Blinding**. The process used in epidemiological studies and clinical trials in which the participants, investigators, and/or assessors remain ignorant concerning the treatments which participants are receiving. In single-blind studies only participants are blind to their allocations, while in double-blind studies at minimum the participants and assessors are blind to their allocations. Occasionally, even higher levels of blinding are found, when exigencies of design demand it.

**Care pathway (or integrated care pathway)**. An integrated care pathway (ICP) is a multidisciplinary outline of anticipated care, placed in an appropriate timeframe, to help a patient with a specific condition or set of symptoms move progressively through a clinical experience to positive outcomes. Variations from the pathway may occur as clinical freedom is exercised to meet the needs of the individual patient.

ICPs are important because they help to reduce unnecessary variations in patient care and outcomes. They support the development of care partnerships and can empower patients and their carers. ICPs can also be used as a tool to incorporate local and national guidelines into everyday practice, manage clinical risk, and meet the requirements of clinical governance. When designing and introducing ICPs, it is important to incorporate them into organizational strategy and choose appropriate topics that will provide opportunities for improvement.

**Case-control study**. A study that involves identifying patients who have the outcome of interest (cases) and control patients who do not have that same outcome and looking back to see if they had the exposure of interest. The exposure could be some environmental factor, a behavioural factor, or exposure to a drug or other therapeutic intervention.

**Case report**. A report on a single patient with an outcome of interest.

**Case series**. A report on a series of patients with an outcome of interest. No control group is involved. For both case reports and case series there are useful guidelines about maximizing their evidential value.

**Class effect**. When it is assumed that all interventions of the same sort or with the same mechanism of action generate rather similar effects, or that particular effects both in nature and extent are associated with interventions of that type. Criteria for drugs to be grouped together as a class involve some or all of the following:

- drugs with similar chemical structure;
- drugs with similar mechanism of action;
- drugs with similar pharmacological effects.

Guidelines have been set out for what constitutes a class effect.

**Clinical practice guideline**. A systematically developed statement designed to assist clinician and patient decisions about appropriate health-care for specific clinical circumstances. Guidelines should be based on evidence, combined with local knowledge to ensure that they are appropriate for local conditions.

**Clinical trial**. A research study conducted with patients that tests out a drug or other intervention to assess its effectiveness and safety. Each trial is designed to answer scientific questions and to find better ways to treat individuals with a specific disease. This general term encompasses controlled clinical trials and randomized controlled trials.

A controlled clinical trial (CCT) is a study testing a specific drug or other treatment involving two (or more) groups of patients with the same disease. One (the experimental group) receives the treatment that is being tested, and the other (the comparison or control group) receives an alternative treatment, a placebo (dummy treatment), or no treatment. The two groups are followed up to compare differences in outcomes to see how effective the experimental treatment was. A CCT where patients are randomly allocated to treatment and comparison groups is called a randomized controlled trial.

**Clouded thinking**. A form of innumeracy, in which a person knows about the risks but not how to draw conclusions or inferences from them. For instance, physicians often know the error rates of mammography and the base rate of breast cancer, but not how to infer from this information the chances that a woman with a positive test actually has breast cancer.

Mind tools for overcoming clouded thinking, such as natural frequencies, are representations that facilitate drawing conclusions.

**Cohort study**. Involves identification of two groups (cohorts) of patients —one that received the exposure of interest and one that did not—and following these cohorts forward for the outcome of interest.

**Concealment of allocation**. The process used to prevent foreknowledge of group assignment in a randomized controlled trial, which should be seen as distinct from blinding. The allocation process should be impervious to any influence by the individual making the allocation by having the randomization process administered by someone who is not responsible for recruiting participants, for example, a hospital pharmacy or a central office. Methods of assignment such as date of birth and case record numbers (see quasi-random allocation) are open to manipulation. Adequate methods of allocation concealment include: centralized randomization schemes; randomization schemes controlled by a pharmacy; numbered or coded containers in which capsules from identical-looking, numbered bottles are administered sequentially; on-site computer systems, where allocations are in a locked unreadable file; and sequentially numbered opaque, sealed envelopes.

**Confidence interval (CI)**. Quantifies the uncertainty in measurement. It is usually reported as 95% CI, which is the range of values within which we can be 95% sure that the true value for the whole population lies. For example, for an NNT of 10 with a 95% CI of 5–15, we would have 95% confidence that the true NNT value was between 5 and 15.

A caveat is that the confidence interval relates to the population sampled. If we have a small sample of part of a population, or a very small sample of the whole population, then the confidence interval that is generated is not necessarily that for the whole population.

**Conflict of interest**. A conflict of interest occurs when those who are involved with the conduct or reporting of research also have financial or other interests, or where they can benefit in some other way, depending on the results of the research. The obvious example is where a company reports results of a trial of its product.

Conflict of interest statements often accompany published papers. They consist of a statement by a contributor to a report or review of personal, financial, or other interests that could have influenced the findings or their interpretation. Conflicts of interest are the norm, and not the exception.

The point about a conflict of interest is that a reader needs to know that it is there. It should not, and probably most of the time does not, impart any effect on the results of a trial. But it might, and if we discovered a conflict of interest at some later time, when it had been hidden, we would be concerned.

In relationships with industry, which often funds clinical trials or reviews, there are some things to look for. Most important is freedom to publish, whatever the result, the result of a trial or a review. That is the key element that most folks forget. If it is a review of otherwise unpublished material, it is worth looking for a declaration that all available trials had been made available.

**Confounding**. Confounding refers to a situation in which a measure of the effect of an intervention or exposure is distorted because of the association of exposure with other factor(s) that influence the outcome under investigation. This can lead to erroneous conclusions being drawn, particularly in observational studies.

**Confounding by indication**. This bias can arise in observational studies when patients with the worst prognosis are allocated preferentially to a particular treatment. These patients are likely to be systematically different from those not treated, or treated with something else.

**CONSORT**. The CONSORT statement is an important research tool that takes an evidence-based approach to improve the quality of reports of randomized trials. The statement is available in six languages and has been endorsed by prominent medical journals such as *The Lancet, Annals of Internal Medicine*, and the *Journal of the American Medical Association*. Its critical value to researchers, health-care providers, peer reviewers, journal editors, and health policy-makers is the guarantee of integrity in the reported results of research.

CONSORT comprises a checklist and flow diagram to help improve the quality of reports of randomized controlled trials. It offers a standard way for researchers to report trials. The checklist includes items, based on evidence, that need to be addressed in the report; the flow diagram provides readers with a clear picture of the progress of all participants in the trial, from the time they are randomized until the end of their involvement. The intent is to make the experimental process more clear, flawed or not, so that users of the data can more appropriately evaluate its validity for their purposes.

**Control**. A control is something against which we make a comparison. If we put large amounts of manure on our roses (an experimental group), we might want to find out what happened to roses on which no manure was used (control group). There can be all sorts of types and names for controls, some appropriate, others not.

- In clinical trials comparing two or more interventions, a control is a person in the comparison group who receives a placebo, no intervention, usual care, or another form of care.
- In case-control studies a control is a person in the comparison group without the disease or outcome of interest.
- In statistics control means to adjust for or take into account extraneous influences or observations.
- Control can also mean programmes aimed at reducing or eliminating the disease when applied to communicable (infectious) diseases.

**Control event rate (CER)**. The rate at which events occur in a control group. It may be represented by a percentage (say, 10%) or as a proportion (when it is 0.1).

**Cost–benefit analysis**. Assesses whether the cost of an intervention is worth the benefit by measuring both in the same units; monetary units are usually used.

**Cost-effectiveness analysis**. Measures the net cost of providing a service as well as the outcomes obtained. Outcomes are reported in a single unit of measurement.

**Cost minimization analysis**. If health effects are known to be equal, only costs are analysed and the least costly alternative is chosen.

**Cost utility analysis**. Converts effects into personal preferences (or utilities) and describes how much it costs for some additional quality gain (e.g. cost per additional quality-adjusted life-year, or QALY).

**Cox model**. A Cox model is a well-recognized statistical technique for exploring the relationship between the survival of a patient and several explanatory variables.

- Survival analysis is concerned with studying the time between entry to a study and a subsequent event (such as death). Censored survival times occur if the event of interest does not occur for a patient during the study period.
- A Cox model provides an estimate of the treatment effect on survival after adjustment for other explanatory variables. It allows us to estimate the hazard (or risk) of death, or other event of interest, for individuals, given their prognostic variables.
- Even if the treatment groups are similar with respect to the variables known to affect survival, using the Cox model with these prognostic variables may produce a more precise estimate of the treatment effect (for example, by narrowing the confidence interval).
- Interpreting a Cox model involves examining the coefficients for each explanatory variable. A positive regression coefficient for an explanatory variable means that the hazard is higher, and thus the prognosis worse, for higher values. Conversely, a negative regression coefficient implies a better prognosis for patients with higher values of that variable.

**Critical appraisal**. The process of assessing and interpreting evidence by systematically considering its validity, results, and relevance. This sounds great, and often is. Of course, one needs to look at different forms of evidence differently—controlled trials versus observational studies, for instance, or diagnostic studies, or health economic studies. A number of schema have been developed for doing this, and are useful. The trouble is that any one of them can be wrong for a given paper, because some things are hard to define, such as what constitutes a valid or relevant study.

For evidence to be strong, it has to fulfil the requirements of all three of the following criteria—quality, validity, and size.

- Quality. Trials that are randomized and double-blind, to avoid selection and observer bias, and where we know what happened to most of the subjects in the trial.
- Validity. Trials that mimic clinical practice, or could be used in clinical practice, and with outcomes that make sense. For instance, in chronic disorders we want long—not short—term trials. We are not interested in small but marginally statistically significant ($p < 0.05$, say, or a 1 in 20 chance of being wrong) outcomes, but rather outcomes that are large, useful, and statistically very significant ($p < 0.01$, a 1 in 100 chance of being wrong).
- Size. Trials (or collections of trials) that have large numbers of patients, to avoid being wrong because of the random play of chance. For instance, be sure that a number needed to treat (NNT) of 2.5 is really between 2 and 3, we need results from about 500 patients. If that NNT is above 5, we need data from thousands of patients.

**Cross-over study design**. The administration of two or more experimental therapies one after the other in a specified or random order to the same group of patients. There are some important issues with cross-over designs. Two in particular often crop up.

- First is the issue of order effects, in which the order in which treatments are administered may affect the outcome. An example might be a drug with many adverse events given first making patients taking a second, less harmful medicine more sensitive to any adverse effect.
- Second is the issue of carry-over between treatments. In practice carry-over can be dealt with by use of a wash-out period between treatments, or by making observations sufficiently later after the start of a treatment period that any carry-over effect is minimized.

**Cross-sectional study**. The observation of a defined population at a signal point in time or time interval. Exposure and outcome are determined simultaneously.

**Cumulative meta-analysis**. In cumulative meta-analysis, studies are added one at a time in a specified order (e.g. according to date of publication or quality) and the results are summarized as each new study is added. In a graph of a cumulative meta-analysis, each horizontal line represents the summary of the results as each study is added, rather than the results of a single study.

**Decision analysis (or clinical decision analysis)**. The application of explicit, quantitative methods that quantify prognoses, treatment effects, and patient values in order to analyse a decision under conditions of uncertainty.

**Duplication**. Trials can be reported more than once, a process known as duplication. Duplication can be justified, for instance, where results from a study at 2 years are followed later by results at 4 years. Another example might be reporting different results from a single trials (clinical or economic, for instance). But multiple publication can also be covert, and lead to overestimation of the amount of information available.

**Ecological survey**. A survey based on aggregated data for some population as it exists at some point or points in time: to investigate the relationship of an exposure to a known or presumed risk factor for a specified outcome.

**Effect size**. This is the standardized effect observed. By standardizing the effect, the effect size becomes dimensionless (and that can be helpful when pooling data). The effect size then becomes:

- a generic term for the estimate of effect for a study;
- a dimensionless measure of effect that is typically used for continuous data when different scales (e.g. for measuring pain) are used to measure an outcome and is usually defined as the difference in means between the intervention and control groups divided by the standard deviation of the control or both groups.

The effect size can be just the difference between the mean values of the two groups, divided by the standard deviation, as below, but there are other ways to calculate effect size in other circumstances.

Effect size = (mean of experimental group − mean of control group)/ standard deviation.

Generally, the larger the effect size, the greater is the impact of an intervention. Jacob Cohen has written the most on this topic. In his well-known book he suggested, a little ambiguously, that a correlation of 0.5 is large, 0.3 is moderate, and 0.1 is small (Cohen, J. (1988). *Statistical power analysis for the behavioral sciences*, 2nd edn. Lawrence Erlbaum, New Jersey). The usual interpretation of this statement is that anything greater than 0.5 is large, 0.5–0.3 is moderate, 0.3–0.1 is small, and anything smaller than 0.1 is trivial. There is a good site that describes all this and is worth a visit for those really interested (*http://davidmlane.com/hyperstat/effect_size.html*).

**Empirical**. Empirical results are based on experience (or observation) rather than on reasoning alone.

**Epidemiology**. The study of the distribution and determinants of health-related states or events in specified populations.

**Error**. A test can result in one of two errors, a false-positive or a false-negative. These errors can result from various sources, including human error (for example, the laboratory assistant confuses two samples or labels, or enters the wrong result on the computer) and medical conditions (for example, a positive HIV test can result from rheumatological diseases and liver diseases that have nothing to do with HIV). Errors can be reduced but not completely eliminated, and they may even be indispensable to adaptation and survival, as the copying errors (mutations) in DNA illustrate.

**Event rate**. The proportion of patients in a group in whom the event is observed. Thus, if out of 100 patients the event is observed in 27, the event rate is 0.27 or 27%. Control event rate (CER) and experimental event rate (EER) are used to refer to this in control and experimental groups of patients, respectively.

The patient expected event rate (PEER) refers to the rate of events we would expect in a patient who received no treatment or conventional treatment.

**Evidence-based health-care**. Extends the application of the principles of evidence-based medicine to all professions associated with health-care, including purchasing and management.

**Evidence-based medicine**. The conscientious, explicit, and judicious use of current best evidence in making decisions about the care of individual patients. The practice of evidence-based medicine means integrating individual clinical expertise with the best available external clinical evidence from systematic research. Evidence-based medicine does not mean 'cook-book' medicine, or the unthinking use of guidelines. It does imply that evidence should be reasonably readily available in an easily understood and useable form.

**Experimental event rate (EER)**. The rate at which events occur in an experimental group. It may be represented by a percentage (say, 50%) or as a proportion (when it is 0.5).

**False-negative**. A test result in which the test is negative (for example, a pregnancy test finds no sign of pregnancy) but the event is actually there (the woman is pregnant)—also called a 'miss'. The proportion of negative tests among people with the disease of the condition. It is typically expressed as a conditional probability or a percentage. For instance, mammography screening has a false-negative rate of 5–20% depending on age, that is, 5–20% of women with breast cancer receive a negative test result. The false-negative rate and the sensitivity (hit rate) of a test add up to 100%. The false-negative rate and the false-positive rate are dependent: to decrease one is to increase the other.

**False-positive**. A test result in which the test is positive (for example, a positive pregnancy test) but the event is not extant (the woman is not pregnant)—also called a 'false alarm'. The trouble with false-positives is that the more you test the more apparent disease you find, also called a *false-positive explosion*. The proportion of positive tests among people without the disease or condition. It is typically expressed as a conditional probability or a percentage. For instance, mammography screening has a false-negative rate of 5–10% depending on age, that is, 5–10% of women without breast cancer nevertheless receive a positive test result. The false-positive rate and the specificity (power) of a test add up to 100%. The false-positive rate and the false-negative rate are dependent: to decrease one is to increase the other.

**Fixed effects model**. This is a statistical model that stipulates that the units under analysis (people in a trial or study in a meta-analysis) are the ones of interest and thus constitute the entire population of units. Only within-study variation is taken to influence the uncertainty of results (as reflected in the confidence interval) of a meta-analysis using a fixed effect model. Variation between the estimates of effect from each study (heterogeneity) does not affect the confidence interval in a fixed effect model.

**Framing**. There has been research on the interpretation of numerical information and how that depends on the presentation of the information. Technically this is known as framing, and the effects of framing generally show that relative outputs, such as relative risk, odds ratios, or NNTs, are more likely to be influential than absolute outputs such as percentages or proportions of patients who benefit, or absolute risk reduction or increase.

**Franklin's law**. 'Nothing is certain but death and taxes.' A reminder that, in all human contact, uncertainty is prevalent as the result of human and technical errors, limited knowledge, unpredictability, deception, or other causes. Always useful to bear in mind when people talk glibly about reducing mortality: we may put it off, but the rate stubbornly stays close to 100% if you wait long enough.

**Frequencies**. A number of observations in a class of events. Frequencies can be expressed as relative frequencies, absolute frequencies, or natural frequencies.

Natural frequencies are numbers that correspond to the way humans encountered information before the invention of probability theory. Unlike probabilities and relative frequencies, they are raw observations that have not been normalized with respect to the base rates of the event in question.

Relative frequencies are one of the three major interpretations of probability (the others are degrees of belief and propensities). The probability of an event is defined as its relative frequency in a reference class. Historically, frequencies entered probability theory through mortality tables that provided the basis for calculating life insurance rates. Relative frequencies are constrained to repeated events that can be observed in large numbers.

**Gold standard**. A method, procedure, or measurement that is widely accepted as being the best available.

**Heterogeneity**. In systematic reviews heterogeneity refers to variability or differences between studies in the estimates of effects. A distinction should made between 'statistical heterogeneity' (differences in the reported effects), 'methodological heterogeneity' (differences in study design), and 'clinical heterogeneity' (differences between studies in key characteristics of the participants, interventions, or outcome measures). Where there are large differences in clinical or methodological nature between studies, the simplest question to ask is whether there is any good reason for pooling data from these studies in a meta-analysis where heterogeneity is known to exist.

More difficult is the occurrence of statistical heterogeneity where there is methodological and clinical homogeneity. Statistical tests of heterogeneity are used to assess whether the observed variability in study results (effect sizes) is greater than that expected to occur by chance. These tests have low statistical power, and the boundary for statistical significance is usually set at 10%, or 0.1. Some people think that if these tests are used, then a value of 1%, or 0.01 makes more sense.

An analysis of the performance of commonly used tests shows that the Breslow–Day test performs most consistently (Gavaghan, D.J. et al. (2000). An evaluation of homogeneity tests in meta-analysis in pain using simulations of individual patient data. *Pain* **85**, 415–24).

**Homogeneity**. In systematic reviews homogeneity refers to the degree to which the results of studies included in a review are similar. Clinical homogeneity means that, in trials included in a review, the participants, interventions, and outcome measures are similar or comparable. Studies are considered statistically homogeneous if their results vary no more than might be expected by the play of chance, though most statistical tests would say that 10% of a perfectly homogeneous data set was heterogeneous, because that is the usual set-point for the tests.

**Impact factor**. An impact factor for a journal attempts to provide a measure of how frequently papers published in a journal are cited in the scientific literature. It is derived by dividing the number of citations in any 1 year with items published in the journal in the previous 2 years. The calculation is as follows:

A   Total literature citations to substantive items published in a journal in 2003.

B   Number of citations in A that refer to articles published in 2001 and 2002.

C   Number of substantive articles published in the journal in 2001 and 2002.

The impact factor is then B divided by C, and gives the average number of times an article published in the journal in 2001 and 2002 has been cited in 2003. Thus, if there were 1000 citations in 2003 for 100 articles published in a journal in 2001 and 2002, the impact factor would be 10. Most journals (and there are many, many journals) have impact factors that are below 2. Journals with impact factors above 4 tend to be regarded as having a high impact factor, and those above 10 are stellar (see Garfield, E. (1994). The impact factor. *Current Contents* **20**, 3–7).

**Inception cohort**. A group of patients who are assembled near the onset of the target disorder.

**Incidence**. The proportion of new cases of a particular disease or condition in a population during a specified time interval. It is usual to define the disorder, and the population, and the time, and report the incidence as a rate.

**Individual patient data**. In systematic reviews this term refers to the availability of raw data for each study participant in each included trial, as opposed to aggregate data (summary data for the comparison groups in each study). Reviews using individual patient data require collaboration of the investigators who conducted the original trials, who must provide the necessary data.

**Intention-to-treat analysis (ITT)**. A method of analysis for randomized trials in which all patients randomly assigned to one of the treatments are analysed together, regardless of whether or not they completed or received that treatment. This is a complex area, and there are many definitions of what constitutes ITT. Consider a typical migraine trial, in which patients are randomized in groups, given a tablet, and told to take it if they have a migraine. Some people have a migraine and take the tablet. Some do not have a migraine and do not take the tablet. Is the proper analysis on the number randomized or the number of those randomized who actually had a migraine? There is no simple answer as to what is correct.

**Independence**. Two events are independent if knowing the outcome of one does not inform us about the outcome of the other. Formally, two events A and B are independent if the probability $p(A \& B)$ that A and B occur together is the product of $p(A)$ times $p(B)$. The concept of independence is crucial, for instance, to evaluating a match between a defendant's DNA and that found on a victim.

Assume only 1 out of 1 million men show such a match. If the DNA of all of a country's citizens are in a data bank, and one citizen's DNA is randomly selected, then the probability of a match is about 1 in a million. If the defendant, however, has an identical twin, the probability that the twin also shows a match is 1 (except for procedural errors), not 1 in 1 million. Similarly, if the defendant has brothers, the probability that they match is considerably higher than for the general population. The DNA of relatives is not independent; knowing that one matches increases the chances that the relative also matches.

**L'Abbé plot**. A first stage in any review is to look at a simple scatter plot, which can yield a surprisingly comprehensive qualitative view of the data. Even if the review does not show the data in this way you can do it from information on individual trials presented in the review tables. A L'Abbé plot simply shows the scatter of trials according to outcomes for intervention and control. Visual inspection gives a quick and easy indication of the level of agreement among trials. Heterogeneity is often assumed to be due to variation in the experimental and control event rates, but that variation is often due to the small size of trials.

**Likelihood ratio**. The likelihood that a given test result would be expected in a patient with the target disorder compared with the likelihood that the same result would be expected in a patient without the target disorder.

**Longitudinal study**. A study of the same group of people at more than one point in time. (This type of study contrasts with a cross-sectional study, which observes a defined set of people at a single point in time.)

**Mean**. The average value, calculated by adding all the observations and dividing by the number of observations.

**Median**. Middle value of a list. If you have numbers 2, 3, 4, 5, 6, 7, and 8, the median is 5. Medians are often used when data are skewed, meaning that the distribution is uneven. In that case, a few very high numbers could, for instance, change the mean, but they would not change the median.

Other definitions include the smallest number such that at least half the numbers in the list are no greater than it. If the list has an odd number of entries, the median is the middle entry in the list after sorting the list into increasing order. If the list has an even number of entries, the median is equal to the sum of the two middle (after sorting) numbers divided by two. The median can be estimated from a histogram by finding the smallest number such that the area under the histogram to the left of that number is 50%. But all mean the same thing in the end.

**Meta-analysis**. A systematic review that uses quantitative methods to summarize the results. A meta-analysis is where we pool all the information we have from a number of different (but similar) studies. It should not be about adding small piles of rubbish together to make a big pile of rubbish. It is only worth doing when individual trials are themselves of sufficient quality and validity. What meta-analysis does is to give enough size to have the power to see the result clearly, without the noise of the random play of chance.

Any meta-analysis must have enough events to make sense. Combining small, poor, trials with few events will mislead.

**Mode**. For lists, the mode is the most common (frequent) value.

**MOOSE**. Guidelines for reporting meta-analysis of observational studies.

**N-of-1 trials**. In such trials, the patient undergoes pairs of treatment periods organized so that one period involves the use of experimental treatment and the other involves the use of an alternate or placebo therapy. The patient and physician are blinded, if possible, and outcomes are monitored. Treatment periods are replicated until the clinician and patient are convinced that the treatments are definitely different or definitely not different.

**Negative predictive value**. Proportion of people with a negative test who are free of the target disorder.

**Null hypothesis**. In simplest terms, the null hypothesis states that the results observed in a study are no different from what might have occurred as a result of the play of chance. More formally, the statistical hypothesis that one variable (e.g. whether or not a study participant was allocated to receive an intervention) has no association with another variable or set of variables (e.g. whether or not a study participant died) or that two or more population distributions do not differ from one another.

**Number needed to harm (NNH)**. This is calculated in the same way as for NNT (see next entry), but used to describe adverse events. For NNH, large numbers are good, because they mean that adverse events are rare. Small values for NNH are bad, because they mean adverse events are common.

**Number needed to treat (NNT)**. The inverse of the absolute risk reduction or increase and the number of patients that need to be treated for one to benefit compared with a control. The ideal NNT is 1, where everyone has improved with treatment and no one has with control. The higher the NNT, the less effective is the treatment. But the value of an NNT is not just numeric. For instance, NNTs of 2–5 are indicative of effective therapies, such as analgesics for acute pain. NNTs of about 1 might be seen by treating sensitive bacterial infections with antibiotics, while an NNT of even 40 or more might be useful, as when using aspirin after a heart attack.

**Observational study**. In research about diseases or treatments, this refers to a study in which nature is allowed to take its course. Changes or differences in one characteristic (e.g. whether or not people received a specific treatment or intervention) are studied in relation to changes or differences in other(s) (e.g. whether or not they died) without the intervention of the investigator. There is a greater risk of selection bias than in experimental studies.

**Odds**. A ratio of the number of people incurring an event to the number of people who have no events.

**Odds ratio**. The ratio of the odds of having the target disorder in the experimental group relative to the odds in favour of having the target disorder in the control group (in cohort studies or systematic reviews) or the odds in favour of being exposed in subjects with the target disorder divided by the odds in favour of being exposed in control subjects (without the target disorder).

**p-value**. The probability (ranging from zero to one) that the results observed in a study (or results more extreme) could have occurred by chance. Convention is that we accept a p-value of 0.05 or below as being statistically significant. That means a chance of 1 in 20, which is not very unlikely. This convention has no solid basis, other than being the number chosen many years ago. When many comparisons are being made, statistical significance can occur just by chance. A more stringent rule is to use a p-value of 0.01 (1 in 100) or below as statistically significant, though some folk get hot under the collar when you do it.

**Peer review**. Review of a study, service, or recommendations by those with similar interests and expertise to the people who produced the study findings or recommendations. Peer reviewers can include professional, patient, and carer representatives. The trouble is that peer review does not always (or even frequently) work very well. Many poor papers are published, and even papers published in top medical journals can have major flaws. Just because something is found in a peer-reviewed journal does not mean it is right, or good, or sensible.

## Phases in drug development

- Phase I studies. The first stage in testing a new drug in humans. Usually performed on healthy volunteers without a comparison group.
- Phase II studies. Second stage in testing a new drug in humans. These are often randomized controlled trials, and often performed in patients with the condition of interest. Typically they will be studies of shorter duration or will examine dose–response relationships.

- Phase III studies. Studies that are a full-scale evaluation of treatment. After a drug has been shown to be reasonably effective, it is essential to compare it to the current standard treatments for the same condition. Phase III studies are usually randomized controlled trials, and are of longer duration, and larger than phase II studies.
- Phase IV studies. Studies that are concerned with post-marketing surveillance. They are often promotional exercises aimed at bringing a new drug to the attention of a large number of clinicians, and may be of limited scientific value. Phase IV studies may also be conducted in slightly different populations for licence extensions.

**Placebo**. A placebo is a fake or inactive intervention, received by the participants allocated to the control group in a clinical trial, that is indistinguishable from the active intervention received by patients in the experimental group. One definition is that use of a placebo describes what happens when you do nothing so that, in the context of a clinical trial, for instance, a placebo group could describe the natural history of a disorder without the intervention under test.

**Point estimate**. The results (e.g. mean, weighted difference, odds ratio, relative risk, or risk difference) obtained in a sample (a study or a meta-analysis), which are used as the best estimate of what is true for the relevant population from which the sample is taken. A confidence interval is a measure of the uncertainty (due to the play of chance) associated with that estimate.

**Positive predictive value**. Proportion of people with a positive test who have the target disorder.

**Pre- and post-test odds**
- Pre-test odds. The odds that the patient has the target disorder before the test is carried out (pre-test probability/[1 − pre-test probability]).
- Post-test odds. The odds that the patient has the target disorder after the test is carried out (pre-test odds × likelihood ratio).

**Pre- and post-test probability**
- Pre-test probability. The proportion of people with the target disorder in the population at risk at a specific time (point prevalence) or time interval (period prevalence). Prevalence may depend on how a disorder is diagnosed.
- Post-test probability. The proportion of patients with that particular test result who have the target disorder (post-test odds/[1 + post-test odds]).

**Precision**. Precision is a term that can have slightly different meanings, depending on the context in which it is used. Some would argue that what we should be talking about is imprecision—the propensity of any series of measurements to get different answers. If we measure the same thing in the same (or different) ways, we expect to get the same answer. Often we do not. Here are some definitions.

1. A measure of the closeness of a series of measurements of the same material. In laboratories precision is expressed as a coefficient of variation, which is nothing more than the standard deviation divided by the mean and expressed as a percentage.
2. A measure of the likelihood of random errors in the results of a study, meta-analysis, or measurement. Confidence intervals around the estimate of effect from each study are a measure of precision, and the weight

given to the results of each study in a meta-analysis (typically the inverse of the variance of the estimate of effect) is a measure of precision (i.e. the degree to which a study influences the overall estimate of effect in a meta-analysis is determined by the precision of its estimate of effect). (Note: faked studies are often very precise, and can be given disproportionate weight in meta-analysis. Very great precision is not a feature of biological systems, and should be looked at with a cold and fishy eye.)

3. The proportion of relevant citations located using a specific search strategy (i.e. the number of relevant studies meeting the inclusion criteria for a trials register or a review) divided by the total number of citations retrieved.

**Prevalence**. This is a measure of the proportion of people in a population who have a particular disease at a point in time, or over some period of time.

**Probability**. A measure that quantifies the uncertainty associated with an event.

- If an event A cannot happen, the probability $p(A)$ is zero.
- If an event happens with certainty, $p(A)$ is 1.
- Otherwise the values of $p(A)$ are between zero and 1.

For a set of events, A and B that are mutually exclusive and exhaustive, the probabilities of the individual events add up to 1. Probabilities can also be expressed as percentages, when the sum of all probabilities is 100%.

- Prior probability. The probability of an event before new evidence. Bayes's rule specifies how prior probabilities are updated in the light of new evidence.
- Posterior probability. The probability of an event after a diagnostic result, that is, the updated prior probability. It can be calculated from the prior probability using Bayes's rule.
- Conditional probability. The probability that an event A occurs given event B, usually written $p(A|B)$. An example of a conditional probability is the probability of a positive screening mammogram given breast cancer, which is around 0.9. The probability $p(A)$, for instance, is not a conditional probability. Conditional probabilities are notoriously misunderstood, and that in two different ways. One is to confuse the probability of A given B with the probability of A and B; the other is to confuse the probability of A given B with the probability of B given A. One can reduce this confusion by replacing conditional probabilities with **natural frequencies**.

**Programme budgeting and marginal analysis**. Programme budgeting and marginal analysis (PBMA) is a process that helps decision-makers maximize the impact of health-care resources on the health needs of a local population.

Programme budgeting is an appraisal of past resource allocation in specified programmes, with a view to tracking future resource allocation in those same programmes. Marginal analysis is the appraisal of the added benefits and added costs of a proposed investment (or the lost benefits and lower costs of a proposed disinvestment).

**Prospective study**. In evaluations of the effects of health-care interventions, a study in which people are divided into groups who are exposed or not exposed to the intervention(s) of interest before the outcomes have occurred. Randomized controlled trials are always prospective studies and case-control studies never are. Concurrent cohort studies are prospective studies, whereas historical cohort studies are not (see cohort study), although in epidemiology a prospective study is sometimes used as a synonym for cohort study.

**Protocol**. This is the plan or set of steps to be followed in a study. In a clinical trial the protocol should, as a minimum, set out the study design, the entry criteria for patients and any exclusion criteria, the treatments, dose, duration, outcomes (both efficacy and adverse events, and how they are to be measured), and analysis plan.

A protocol for a systematic review should describe the rationale for the review; the objectives; and the methods that will be used to locate, select, and critically appraise studies and to collect and analyse data from the included studies.

Protocols can, and probably should, be amended. A plan may change because the nature of a trial or review changes. The key thing is that the amendments to the protocol need to be noted, together with the reasons. Protocols are good things because they make you think about what you are going to do, and why.

**QALY**. Quality-adjusted life year.

**Qualitative and quantitative research**

- Qualitative research is used to explore and understand people's beliefs, experiences, attitudes, behaviour, and interactions. It generates non-numerical data, e.g. patients' descriptions of their pain rather than a measure of pain. In health-care, qualitative techniques have been commonly used in research documenting the experience of chronic illness and in studies about the functioning of organizations. Qualitative research techniques such as focus groups and in-depth interviews have been used in one-off projects commissioned by guideline development groups to find out more about the views and experiences of patients and carers.
- Quantitative research generates numerical data or data that can be converted into numbers, for example, clinical trials or the National Census, which counts people and households.

**Quality of life**. Quality of life is a descriptive term that refers to an individual's emotional, social, and physical well-being, and his/her ability to function in the ordinary tasks of living.

**Quality scoring**. If studies are not done properly, any results they produce will be worthless. We call this validity. What constitutes a valid study depends on many factors; there are no absolute hard and fast rules that can cover every clinical eventuality. Validity has a dictionary definition of 'sound and defensible'. But the quality of study conduct and reporting is also important, because incorrect conduct can introduce bias. Bias has a dictionary definition of a one-sided inclination of the mind, and studies with bias may be wrong even if the study is valid.

**Random effect mode**. This is a statistical model sometimes used in meta-analysis in which both within-study sampling error (variance) and between-studies variation are included in the assessment of the uncertainty (confidence interval) of the results of a meta-analysis. If there is significant heterogeneity among the results of the included studies, random-effect models will give wider confidence intervals than fixed effect models.

**Randomization (or random allocation)**. Method analogous to tossing a coin to assign patients to treatment groups (the experimental treatment is assigned if the coin lands heads and a conventional, control, or placebo treatment is given if the coin lands tails). Usually done by using a computer that generates a list of random numbers that can then be used to generate a treatment allocation list.

- Randomized controlled clinical trial (RCT). A group of patients is randomized into an experimental group and a control group. These groups are followed up for the variables/outcomes of interest. The point about using randomization is that it avoids any possibility of selection bias in a trial. The test that randomization has been successful is that different treatment groups have the same characteristics at baseline. For instance, there should be the same number of men and women, or older or younger people, or different degrees of disease severity.

- Quasi-random allocation. A method of allocating participants to different forms of care that is not truly random—for example, allocation by date of birth, day of the week, medical record number, month of the year, or the order in which participants are included in the study (alternation). A quasi-randomized trial uses a quasi-random method of allocating participants to different interventions. There is a greater risk of selection bias in quasi-random trials where allocation is not adequately concealed compared with randomized controlled trials with adequate allocation concealment.

- Stratified randomization. In any randomized trial it is desirable that the comparison groups should be as similar as possible as regards those characteristics that might influence the response to the intervention. Stratified randomization is used to ensure that equal numbers of participants with a characteristic thought to affect prognosis or response to the intervention will be allocated to each comparison group. For example, in a trial of women with breast cancer, it may be important to have similar numbers of pre-menopausal and post-menopausal women in each comparison group. Stratified randomization could be used to allocate equal numbers of pre- and post-menopausal women to each treatment group. Stratified randomization is performed either by performing separate randomization (often using random permuted blocks) for each strata, or by using minimization.

**Relative risk**. The ratio of risk in the treated group (EER) to risk in the control group (CER). Relative risk = EER/CER. It is used in randomized trials and cohort studies.

**Relative risk reduction**. The relative risk reduction is the difference between the EER and CER (EER − CER) divided by the CER, and usually expressed as a percentage.

**Retrospective study**. A retrospective study deals with the present and past and does not involve studying future events. This contrasts with studies that are prospective.

**Risk factor**. An aspect of a person's condition, lifestyle, or environment that increases the probability of occurrence of a disease. For example, cigarette smoking is a risk factor for lung cancer.

**Screening**. The testing of a symptomless population in order to detect cases of a disease at an early stage. The basic principles of screening are:
- The condition is common and disabling, the natural history is known, and there is a recognizable latent or pre-symptomatic phase.
- The screening test is reliable, valid, and repeatable; is acceptable and easy to perform; and is sensitive, specific, and low-cost.
- The treatment should be effective and available, and there should be an agreed policy on whom to treat.

The term screening is also used outside of medicine, for instance, when a population is screened for a DNA profile.

**Selection bias**. In assessments of the validity of studies of health-care interventions, selection bias refers to systematic differences between comparison groups in prognosis or responsiveness to treatment. Random allocation with adequate concealment of allocation protects against selection bias. Other means of selecting who receives the intervention of interest, particularly leaving it up to the providers and recipients of care, are more prone to bias because decisions about care can be related to prognosis and responsiveness to treatment.

Selection bias is sometimes used to describe a systematic error in reviews due to how studies are selected for inclusion. Publication bias is an example of this type of selection bias.

Selection bias, confusingly, is also sometimes used to describe a systematic difference in characteristics between those who are selected for study and those who are not. This affects the generalizability (external validity) of a study but not its (internal) validity.

**Selection criteria**. Explicit standards used by reviewers to decide which studies should be included and excluded from consideration as potential sources of evidence.

**Sensitivity**. Proportion of people with the target disorder who have a positive test. It is used to assist in assessing and selecting a diagnostic test/ sign/symptom.

**Sensitivity analysis**. An analysis used to determine how sensitive the results of a study or systematic review are to changes in how it was done, such as using only randomized trials compared with non-randomized, or double-blind compared with open, or large versus small studies. Sensitivity analyses are used to assess how robust the results are to uncertain decisions or assumptions about the data and the methods that were used. Criteria on which sensitivity analysis may be based include (but are not limited to):
- random versus non-random studies;
- blind versus open studies;
- dose of intervention;
- duration of intervention;
- duration of observations;
- severity of condition at start of a trial;
- magnitude of outcome;
- size of trial;
- geographical location of study;
- quality of study;
- validity of study.

**SnNout**. When a sign/test/symptom has a high *sensitivity*, a *negative* result rules out the diagnosis. For example, the sensitivity of a history of ankle swelling for diagnosing ascites is 93%; therefore, if a person does not have a history of ankle swelling, it is highly unlikely that the person has ascites.

**Specificity**. Proportion of people without the target disorder who have a negative test. It is used to assist in assessing and selecting a diagnostic test/sign/symptom.

**Spectrum bias**. An unrecognized (but probably very real) problem is that of spectrum bias. This is the phenomenon of the sensitivity and/or specificity of a test varying with different populations tested—populations who might vary in sex ratios, age, or severity of disease as three simple examples.

**SpPin**. When a sign/test/symptom has a high *specificity*, a *positive* result rules in the diagnosis. For example, the specificity of a fluid wave for diagnosing ascites is 92%; therefore, if a person does have a fluid wave, it rules in the diagnosis of ascites.

**Statistical power**. The ability of a study to demonstrate an association or causal relationship between two variables, given that an association exists. For example, 80% power in a clinical trial means that the study has a 80% chance of ending up with a *p*-value of less than 5% in a statistical test (i.e. a statistically significant treatment effect) if there really was an important difference (e.g. 10% versus 5% mortality) between treatments. If the statistical power of a study is low, the study results will be questionable (the study might have been too small to detect any differences). By convention, 80% is an acceptable level of power.

**Surrogate endpoints**. Outcome measures that are not of direct practical importance but are believed to reflect outcomes that are important are called surrogate outcomes. For instance, cholesterol is used as a surrogate endpoint in many trials where cholesterol reduction is used as a surrogate for reduced mortality. The trouble is that trials to demonstrate mortality reduction have to be large and long. Cholesterol reduction is known to be strongly associated with mortality benefits, and can be measured easily in smaller numbers of patients. In another example, blood pressure is not directly important to patients but it is often used as an outcome in clinical trials because it is a risk factor for stroke and heart attacks.

Surrogate endpoints are often physiological or biochemical markers that can be relatively quickly and easily measured, and that are taken as being predictive of important clinical outcomes. They are often used when observation of clinical outcomes requires long follow-up. The main thing to remember is that there has to be a good reason to accept a surrogate endpoint. We have to be sure that the utility of the surrogate is well established.

**Systematic review**. A summary of the medical literature that uses explicit methods to perform a thorough literature search and critical appraisal of individual studies and that uses appropriate statistical techniques to combine these valid studies.

**Uncertainty**. An event or outcome that is not certain but may or may not happen is uncertain. When the uncertainty is quantified on the basis of empirical observations, it is called risk.

**Utility**. In economic and decision analysis, the desirability of an outcome, usually expressed as being between zero and one (e.g. death typically has a utility value of zero and a full healthy life has a value of one).

**Validity**. This term is a difficult concept in clinical trials, but refers to a trial being able to measure what it sets out to measure. A trial that set out to measure the analgesic effect of a procedure might be in trouble if patients had no pain. Or in a condition where treatment is life-long, evaluating an intervention for 10 minutes might be seen as silly.

**Variable**. A measurement that can vary within a study, e.g. the age of participants. Variability is present when differences can be seen between different people or within the same person over time, with respect to any characteristic or feature that can be assessed or measured.

**Variance**. A measure of the variation shown by a set of observations, defined by the sum of the squares of deviations from the mean, divided by the number of degrees of freedom in the set of observations.

**Weighted mean or weighted mean difference**

In meta-analysis, information to be pooled can either be dichotomous (how many patients die, say, out of a total number) or continuous (the mean cholesterol was $X$ mmol/L, with some estimate of variance).

For continuous variables we need to combine measures, where the mean, standard deviation and sample size in each group are known. The weight given to each study (how much influence each study has on the overall results of the meta-analysis) is determined by the precision of its estimate of effect and, in the statistical software in RevMan, is equal to the inverse of the variance. This method assumes that all of the trials have measured the outcome on the same scale.

The weighted mean could be calculated for groups before and after an intervention (such as blood pressure lowering), and the weighted mean difference would be the difference between start and finish values. For this, though, the difference would usually be calculated not as the difference between the overall start value and the overall final value, but rather as the sum of the differences in the individual studies, weighted by the individual variances for each study.

Precision is not the only way of calculating a weighted mean or weighted mean difference. Another, simpler, way is to weight by the number in the study. This is a defence against giving undue weight to small studies of low variance where there may have been less than robust treatment of data and where people could have cheated.

# Index